Does Consciousness Cause Behavior?

edited by Susan Pockett, William P. Banks, and Shaun Gallagher

The MIT Press
Cambridge, Massachusetts
London, England

MIT Press books may be purchased at special quantity discounts for business or sales promotional use. For information, please email special_sales@mitpress.mit.edu or write to Special Sales Department, The MIT Press, 55 Hayward Street, Cambridge, MA 02142.

Set in Times by SNP Best-set Typesetter Ltd., Hong Kong.
Printed and bound in the United States of America.

Library of Congress Cataloging-in-Publication Data

Does consciousness cause behavior? / edited by Susan Pockett, William P. Banks, and Shaun Gallagher.
   p. ; cm.
Includes bibliographical references and index.
ISBN 0-262-16237-7 (hc : alk. paper)
1. Consciousness. 2. Neuropsychology. 3. Mind and body. 4. Intention. I. Pockett, Susan.
II. Banks, William P. III. Gallagher, Shaun, 1948–
[DNLM: 1. Neuropsychology—methods. 2. Consciousness. 3. Personal Autonomy.
4. Philosophy. WL 103.5 D653   2006]
QP411.D54   2006   153–dc22   2005052116

10 9 8 7 6 5 4 3 2 1

Contents

Does Consciousness Cause Behavior?

Introduction

Susan Pockett, William P. Banks, and Shaun Gallagher

All normal humans experience a kind of basic, on-the-ground certainty that we, our conscious selves, cause our own voluntary acts. When this certainty is removed (for example, by whatever brain dysfunction causes schizophrenia), its loss tends to be very upsetting. Yet, despite the compelling nature of the raw experience that consciousness does cause behavior, the counterintuitive question "[Yes but] Does consciousness [really] cause behavior?" is by no means a new one. William James spends a whole chapter of his classic *The Principles of Psychology* (1890) arguing against what he calls "the automaton theory" of Thomas Huxley, who had earlier compared mental events to a steam whistle that contributes nothing to the work of a locomotive (Huxley 1874). Many of the intelligentsia of Victorian England ignored the colonial James and continued to support Huxley's notion that humans are indeed nothing more than "conscious automata." This idea was elaborated further by Sigmund Freud, who famously suggested that much of our everyday behavior is not even acknowledged, let alone caused, by consciousness (Freud 1954). Freud's work may be now largely discredited as science, but this has not prevented its exerting a remarkable influence on all aspects of Western culture. Apparently the idea that consciousness does *not* cause our voluntary behavior is not quite as counterintuitive and aversive as it may at first appear.

In more recent times, the wide promulgation of two new lines of genuinely scientific (that is to say, experimental) evidence has seized the philosophical and scientific imagination and again brought the whole question to the forefront of intellectual debate. This book springs from a desire to examine, place in context, and discuss the implications for society of those lines of evidence.

The first is due to Benjamin Libet (Libet et al. 1983). Libet recorded the EEG event-related potential that was already known to precede a voluntary finger movement and compared the onset time of this potential with the time at which his subjects reported becoming conscious that they were about to make each movement (figure I.1). He found that the conscious awareness came before the actual movement, but after the start of the brain activity leading up to it. While Libet

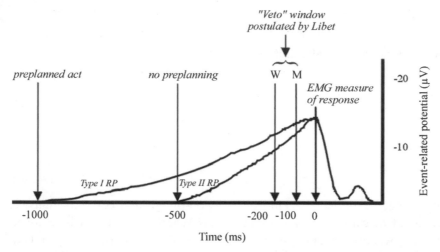

Figure I.1
Diagram illustrating results of Libet experiment. W indicates time at which subjects reported having experienced the urge, desire or intention to move their finger. This time was determined by having them watch a revolving spot of light and indicate the position on a clock-face where the spot was at the instant they became conscious that they were about to move. M indicates the time at which they reported that they actually made the movement (determined similarly). "EMG measure of response" shows the time at which they objectively made the movement (that is, the time at which their muscles became measurably active). Type I and Type II RPs (readiness potentials) are EEG event-related potentials measured while the subject was preparing to make and making the finger movement. Type I RPs occurred when subjects admitted to having preplanned some of their movements and Type II RPs when they did not preplan any of the movements. The main point to observe is that even with Type II RPs, the reported time of consciously intending to move is well after the time at which the RP began.

acknowledged that this result meant the consciousness could not have caused the movement in this particular case, he could not bring himself to accept that it meant consciousness is entirely epiphenomenal or acausal—even for this specific movement, let alone for all movements. His proposal was that, since consciousness did arise slightly in advance of the movement, it might still be capable of exerting a veto in the fraction of a second before the movement was carried out. The causal power of consciousness is thus rescued, if seriously constrained. Quite how this veto might be accomplished by a dualist consciousness of the sort that Libet later proposes (Libet 1994) is not clear, but probably not relevant either. The main point is that these elegant experiments do show quite clearly that at least some simple, but definitely self-initiated and voluntary, movements are triggered not by consciousness, but by the subconscious workings of the brain.

The second new line of experimental evidence is ascribed to Daniel Wegner (2002). Wegner started with the hypothesis that the experience of having personally caused an action is no different from any other experience of cause and effect—we think that something causes something else if and only if what we think of as the causal event occurs just before what we think of as the effect (the priority principle), is consistent with the putative effect (the consistency principle), and is the only apparent cause of the putative effect (the exclusivity principle).

Wegner arranged two experiments to test these principles. In the first (Wegner and Wheatley 1999), the subjects were asked to move a cursor randomly around a computer screen and every 30 seconds or so to stop the cursor over some object depicted on the screen. After each stop, subjects gave an "intentionality" rating, ranging from feeling completely sure that they had caused the cursor to stop (100 percent) to feeling completely sure that the experimenter had caused the cursor to stop (0 percent). Surprisingly, they proved to be quite bad at telling whether they or the experimenter had caused the cursor to stop. When the subject had really caused all of the stops, the average intentionality rating was only 56 percent. When the stops were actually forced by the experimenter, the intentionality rating was 52 percent if the subjects heard the name of the object over which the cursor stopped spoken through headphones 30 seconds before or 1 second after each stop. It was 56 percent—the same as if they really had caused the stops themselves—if they heard the name of the object either 5 seconds or 1 second before each forced stop. These results were interpreted as showing that subjects could be fooled into wrongly believing that that they had caused the cursor to stop over a particular object when in fact the experimenter had caused the stop, if the subject simply heard the name of the object just before the cursor stopped. This was taken as evidence supporting the priority principle. If you think about an entity just before some event happens to it, you tend to believe that your thought caused the event.

A second experiment involved subjects who viewed other people's gloved hands in the position where their own hands would normally be (Wegner et al. 2004). The viewed hands performed a series of actions, and the subjects were asked to rate on a scale from 1 to 7 the extent to which they felt they had controlled the actions, a rating of 1 meaning "not at all" and a rating of 7 meaning "very much." Again, in the baseline condition subjects were not entirely sure they had not controlled the hand movements, returning a score of 2.05 ± 1.61 (SD). When the owner of the hands was moving them according to a set of instructions that were also heard by the subject, the subject's rating of their control over the hands rose to 3.00 ± 1.09, a significant increase. This is cited (Wegner 2002) as evidence in favor of the consistency principle. If your thoughts about an entity are consistent with what happens to it, you tend to believe that you caused what happens to it.

These and numerous other observations lead Wegner to the model summarized in figure I.2. In this model, actions and conscious thoughts are represented as being produced in parallel—both generated by the real driving force, which is unconscious neural events. The dotted arrow from conscious thought to action represents a

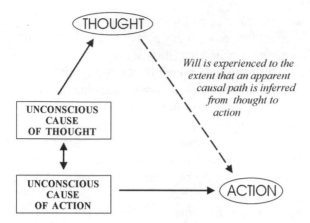

Figure I.2
Wegner's model of the relationship between conscious and unconscious processes in relation to the generation of voluntary actions. Unconscious events are shown in rectangular boxes and conscious events in ellipses.

causal path that does not occur in reality, but may be erroneously inferred, in the same way as any external causal relationship (the wind's causing the movement of a tree branch, for example) is inferred.

These two lines of evidence, though perhaps the most widely known, are by no means the only experiments suggesting that consciousness does not cause behavior. Part I of this volume (Neuroscience) begins with a chapter in which Susan Pockett outlines an empirically based model of how the brain causes behavior, and where consciousness presently seems to fit into the picture. In chapter 2, Marc Jeannerod summarizes his accumulated evidence that ongoing actions are generally controlled unconsciously by the brain, with the subject's consciousness being kept informed (if indeed it is informed at all) only after the event, and then more as a professional courtesy than anything else. In chapter 3, Suparna Choudhury and Sarah-Jayne Blakemore examine the neurological mechanisms by which we recognize actions as our own and discuss how a sense of self may emerge from this recognition. In chapter 4, Richard Passingham and Hakwan Lau report new brain imaging experiments. These further our knowledge of the mechanisms by which brains generate actions, but they also emphasize that the question of whether consciousness causes or results from the initiation of actions more complex than Libet's finger movements has not yet been answered. In chapter 5, Walter Freeman, with his usual originality, suggests that we may be looking at the whole thing in completely the wrong way when we ask whether consciousness causes or is caused by neural activity. He suggests that circular causation is a more relevant concept in this regard than linear causation. Consciousness and neural activity are certainly interdependent, but it is impossible in principle to say that either causes the other. Thus the whole concept of consciousness as agent is simply a misreading of the true situation.

The chapters in part II (Philosophy) address the philosophical presuppositions the authors regard as having informed the empirical studies of motor control, action, and intention, and raise questions about what legitimately can be concluded from Libet's and Wegner's experimental results. One of the philosophical outcomes of Libet's experiments is that they might be taken as suggesting we do not have conscious free will. However, in chapter 6 Shaun Gallagher suggests that Libet's results show nothing about whether or not we have free will, because free will is a concept that does not apply to the movements Libet studied. Based on considerations of temporality and levels of description, Gallagher argues for a distinction between the initiation and control of movement, much of which is unconscious, and the conscious exercise of free will in intentional action. In chapter 7, Peter Ross considers what empirical science can contribute to an understanding of free will. He argues that empirical research cannot resolve the dispute between compatibilism and incompatibilism, although it can address the dispute between libertarianism (which claims that indeterminacy is, in certain contexts, sufficient for freedom) and the positions of hard determinism and compatibilism (which deny this). In chapter 8, Elisabeth Pacherie offers a sketch of a dynamic theory of intentions. She argues that several categories of intentions should be distinguished on the basis of their different functional roles and on the basis of the different types of contents they involve. To understand the distinctive nature of actions and intentionality requires a proper understanding of the dynamic transitions among these different categories of intentions. In this context Pacherie argues that the experiments conducted by Libet and Wegner fail to provide conclusive reasons to think that mental causation is generally illusory. In chapter 9, Timothy Bayne also offers a critical evaluation of Wegner's claim that the conscious will is an illusion. He argues that the content of the "experience of conscious will" is more complicated than has been assumed. He concludes that, although the role of the self and intentional states in the genesis of actions requires further explanation, it is unlikely that the phenomenology of agency is systematically misleading. There is little reason to think that our experience of ourselves as agents who do things for reasons leads us into error. In chapter 10, Alfred Mele develops a conceptual analysis of some of the concepts that inform the recent experimental studies of intentional action. Based on a distinction between unconscious urge and conscious decision, he suggests that the neural activity described by Libet's experiments may represent an urge to move rather than a decision to do so, and that the decision to move might be made only when the subject becomes conscious of the urge. If this is the case, then Libet's experiments do not threaten free will. In chapter 11, Bertram Malle provides further conceptual analysis, focusing on skeptical arguments about self-awareness and the awareness of actions and intentional agency. He argues that the skeptics often misrepresent the pertinent folk assumptions about these phenomena. Indeed, scientific discussions about introspection, action explanation, and intentional agency often set up folk psychology as a straw man instead of dealing with the actual and complex array of concepts and assumptions that uniquely characterize human beings.

William Banks kicks off part III (Law and Public Policy) with a wide-ranging chapter in which he examines the concepts of free will and conscious efficacy in light of recent psychological and neuroscientific research, criticizes these results and the inferences drawn from them, and offers a range of ideas, from the reasonable to the frightening, about the impact these developments may have on the whole area of legal, social, and moral judgments of responsibility and blame. In chapter 13, Wolfgang Prinz argues that we should understand consciousness not as a naturally given mental capacity but rather as a social institution. The thesis is that consciousness is not a brute fact of nature, but rather a matter of social construction. In this sense it *is* causally efficacious for the control of behavior, no matter what the neuroscience may say. In chapter 14, Leonard Kaplan points out that if it were to be concluded that consciousness does *not* cause behavior, the Western legal system (which has always relied on the demonstration of conscious intent for an act to be considered punishable) would be seriously compromised. He warns that lawyers will certainly ignore reasonable scientific expressions of caution about such a conclusion when attempting to defend their clients in court. In chapter 15, Susan Hurley discusses whether or not public policy decisions such as the censorship of violent entertainment should be based on scientific evidence that people unconsciously imitate actions they see. In chapter 16, Sabine Maasen provides a sociological analysis of a public debate on these issues which has recently taken place in Germany.

References

Freud, S. 1954. *Psychopathology of Everyday Life.* E. Benn.

Huxley, T. H. 1874. On the hypothesis that animals are automata, and its history. *Fortnightly Review*, n.s. 16: 555–580. Reprinted in *Method and Results: Essays by Thomas H. Huxley* (D. Appleton, 1898).

James, W. 1890. *The Principles of Psychology.* Henry Holt.

Libet, B. 1994. A testable mind-brain field theory. *Journal of Consciousness Studies* 1: 119–126.

Libet, B., Gleason, C. A., Wright, E. W., and Pearl, D. K. 1983. Time of conscious intention to act in relation to onset of cerebral activity (readiness-potential). *Brain* 106: 623–642.

Wegner, D. M. 2002. *The Illusion of Conscious Will.* MIT Press.

Wegner, D. M., and Wheatley, T. 1999. Apparent mental causation: Sources of the experience of will. *American Psychologist* 54: 480–492.

Wegner, D. M., Sparrow, B., and Winerman, L. 2004. Vicarious agency: Experiencing control over the movements of others. *Journal of Personality and Social Psychology* 86: 838–848.

I NEUROSCIENCE

1 The Neuroscience of Movement

Susan Pockett

Over a century ago, T. H. Huxley famously remarked that "the great end of life is not knowledge but action" (1877). It is still reasonable to regard the major job of the human brain—even the brain of those as dedicated to pure thought as philosophers— as being the initiation and control of bodily movements. Thus it is no surprise that the motor system of the brain is extensive. In no particular order, movement-related regions include the primary motor cortex, supplementary and pre-supplementary motor areas, premotor cortex, frontal eye fields, cingulate cortex, posterior parietal cortex, dorsolateral prefrontal cortex, the basal ganglia, thalamus, cerebellum, and, of course, most of the spinal cord. Complex reciprocal communications exist not only among these areas, but also between them and the somatosensory, visual and auditory cortices and various parts of the limbic system. For ease of reference, the physical locations of most these brain areas are shown in figure 1.1. It can be seen that there is relatively little of the brain that is *not* involved in producing movements.

The main aim of this chapter is to provide a short overview of how all these multifarious brain areas interact to initiate and control movement. The hope is that this will provide background information that will be useful not only in understanding the other neuroscientific contributions to this volume, but also in constraining philosophical speculation on the question in the title of the book. Figure 1.2 displays the outline of such an overview.

Clearly, the model shown in figure 1.2 has its flaws. Perhaps inevitably given the complexity of the real system, the model is heavily oversimplified. In the interests of showing the main flow of activity from area to area, it leaves out many known reciprocal connections. Parts of it remain hypothetical—in particular, the idea that the purpose of the frontal cortex/basal ganglia loops is to allow interaction between intention and motivation, and the inclusion of an arrow directly from "willed intentions" to "sensorimotor intentions." A further flaw is probably the lack of a box labeled "action initiation." But in the model's favor, it does represent some attempt to view what is known about the complexities of the motor system and its relationship with the outside world as a whole.

A

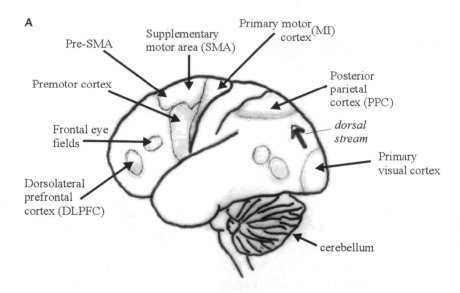

B

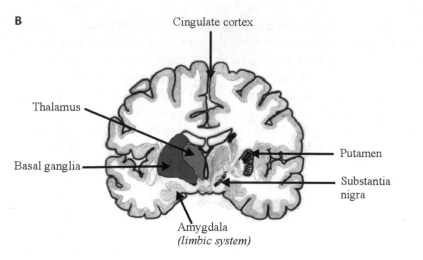

Figure 1.1
Location of brain areas involved in movement. A: Surface of left hemisphere. B: Transverse section in region of SMA.

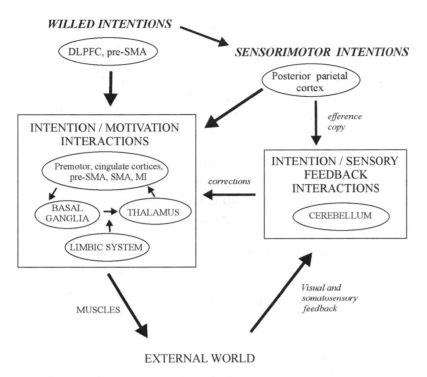

Figure 1.2
Model of anatomical and functional relationships in the motor system. DLPFC: dorsolateral prefrontal cortex. pre-SMA: presupplementary motor area. SMA: supplementary motor area. MI: primary motor cortex.

In what follows, I will first sketch an overview of the model (an overview of the overview, if you like) and then discuss various parts of the model in more detail.

1 Overview of the Model

The model shown in figure 1.2 begins with *intentions*. Intentions are here defined as abstract early plans for movements. They specify the goal and type of movements, but not the detail of how the movements will be carried out. It is possible to have intentions without acting on them—indeed, the road to Hell is said to be paved with good ones. Decisions can be regarded as the outcome of competition between intentions (Platt and Glimcher 1999). No detailed dissection of the internal structure of intentions such as that attempted by Pacherie or Mele (this volume) is represented in figure 1.2, because there is no apparent physiological basis for, or anatomical correlate of, all the various subdivisions of intent proposed by the philosophers. However, there are good neuroscientific reasons to believe in the existence of two basic kinds of intentions, one subsidiary to the other. The two are represented in widely separated regions of the brain, and will be discussed in more detail in section 2.

In the real world, the next step after the formation first of general and then of more detailed intentions or plans for movement must be the *initiation* of the intended actions. Here the first major flaw in our model appears. There is no obvious place in figure 1.2 for neural events dedicated to the initiation of actions. This may be because it is not possible to localize an initiation mechanism. The experience of Parkinson's disease sufferers, who sometimes find that despite willing or intending the immediate performance of a movement they are unable to initiate it, suggests that at least one region important in the initiation of actions must be the substantia nigra of the basal ganglia (the primary lesion site in Parkinson's disease). But, although the basal ganglia are included in figure 1.2, it is not obvious how they fit into any particularly linear pathway from intentions to actions. There are a multitude of interactions between the basal ganglia and the cortex, and Parkinsonism causes a decrease in activity not only in the basal ganglia, but also (and probably consequently) in the prefrontal cortex (Jahanshahi et al. 1995), SMA, pre-SMA, and motor cortex (Buhman et al. 2003). Certainly parallel processing is a major feature of brain function, and perhaps the notion of circular causality (Freeman, this volume) is also more important in the brain than has hitherto been realized.

A further difficulty with the sensible placing of action-initiation in any putative linear chain of causation from intention to action-completion is that the experiments of Libet (1983) suggest the subject's consciousness of initiating at least a simple voluntary act does not appear until the very last step in the chain of neural events leading up to the movement (section 3). This, of course, is one of the main experimental results leading to the suggestion that consciousness is not the true initiator of actions, but is largely epiphenomenal.

After an action has been intended, planned, and initiated (or, as Deecke and Kornhuber (1978) proposed, after the "what to do, how to do and when to do" of the movement have been taken care of), the action must be seen through to its conclusion. There must be ongoing *control and correction* of the movements involved, using feedback both from proprioception and from the effects of the action on the external world, as received by various sensory systems. This ongoing control can be either conscious or, more frequently, unconscious. It is perhaps an overgeneralization to say that unconscious control of ongoing movements is mediated by the cerebellum and conscious control by various parts of the frontal cortex, but there is some evidence pointing in this direction. (See the chapter by Jeannerod.)

This brief introduction has carried us on the surface from intention to the successful conclusion of an intended movement. I will now consider in slightly more detail the neuroscientific evidence underlying the model shown in figure 1.2.

2   Willed and Sensorimotor Intentions

Reading figure 1.2 from the top, we first encounter two widely separated areas of the brain that are marked as encoding intentions. The two areas can be said to support two different types or perhaps levels of intention—using terminology similar to that of Jahanshahi and Frith (1998), these can be called *willed intentions* and *sensorimotor intentions*. The dorsolateral prefrontal cortex (DLPFC) and the adjacent pre-supplementary motor area (pre-SMA) are shown as the source of willed intentions. I define willed intentions as those that are accessible to consciousness.[1]

To be more specific about the definition of willed intentions, they typically consist of general plans to carry out a particular act. One might form a willed intention to phone a friend at 2 o'clock this afternoon, for example.

The second type of intention shown in figure 1.2, neurally located in the posterior parietal cortex, is here called a *sensorimotor intention*. This sort of intention codes for the relatively low-level and immediate motor plans required when 2 o'clock arrives and we want to reach for the telephone and pick it up. In this sense it is subsidiary to the willed intention to make the call at some later time. I call these immediate motor plans *intentions* because this is what Andersen and Buneo (2002) call them, and *sensorimotor intentions* because they integrate sensory information (about the location of the telephone) with motor intentions. However, they might reasonably be equated with the motor representations of Jeannerod (1994) or the stimulus intentions of Jahanshahi and Frith (1998).

Willed Intentions

Data from both brain imaging and subdural recording have suggested that one source of willed intentions is the dorsolateral prefrontal cortex (DLPFC) (Jahanshahi and Dirnberger 1999; Jahanshahi et al. 2001). However, the fMRI measurements of Lau et al. (2004) suggest that conscious intention is mediated specifically by the pre-supplementary motor area (pre-SMA). The experiments of the latter group do show a significant regression coefficient for activity between the pre-SMA and the DLPFC, though, which supports the idea that intention-related activity may have begun in the DLPFC and progressed to involve the pre-SMA.

Sensorimotor Intentions

Sensorimotor intentions are located in the posterior parietal cortex[2] (Andersen and Buneo 2002). Specific varieties of sensorimotor intention are known to be represented in specific areas of the posterior parietal cortex. For example, area LIP is specialized for the planning of saccades (the rapid eye movements used to position the fovea in the optimal place for seeing an object)—after a brief burst of activity

specific to the object, most LIP cells code for the direction of the planned eye movement, not the qualities of the object to be foveated (Zhang and Barash 2000). Areas
MIP, 5, PO, 7m, PRR, and Pec are each specialized for planning different kinds of
reaching movements—activity in these areas also codes mostly for the direction of
the movement rather than the location of the stimulus (Eskandar and Assad 1999;
Kalaska 1996).

In order to form a plan to reach for a particular telephone, one needs to know
exactly where that telephone is. Since sensorimotor intentions code for the direction of particular movements, sensory (usually visual) information is necessary for
their formation. The posterior parietal cortex is perfectly placed anatomically to
receive such information, being located at the end of the dorsal or "where" stream
of the visual system (Milner and Goodale 1995). To summarize the anatomy of
vision in a couple of sentences: Input from the external world enters at the eyes,
flows through the large fiber tract of the optic radiation to the primary visual cortex
at the rear of the brain, and then streams back toward the front of the brain, split-
ting in two as it does so. The ventral of these two streams, originally called the "what"
stream, culminates in the generation of conscious visual sensations/perceptions,
probably in the infratemporal region. The dorsal stream, often called the "where"
stream, is not associated with consciousness. It codes for the location of objects, and
terminates in the posterior parietal cortex, where intentions are (Wise et al. 1997).

The output of the posterior parietal cortex flows in two directions: to the frontal
motor areas and to the cerebellum. The cerebellar stream constitutes a form of efference copy, which enables the comparison of intention with peripheral feedback and
thus the correction of ongoing movements. (This will be discussed in section 4.) The
main stream of posterior parietal output leads to the frontal cortex and the initiation of movements.

3   Initiation of Movements

Figure 1.2 does not show a specific site labeled "initiation of movements." This
reflects the fact that the initiation of movements has not yet been the specific subject
of very much neuroscientific investigation. All we can say at present is that the initiation of movements is probably subserved somewhere in the left half of figure
1.2—either between "willed intentions" and the box labeled "attention/motivation
interactions" or at some point within the complex series of parallel intercortical
interactions and cortical/subcortical loops whose existence is hinted at in that box.

Some movements are initiated in response to external cues. There is a long history
of psychological studies on reaction times, but again, little neuroscience. One
notable exception is the study of Jenkins et al. (2000), which shows that externally
triggered movements are preceded by activity in the contralateral primary sensori-

motor area, the adjacent (caudal) SMA, and the contralateral putamen (part of the basal ganglia). In contrast, self-initiated movements involve activity in each of these areas, and also in the rostral (pre-) SMA, the adjacent anterior cingulate cortex, and the DLPFC bilaterally. Cunnington et al. (2002), who also use fMRI to compare self-initiated and externally triggered movements, emphasize that activity in the basal ganglia occurs for the self-initiated movements only—their tasks activate the pre-SMA and the anterior cingulate equally in both sorts of movements (although the pre-SMA is activated earlier in the self-initiated movements).

Presumably, then, if the initiation of movements can be said to have a specific neural correlate at all, it must reside in one or more of the DLPFC, pre-SMA, SMA proper, basal ganglia, or primary sensorimotor cortex. There is a great deal of parallel processing in this region and the exact temporal order of activation of these areas when a movement starts is still controversial, but it is a reasonable assumption that activity flows from the prefrontal region (DLPFC) in a generally caudal direction to finish in the primary motor area. In between, it reverberates around at least five separate cortico-basal ganglia loops, all of which are probably active in parallel (Jahanshahi and Frith 1998). The output from this region is via the direct connections that exist between most of these areas and the spinal cord, which provides the final common pathway to the muscles.

In order to answer the question posed in the title of this book, we would like to know (a) the site at which a movement can be said to be actually initiated and (b) the site at which the consciousness involved with movement initiation is generated. Although various analytical philosophers have decided that the concept of causation ought to be broad enough to accommodate backwards causation, there is absolutely no physical evidence that causation can operate backwards in time. Thus, if neural activity in area (b) occurs later than that in area (a), it would seem a fair bet that the consciousness of initiating the movement is not causal in the actual initiation of the movement.

Libet's Experiments on the Timing of Consciousness in Relation to Voluntary Movement

It has long been traditional among biologists to elucidate complex physiological processes by working out the simplest possible example first. The simplest possible voluntary act is probably the movement studied by Libet (1983). Libet asked each participant in his experiments to "wait for one complete revolution of the CRO spot [this spot being used for timing the subjective intention] and then, at any time thereafter when he felt like doing so, to perform the quick, abrupt flexion of the fingers and/or wrist of the right hand." To encourage "spontaneity," the subject was instructed to "let the urge to act appear on its own at any time without any preplanning or concentration on when to act." According to Libet, this instruction was "designed to elicit voluntary acts that were freely capricious in origin," but it seems to me that it may actually have resulted in acts that were not so much voluntary as random—in neurophysiological terms, the subjects may have interpreted these instructions as requiring them to form a motor plan, adjust the excitability of the relevant parts of their brain to the very edge of becoming active, and then wait for some random neural event to tip the system over the edge and start the action. Be that as it may, Libet then used an ingenious timing method to elicit subjective reports of exactly when the conscious "urge, intention or decision" to make each of these simple movements arose, and matched the subjective reports up with the objectively measured EEG readiness potential (RP) that preceded the movement. His now well-known finding was that the subjects reported becoming aware of the urge or desire to move only 350 milliseconds *after* the start of the shortest variety of readiness potential he measured, which he called a Type II RP.

All sorts of philosophical implications of this finding are discussed at length elsewhere in the present volume, but for our immediate purposes the importance of the result is that it puts a precise time on the appearance of the consciousness associated with a voluntary movement and thus offers a means of localizing the neural correlate of whatever conscious event was interpreted by these subjects as being "the urge, intention or decision to move." All we need to achieve this localization is an understanding of the temporal evolution of the neural events underlying the RP (a.k.a. Bereitschaftspotential or BP). Inevitably perhaps, this turns out to be not quite as simple as it sounds.

The subjective timing data are clear—Libet's subjects reported experiencing the conscious awareness of an "urge, intention or decision" to move approximately 200 ms before the movement actually took place. This places the appearance of their conscious awareness that they were about to move right in the middle of what Libet calls the Type II RP and other investigators call BP2, NS', or (using a subtraction procedure) the lateralized readiness potential. What are the neural generators of this waveform? It is not entirely clear.

The problem is that non-invasive electrophysiological measurements like EEG and MEG have the requisite time resolution, but very poor spatial resolution (because the electromagnetic fields generated by brain activity spread out spatially within a very short distance, so that by the time they get to the outside of the head seriously problematical reconstruction techniques must be used to determine their source), while brain imaging methods that rely on increased blood flow to active areas of the brain have good spatial resolution but very poor time resolution (simply because it takes a couple of seconds for the blood flow to neurally active regions to increase). The trump technique ought to be intracortical recording, which combines the best in temporal and spatial resolution. But intracortical recording in humans is restricted by very tight ethical guidelines. The usual reason for implanting electrodes in the brain is to locate epileptic foci before their surgical excision, and epileptic foci in the SMA and motor cortex are relatively rare. Thus studies using intracortical recording are mostly restricted to animal subjects, which are unable to report verbally on their conscious experiences.

Enough apologies. What do these various techniques show about the temporal evolution of neural activity underlying RPs? Although Type II RPs can occur on their own if the subject has taken care not to pre-plan a particular movement, they can also be seen as the latter half of Type I RPs. Type I RPs begin a second or more before the movement. Their first segment—from the start of the waveform till about 500 ms before the movement—is probably underpinned by bilateral activity in the midline SMA (Toro et al. 1993; Praamstra et al. 1999; Cui et al. 2000). Type II RPs begin about 500 ms before the movement. Most EEG and MEG measurements put neural activity between −500 ms and the movement as occurring mainly in the contralateral primary sensorimotor area MI, with some residual activity still going on in the SMA (e.g. Toro et al. 1993; Praamstra et al. 1999; Cui et al. 2000). On the other hand, combined MEG and PET recordings (Pedersen et al. 1998) show SMA activity in the interval from −300 ms to −100 ms, premotor cortex activity from −100 ms till the onset of the movement and MI activity only from the onset of the movement till 100 ms *after* the onset of the movement. This would suggest that the neural generators of the Type II RP lie in the SMA rather than in M1. Unfortunately, the few existing accounts of human intracortical recording which could have answered this question definitively have not reported enough detail about the timing of activity in the relevant brain areas to allow any conclusions. Rektor (2002) has recorded intracranial activity in subcortical as well as cortical structures and not unreasonably suggests that scalp-recorded RPs contain contributions from subcortical sources, but his published data do not contain the information needed to determine what brain structures are active specifically at 200 ms before the movement. Shibasaki's group (see e.g. Satow et al. 2003) has also recorded RPs from inside the skull, but again it is impossible to see from their records exactly what areas are active at 200 ms before their subject's movements.

A further complicating factor is that Lau et al. (2004) repeated Libet's experiments and confirmed that their subjects reported consciously experiencing the "intention to move" at about the same time as Libet's subjects did (i.e. a little more than 200 ms before the movement), and yet found that their instruction that the subjects should attend to their "intention to move" resulted in increased activity specifically in the pre-SMA. According to their calculations, the pre-SMA starts to be active 2–3 *seconds* before the movement, not 200–300 milliseconds.

The problem here may be that the word 'intention' has been used in different senses on different occasions. When Libet asked his subjects to report on the time of their intention to move, he made it very clear that they were not to pre-plan exactly when they were going to make any of their movements. On the other hand, the model shown in figure 1.2 of the present chapter uses the word 'intention' precisely to *mean* a pre-plan for movement. Thus it seems fairly clear that when Libet uses the word 'intention', he is using it in a different sense from that meant in figure 1.2. I believe that what Libet's subjects were reporting on was their awareness of an urge or decision (which on the face of it, they would appear immediately to have carried out) to "act-now"—in other words, they are reporting on their consciousness of *initiating* their movements. On a third hand, however, Lau et al. (2004) may be seen as having used 'intention' in both of these senses within the same experiment. These workers replicate Libet's task without mentioning (at least in the published report) that their subjects were to avoid pre-planning movements, and then essentially ask the subjects to do two things: (i) attend to their intention to move and (ii) report using Libet's revolving spot method when they first experienced an intention to move. It seems possible that these subjects may have taken instruction (i) to mean that they *should* pre-plan their movements—and furthermore that they should pay attention to that pre-planning—and instruction (ii) to mean, as did Libet's subjects, that they should report on the time of each of their decisions to "act-now." Two pieces of evidence that may be seen as supporting this interpretation are the following:

(a) When Libet's subjects did admit to having pre-planned some of the movements in particular trials, their reported time of awareness of intention to move was −233 ms, which is almost identical to Lau et al.'s −228 ms. In contrast, Libet's subjects in non-pre-planning mode reported awareness times of −192 ms. The difference may not be statistically significant, but it is suggestive.

(b) The pre-SMA activity recorded by Lau et al. was specifically not due to the initiation of a self-paced action, because it was not present when the subjects were instructed to attend to the movement itself, rather than their intention to make it.

In any case, Lau and Passingham (this volume) report extensive and ingenious further experiments in this area.

Overall, there would appear to be two reasonable conclusions from the work discussed above:

1. However you define intention, the fact remains that the first conscious awareness associated with the initiation of the movements studied here occurs well after the start of the neural activity that culminates in the movement. Even when there is no pre-planning and the first recordable neural events time-locked to the movement happen in what is probably MI (the last cortical way station before transmission to the spinal cord), the conscious event associated with initiating the movement arises only 250–300 ms *after* the start of the neural events. This clearly suggests that

whatever events one might reasonably consider to be the neural initiators of these movements, those events occur pre-consciously.

2. A more practically oriented conclusion might be that it is important to be clear about exactly what experience one wants one's subjects to introspect. Of course, explaining to the subjects exactly what the experimenter wants them to experience can bring its own problems—as Lau and Passingham (this volume) point out, instructions to attend to a particular internally generated experience can easily alter both the timing and the content of that experience and even whether or not it is consciously experienced at all. It seems that study of the consciousness associated with voluntary movements is just as difficult as study of any other conscious experience.

More Complicated Voluntary Movements

As was mentioned earlier, the button-pressing movements discussed above are examples of the simplest possible kind of voluntary movement. Button-pressing ad lib is not something that most of us spend a lot of time doing in everyday life. The next step in extending this sort of work to movements that are of more everyday utility is to investigate the situation when the subjects are asked to make a relatively realistic decision before deciding to press the button. Haggard and Eimer (1999) made a start on developing this paradigm by asking their subjects to choose whether to move their right or left hands. They found no difference in the reported time of intention to move between this and the usual Libet paradigm. Clearly there is great scope for further experimentation in this area.

For example, one tidbit of information along these lines concerns the fact that real-world decisions about whether or not to initiate a particular action are inevitably influenced by whether the subject perceives that the action will be rewarded. Hadland et al. (2003) have shown that in monkeys this aspect of action initiation is mediated by the anterior cingulate area.

4   Control of Ongoing Movements

While sensory intentions (and perhaps particularly those in the left AIP (Rushworth et al. 2001)) may themselves be associated with consciousness, it is fairly clear that their use in ongoing motor control is usually not (Jeannerod, this volume).

When laypersons think about unconscious movements, they normally think of involuntary reflexes and tics, which are not associated with consciousness at all. But in fact, any voluntary or consciously willed act of any complexity—be it as simple as picking up a coffee cup or as complicated as walking down to the beach for a swim or sight-reading a piece of Chopin—is *performed* largely unconsciously. We are (probably) aware of a general intent to perform the act. We may (or may not) be aware of a specific decision to initiate the act. During performance of the movement we are probably aware of some fraction of the multitude of potential sensory experiences generated by that performance. But we are certainly quite unaware of the complex calculations of coordinates and joint angles and forces and the sequential action of muscles that are required to move the arm to the right place, curve the hand in anticipation of the shape of the mug, grasp the mug and lift it to the lips without spilling coffee. We are not conscious at all of the comparisons of performance with intention, the ongoing readjustments to cope with changing environmental circumstances, the automatic alteration of breathing movements, the activation of an innate motor program (perhaps modified by learning) that are necessary to make our way to the water, dive in, avoid breathing water and start swimming. And if we have practiced enough, even the complicated eye-hand coordination needed to translate from observed dot position on a page of music to rule-governed finger movement on the keyboard has become entirely automatic.

This *un*consciousness is undoubtedly a great biological boon. When we are performing the sorts of novel or very difficult acts that do involve the constant presence of consciousness, (a) our movements tend to lack smoothness and precision and (b) the allocation of attention to the ongoing movement means that we are unable to be aware of much else.

The feedback control of ongoing movements using the somatosensory information generated during their execution occurs in the cerebellum. The posterior parietal cortex does not have direct connections through the spinal cord to muscles—rather, its main output flows to the motor areas at the front of the cortex. But importantly, a copy of the intentional plan is also sent via the pons to the cerebellum. This provides what von Holst (1954) called *efference copy*. It allows the cerebellum to calculate the sensory feedback expected from a successfully executed motor plan, compare this calculated feedback with the actual sensory reafference generated during the movement, and issue new instructions to the cortical motor areas for correction of movement errors (Jeuptner et al. 1996).

This feedback control is the particular function of an area of the cerebellum called the *cerebrocerebellum*. Lesions to the cerebrocerebellum cause delays in movement initiation and errors in coordination of limb movements. When this region is damaged, rapid movements are overshot, and over-correction of the overshoot gives rise to a period of instability at the end of the movement which is variously called terminal, action, or intention tremor. The other two main functional regions of the cerebellum are the *vestibulocerebellum*, which receives inputs from the vestibular organs (semicircular canals and otolith organs) and uses this in control of both saccadic and smooth pursuit eye movements (Goldberg et al. 1991) and the limb muscles used to maintain balance, and the *spinocerebellum*, which receives somatosensory, auditory, visual, and vestibular information and integrates this with cortical intention commands to control muscle tone. Damage to the spinocerebellum results in hypotonia, a diminished resistance to passive limb movement. The lateral cerebellum also appears to be a specialized region, in this case for timing: patients with damage to the lateral cerebellum show a sign called dysdiadochokinesia—the inability to sustain a regular rhythm of hand tapping—and the area may also perform a more general timing function that affects cognitive as well as motor performance (Ghez 1991).

Over and above these ongoing control functions, a particular kind of motor learning is also mediated by the cerebellum. As might be expected from the structure's role in correcting ongoing movements in light of sensory feedback, cerebellar learning is of the supervised or error-based type (Doya 2000). The idea that the cerebellum is a supervised learning system dates back to the hypotheses of Marr (1969) and Albus (1971) and the subsequent discovery by Ito (1982) of the synaptic long-term depression that provides a cellular basis for such learning.

One suggestion for a further function of efference copy is made by Choudhury and Blakemore (this volume), who suggest, with Jeannerod, that efference copy may provide the means by which one's own actions are distinguished from the actions of others. In the words of Choudhury and Blakemore, "the conscious awareness of unconsciously monitored actions is the means by which our actions are experienced as subjectively real, willed, and owned."

Conclusions

The above discussion gives only a brief overview of the structure and function of the motor system in the human brain. On the basis of this relatively limited understanding, the answer to the question "Does consciousness cause behavior?" would appear to be "It depends."

In the case of very simple voluntary acts such as pressing a button whenever one feels like it, good experimental evidence shows that the consciousness of being about to move arises before the movement occurs, but after the neural events leading up to the movement have begun. It is a reasonable conclusion that consciousness is not the immediate cause of this simple kind of behavior.

In the case of the correction of ongoing actions, consciousness of having moved more often than not arises actually *after* the correcting movement has been completed (and sometimes does not arise at all). Clearly, consciousness does not cause this extremely complex kind of behavior, either.

In the case of the initiation of actions based on complex decisions or long-term intentions, our question has not yet been answered one way or the other. Neurophysiologically speaking, relatively long-term intentions are formed in the DLPFC and/or pre-SMA, more detailed intentions are (or may not be, depending on the action) formed in the posterior parietal cortex, and any acts that result from these intentions are initiated somewhere in the complex web of parallel processing that goes on in the frontal cortex/basal ganglia loops physically located between the pre-SMA and the primary motor cortex. However, while it is clear that consciousness is generally *associated with* these processes, nobody has yet been able to design experiments that would unequivocally nail down the temporal relationship between the appearance of this consciousness and the onset of whatever neural events underpin the intentions and movement-initiations.

Which comes first in the initiation of complex moves—the consciousness, or the neural events? Given the importance of the answer for our legal system (Kaplan, this volume), our public policies (Hurley, this volume), and our general self-concept as humans (most of the contributors to part II of this volume), finding a solution to this conundrum must be seen as one of the next great challenges in neuroscience.

Acknowledgments

Thanks to Dick Passingham and Shaun Gallagher for comments on the manuscript. The author's research is supported by the University of Auckland Research Committee.

Note

1. The notion that intentions are "located" in the posterior parietal cortex may annoy some philosophers, but the word is chosen quite deliberately. Intentions in this sense are not abstract entities—they are patterns of neural activity; or perhaps patterns of synaptic strength which are eventually played out into patterns of neural activity. Either kind of pattern clearly has both temporal and spatial extension, which means it must be located somewhere.

References

Albus, J. S. 1971. A theory of cerebellar function. *Mathematical Biosciences* 10: 25–61.

Andersen, R. A., and Buneo, C. A. 2002. Intentional maps in posterior parietal cortex. *Annual Review of Neuroscience* 25: 189–220.

Buhmann, C., Glauche, V., Sturenburg, H. J., Oechsner, M., Weiller, C., and Buchel, C. 2003. Pharmacologically modulated fMRI—cortical responsiveness to levodopa in drug-naïve hemiparkinsonian patients. *Brain* 126: 451–461.

Cui, R. Q., Huter, D., Egkher, A., Lang, W., Lindinger, G., and Deecke, L. 2000. High-resolution DC-EEG mapping of the Bereitschaftspotential preceding simple or complex bimanual sequential finger movement. *Experimental Brain Research* 134: 49–57.

Cunnington, R., Windischberger, C., Deecke, L., and Moser, E. 2002. The preparation and execution of self-initiated and externally-triggered movement: a study of event-related fMRI. *Neuroimage* 15: 373–385.

Deecke, L. 2000. The Bereitschaftspotential as an electrophysiological tool for studying the cortical organization of human voluntary action. In *Clinical Neurophysiology at the Beginning of the 21st Century*, ed. Z. Ambler et al. Elsevier Science.

Deecke, L., and Kornhuber, H. 1978. An electrical sign of participation of the mesial 'supplementary' motor cortex in human voluntary finger movements. *Brain Research* 159: 473–476.

Doya, K. 2000. Complementary roles of basal ganglia and cerebellum in learning and motor control. *Current Opinion in Neurobiology* 10: 732–739.

Eskandar, E. N., and Assad, J. A. 1999. Dissociation of visual, motor and predictive signals in parietal cortex during visual guidance. *Nature Neuroscience* 2: 88–93.

Ghez, C. 1991. The cerebellum. In *Principles of Neural Science*, third edition, ed. E. Kandel et al. Prentice-Hall.

Goldberg, M. E., Eggers, H. M., and Gouras, P. 1991. The ocular motor system. In *Principles of Neural Science*, third edition, ed. E. Kandel et al. Prentice-Hall.

Haggard, P., and Eimer, M. 1999. On the relation between brain potentials and the awareness of voluntary movements. *Experimental Brain Research* 126: 128–133.

Hadland, K. A., Rushworth, M. F. S., Gaffan, D., and Passingham, R. E. 2003. The anterior cingulate and reward-guided selection of actions. *Journal of Neurophysiology* 89: 1161–1164.

Huxley, T. H. 1877. *A Technical Education*. Quoted in Milner and Goodale 1995.

Ito, M., Sakurai, M., and Tongroach, P. 1982. Climbing fibre induced depression of both mossy fibre responsiveness and glutamate sensitivity of cerebellar Purkinje cells. *Journal of Physiology* 324: 113–134.

Jahanshahi, M., Jenkins, I. H., Brown, R. G., Marsden, C. D., Passingham, R. E., and Brooks, D. J. 1995. Self-initiated versus externally triggered movements. I. An investigation using measurement of regional cerebral blood flow with PET and movement-related potentials in normal and Parkinson's disease subjects. *Brain* 118: 913–933.

Jahanshahi, M., and Dirnberger, G. 1999. The left dorsolateral prefrontal cortex and random generation of responses: Studies with transcranial magnetic stimulation. *Neuropsychologia* 37: 181–190.

Jahanshahi, M., and Frith, C. D. 1998. Willed action and its impairments. *Cognitive Neuropsychology* 15, no. 6–8: 483–533.

Jahanshahi, M., Dirnberger, G., Liasis, A., Towell, A., and Boyd, S. 2001. Does the pre-frontal cortex contribute to movement-related potentials? Recordings from subdural electrodes. *Neurocase* 7: 495–501.

Jeannerod, M. 1994. The hand and the object: The role of posterior parietal cortex in forming motor representations. *Canadian Journal of Physiology and Pharmacology* 72: 535–541.

Jenkins, I. H., Jahanshahi, M., Jueptner, M., Passingham, R. E., and Brooks, D. J. 2000. Self-initiated versus externally triggered movements. II. The effect of movement predictability on regional cerebral blood flow. *Brain* 123: 1216–1228.

Jueptner, M., Jenkins, I. H., Brooks, D. J., Frackowiak, R. S., and Passingham, R. E. 1996. The sensory guidance of movement: A comparison of the cerebellum and basal ganglia. *Experimental Brain Research* 112: 462–474.

Kalaska, J. F. 1996. Parietal cortex area 5 and visuomotor behavior. *Canadian Journal of Physiology and Pharmacology* 74: 483–498.

Lau, H. C., Rogers, R. D., Haggard, P., and Passingham, R. E. 2004. Attention to intention. *Science* 303: 1208–1210.

Libet, B. 1983. Time of conscious intention to act in relation to onset of cerebral activity (readiness-potential): The unconscious initiation of a freely voluntary act. *Brain* 106: 623–642.

Marr, D. 1969. A theory of cerebellar cortex. *Journal of Physiology* 202: 437–470.

Milner, A. D., and Goodale, M. A. 1995. *The Visual Brain in Action*. Oxford University Press.

Pedersen, J. R., Johannsen, P., Bak, C. K., Kofoed, B., Saermark, K., and Gjedde, A. 1998. Origin of human motor readiness field linked to left middle frontal gyrus by MEG and PET. *Neuroimage* 8: 214–220.

Platt, M. L., and Glimcher, P. W. 1999. Neural correlates of decision variables in parietal cortex. *Nature* 400: 233–238.

Praamstra, P., Schmitz, F., Freund, H.-J., and Schnitzler, A. 1999. Magneto-encephalographic correlates of the lateralized readiness potential. *Cognitive Brain Research* 8: 77–85.

Rektor, I. 2002. Scalp-recorded Bereitschaftspotential is the result of the activity of cortical and subcortical generators—a hypothesis. *Clinical Neurophysiology* 113: 1998–2005.

Rushworth, M. F. S., Krams, M., and Passingham, R. E. 2001. The attentional role of the left parietal cortex: The distinct lateralization and localization of motor attention in the human brain. *Journal of Cognitive Neuroscience* 13: 698–710.

Satow, T., Matsuhashi, M., Ikeda, A., Yamamoto, J., Takayama, M., Begum, T., Mima, T., Nagamine, T., Mikuni, N., Miyamoto, S., Hashimoto, N., and Shibasaki, H. 2003. Distinct cortical areas for motor preparation and execution in human identified by Bereitschaftspotential recording and EcoG-EMG coherence analysis. *Clinical Neurophysiology* 114: 1259–1264.

Toro, C., Matsumoto, J., Deuschl, G., Roth, B. J., and Hallett, M. 1993. Source analysis of scalp-recorded movement-related electrical potentials. *Electroencephalography and Clinical Neurophysiology* 86: 167–175.

von Holst, E. 1954. Relations between the central nervous system and the peripheral organ. *British Journal of Animal Behaviour* 2: 89–94.

Wise, S. P., Boussaoud, D., Johnson, P. B., and Caminiti, R. 1997. Premotor and parietal cortex: Cortico-cortical connectivity and combinatorial computations. *Annual Review of Neuroscience* 20: 25–42.

Zhang, M., and Barash, S. 2000. Neuronal switching of sensorimotor transformations for antiscaccades. *Nature* 408: 971–975.

2 Consciousness of Action as an Embodied Consciousness

Marc Jeannerod

We usually remain unaware of many of our own actions. One reason is that, even when an action is consciously executed, its memory trace is of a very short duration, and so it is rapidly forgotten. It is indeed a common experience when leaving home to ask oneself "Did I lock the door?" or "Did I turn off the light?" immediately after doing it. One may also drive home and suddenly realize that one has arrived there without having the least idea how one did it. This is not true for all actions, however. Some actions (for example, "I paid the bill at the restaurant last night") leave very vivid memories. The difference between actions that rapidly disappear from memory and those that remain is in the degree of awareness of the agent at the time where the action was performed. Some actions are executed under conscious control, some are executed automatically. In this chapter I will concentrate on those actions that are executed automatically, with the aim of understanding why and how a given action does or does not become conscious. This program, though arguably quite ambitious, is open to empirical analysis. I will use experimental data to evaluate the degree of consciousness involved in a given action, to examine the factors and the constraints for consciousness of an action to appear or not, and to identify some of the neural mechanisms that are involved in this process of access or non-access to consciousness. Before proceeding, however, it seems in order to clarify what is meant by "consciousness of action."

What is consciousness of action about? In other words, what is the content of consciousness when this term refers to an action? In trying to analyze this concept, several possible answers come to mind. The first one is that consciousness of action should refer to what the action is about. Actions have goals. To be aware of the goal one reaches for is one way of being conscious of the action undertaken to reach that goal. Being aware of the goal, however, does not imply awareness of, or conscious knowledge of, how that goal is reached. This is the second possible answer to the question, namely that consciousness of an action can also refer to how that action is (or was) performed. Can these two aspects, what and how, be dissociated from each other? This is obviously one of the empirical questions that will have to be considered in this chapter. In fact, there is still a third possible answer to the question of what consciousness of an action is about: Consciousness of an action can be about who is doing the action. However, I will keep this point outside the scope of this chapter. Questions about the agent of an action ("Did I do that?" or "Who did that?") do not refer to the action itself; rather, they are questions about the self. Being conscious of who did an action (of being the author of an action) corresponds to being conscious of oneself as a causal self, as opposed to other selves. Restricting the investigation to the action without raising the question of the self avoids the problem of self-identification. I will stick to the notion that pure, unambiguous first-person actions (I-actions), such as will be studied here, should be readily perceived as originating from the self, and should normally not pose the problem of identifying the agent. In other words, they should be seen as immune to errors through misidentification (Shoemaker 1963). This problem has been fully addressed elsewhere (Jeannerod 2003a,b; Jeannerod and Pacherie 2004; de Vignemont and Fourneret 2004).

1   The Content of the Consciousness of an Action

Consciousness of the Goal

The first aspect of action consciousness to be considered is what the action is about. This issue of the awareness of the goal of simple goal-directed actions has been extensively considered within the framework of the dual processing of visual information. Simple visually goal-directed movements, whether they are executed in isolation (like grasping and handling an object) or are embedded into a more complex action, have a well-defined status. They are relatively rapid (they typically last less than a second), and their course is almost entirely centrally determined (except for their terminal accuracy, which is improved by direct visual control). They are framed within an egocentric framework; that is, the location of the goal (the object) at which they are directed is coded in coordinates that arise from the subject's body. As such, these movements would be better described as target-directed than as goal-directed. The visuomotor system selects in the goal a small number of parameters that will be transformed into motor commands that will ensure compliance of the effector (e.g., the hand) with the object. In other words, there is nothing to be conscious of in such movements, except that the target has been correctly reached and that the goal has been ultimately achieved. Together with the short duration of the movement, the fact that its target is only a selected part of the goal (the part that is motorically defined), makes it automatic and non-conscious. This mode of processing of visual input (which has been characterized as "pragmatic processing"—see Jeannerod 1997) does not require consciousness. I will come back to this point later, in the context of how and when non-required consciousness may nevertheless arise.

The pragmatic mode of visual processing opposes another mode of processing for identification, whereby the goal is perceived as an entity with all its attributes, including those that are not immediately relevant for the movement (its color, for example). This semantic mode of visual processing, as we may call it, describes objects by their identity and their function, not as mere targets for the motor commands of reaching and grasping. This distinction has been the subject of controversies, mainly bearing on the actual limitations of pragmatic processing. For example, the suggestion has been made that pragmatic processing should only concentrate on the target itself and should disregard the context surrounding the target (Milner and Goodale 1993). An illustration of this point is the case where the context in which an object is perceived causes an illusion about the size or the shape of that object. Because illusions are attributes of conscious perception, they should not influence an automatic movement. A series of experiments by Melvyn Goodale and his co-workers tend to confirm this point. (See Jacob and Jeannerod 2003 for a review.)

These considerations reveal a contrast between overt and covert aspects of the goal. Whereas the detailed target of the movement remains outside awareness, the overt goal of the action, concerning the selection of objects, their use, their adequacy for the task under execution, and so on, can be consciously represented. The conclusion should not be drawn, however, that the covert aspects of the goal cannot be consciously accessed. Here I describe a set of experiments in which this point was specifically tested—that is, subjects were instructed to indicate the moment at which they became aware of a change in the configuration of the target occurring during their movement.

There are situations in everyday life where actions in response to visual events are clearly dissociated from the conscious experience of the same events. We respond first and become aware later. For example, when driving a car, we have to make a change in trajectory because of a sudden obstacle on our way: we consciously see the obstacle after we have avoided it. Castiello et al. (1991) designed a series of experiments to measure this temporal dissociation. Subjects were instructed to reach by hand and grasp an object (a vertical dowel) placed in front of them, as soon as it became illuminated. They also received the instruction to signal, by a vocal utterance, at what time they became aware of the illumination of the object. The onset of the hand movement aimed at the object preceded by about 50 milliseconds the vocal response signaling the subject's awareness of its change in visual appearance. This difference was not noticed by the subjects, who felt their hand movements in coincidence with their perception of the illumination of the object. In the same experiment, the illuminated object jumped by 10° on either side at the time where the reaching movement started. The first sign of correction of the hand trajectory appeared shortly (about 100 ms) after the shift in target position. In contrast, the vocal utterance corresponding to this same event came much later, some 300 ms after the beginning of the change in movement trajectory. The subjects' reports were in accordance with this temporal dissociation between the two responses: they reported that they saw the object jumping to its new position near the end of their movement, just at the time they were about to take the object (sometimes even after they took it).

The main result of this experiment is that the time to awareness of a visual event, as inferred from the vocal response, keeps a relatively constant value across different conditions. Under normal circumstances, when the target object remains stationary and no time pressure is imposed on performing the task, this time is roughly compatible with the duration of motor reaction times: when we make a movement toward an object, we become aware of this object near the time when the movement starts, or shortly after it has started, hence the apparent consistency between our actions and the flow of our subjective experience. This consistency breaks down when the motor reaction time shortens under conditions of time pressure, such as avoiding sudden obstacles or tracking unexpected object displacements, so that the conscious awareness becomes dissociated from the movement. One might suggest that the normally long reaction times (ca. 300 ms) of reaching movements have the function of keeping our subjective experience in register with our actions. Imagine what life would be like if the above temporal dissociation were the usual case, and if our awareness of the external events were systematically delayed from our actions in response to these events!

Observations made in patients with lesion of primary visual cortex and showing the "blindsight" phenomenon add further arguments for this notion of a dual processing of visual information (Weiskrantz 1986). These patients appear to reach consciously for non-conscious goals. For example, patient PJG described by Perenin and Rossetti (1996) correctly adjusted his hand movements at objects of varying size or orientation presented in his blind hemifield without being able to consciously report about the presence of these objects within his visual field.

The dissociation between motor responses and subjective experience, when it happens, as well as the more usual synchrony between the two, reflects the constraints imposed by brain circuitry during the processing of neural information. Different aspects of the same event are processed at different rates, and the global outcome is constrained by the slowness of the process that builds up awareness. Consciousness of the goal of an action is not immediate, it takes time to appear (the Time-On Theory; see Libet 1992). Adequate timing of neuronal activity in different brain areas is a critical condition for achieving subjective temporal consistency between external events. Indeed, it is common experience that goal-directed movements executed under conscious control are usually slow and inaccurate, e.g., during the first attempts at learning a new skill. This effect can be shown experimentally by delaying the onset of a goal-directed movement by only a few seconds after the presentation of the stimulus: this delay results in a severe degradation of the accuracy of the movement (Jakobson and Goodale 1991). In this condition, according to the above hypothesis, it is likely that the representation of the movement deteriorates rapidly and the fast automatic mechanism cannot operate.

In this section, two main points have been made. First, it has been made clear that some of the covert aspects of a goal-directed movement can become conscious in a condition where the subject is specifically instructed to attend to his/her subjective experience. In the above experiments, the subjects were able to report their awareness of the goal of an automatic movement directed at a luminous target. Second, the consciousness of the goal has a different timing from that of the movement itself. At this point, an interpretation of the automaticity of automatic movements can be proposed. This interpretation relies on several assumptions which are supported by experimental data. One has to assume, first, that most of the movement course is represented prior to its execution; second, that the representation coding for a goal-directed movement must have a short life span, that should not exceed the duration of the movement itself, so that the representation of that goal can be erased before another segment of the action starts; and, third, that consciousness is a slow process, and that the above temporal constraint does not leave enough time for consciousness to appear. If these assumptions are correct, it follows that a fast accurate movement can only be executed automatically.

Awareness of How a Movement Is Performed

The next question is about the knowledge of the content of the action itself. Forces and torques are applied automatically to the joints. Yet they can be consciously controlled and modulated, e.g., during learning a new skill. In the experiments reported here, subjects have been placed in situations where what they see or feel from their actions does not correspond to what they actually do. Such situations produce a conflict between the normally congruent signals (e.g., visual, proprioceptive, central motor commands) which are generated at the time of execution of an action. Subjects' reports about their feelings provide a direct insight into their conscious monitoring of these signals.

Since its initial version (Nielsen 1963), this paradigm has greatly contributed to our knowledge of the mechanisms of action recognition. In a more recent version, Fourneret and Jeannerod (1998) instructed subjects to draw straight lines between a starting position and a target, using a stylus on a digital tablet. The output of the stylus and the target were displayed on a computer screen. The subjects saw the computer screen in a mirror placed so as to hide their hand. On some trials, the line seen in the mirror was electronically made to deviate from the line actually drawn by the subject. Thus, in order to reach the target, the subject had to deviate his or her movement in the direction opposite to that of the line seen in the mirror. At the end of each trial, the subject was asked to indicate verbally in which direction he thought his hand had actually moved. The results were twofold. First, the subjects were consistently able to trace lines that reached the target, that is, they accurately corrected for the deviation. Second, they gave verbal responses indicating that they thought their hand had moved in the direction of the target, hence ignoring the actual movements they had performed. Thus, the subjects were unable to consciously monitor the discordance between the different signals generated by their own movements and falsely attributed the drawing of the line to their hand. In other words, they tended to adhere to the visible aspect of their performance, and to ignore the way it had been achieved.

In the experiment of Fourneret and Jeannerod, however, the deviation of the line was limited to 10°, a deviation that apparently remained compatible with the possibilities of the automatic correction mechanism. In a subsequent experiment, Slachevsky et al. (2001), using the same apparatus, introduced deviations of increasing amplitude up to 40°. They found that, as movement accuracy progressively deteriorated, the larger discordance between what subjects did and what they saw made them to become aware of the deviation at an average value of 14°. Beyond this point, they were able to report that the movement of their hand erred in a direction different from that seen on the screen and that, in order to fulfill the instruction of reaching the target, they had to deliberately orient their hand movement in a direction different from that of the target.

Thus, the awareness of a discordance between an action and its sensory consequences emerges when the magnitude of the discordance exceeds a certain amount. This point was recently confirmed by Knoblich and Kircher (2004). In their experiment, the subjects had to draw circles on a writing pad at a certain rate. As in the previous experiments, subjects saw on a computer screen an image of their movement, represented by a moving dot. The velocity of the moving dot could be either the same as that of the subject's movement, or it could be unexpectedly accelerated by up to 80 percent. To compensate for the change in velocity and to keep the dot move in a circle, as requested by the instruction, subjects had to decrease the velocity of their hand movement by a corresponding amount. Subjects were instructed to indicate any perceived change in velocity of the moving dot by lifting their pen. The results showed that the subjects failed to detect the smaller changes in velocity. For example, they could detect only half the changes when the velocity was increased by 40 percent, whereas the detection rate increased for faster velocity changes. Yet subjects were found to be able to compensate for all changes in velocity, including those that they did not consciously detect.

The results reported in this section indicate that subjects, even when they are involved in a conscious task like reaching for a target in an unusual condition, tend to ignore in which direction and at which velocity they actually move. Yet these covert aspects of their action may become accessible to their consciousness if and when a discordance appears between the different signals generated by the movement or, more generally, between the aim of the movement and its outcome. The mechanism underlying this phenomenon is considered in the next section.

2 From Automaticity to Conscious Control: Discordance between an Action and Its Perceived Outcome as a Factor of Its Conscious Access

Introspective Evidence

Consider these three situations:

Situation 1: I am engaged in the complex action of getting a cup of tea. I go through all the constituent actions in the proper sequence: I walk to the room while talking with a colleague, get to the place where the teapot is on the table, reach to it with my right arm, and grasp it. Suppose the teapot's handle is too hot: at the time of contact with my hand, I stop the grasping movement and withdraw my hand. Although the sequence was unfolding automatically, it is now interrupted because of the failure of one of its constituents. In the meantime, I become aware of the cause of the failure, of the fact that I was indeed in the process of getting a cup of tea, and that I will have to start another sequence to overcome the problem of the hot handle.

Situation 2: I have a case of mild tennis elbow in my right arm. I experience no pain when my arm is immobile and my elbow is flexed in the middle of its range. While looking at my computer screen, I reach for my cup of tea on the right side of the computer. Pain arises during the completion of the movement. I suddenly become aware of the fact that I was reaching for the cup and that I cannot do it with my right arm because it would be too painful. I use my left arm to take the cup and drink, and transfer the cup to the left of the computer to avoid repetition of the same painful experience.

Situation 3: This situation is borrowed from the neuroscientist Alf Brodal, who described his experience of his own movements after a stroke had affected the movements of his left arm. He reported the difficulty he experienced for skilled actions like tying his bow (Brodal 1973). Whereas before the stroke, he says in this paper, the action was executed rapidly and automatically, after the stroke he felt as if his fingers did not know the next move. What was apparently defective in the action of tying, Brodal continues, was not the triggering off of the act. There appeared to be a lacking of capacity to let the movements proceed automatically when the pattern is triggered because they could not be performed at the usual speed.

What is common to these three veridical (or at least plausible) situations is that a goal-directed movement, a constituent of a broader intentional action, could not reach its goal because of an intervening or unexpected event: an obstacle to completion of the movement in situation 1, an abnormal sensation in situation 2, and a paralysis in situation 3. In all three cases, the action was unfolding automatically and outside the subject's awareness. The failure triggered a "prise de conscience" of the ongoing action and a reconsideration of the strategy to obtain the final goal (or, in the case of paralysis, a detailed analysis of the sensations arising from the attempt to move). The impression is that the agent, who suddenly becomes aware of an action that he was doing automatically immediately before, has shifted to a different state of consciousness, as if the intervening event had acted as a "stimulus" and triggered consciousness of the action as a "response" to that stimulus. The more likely possibility, already suggested in section 1, is that consciousness was there all the time, but was lagging behind the action execution processes. In the next section, I propose a model that accounts for this possibility.

A Possible Neural Model for Consciousness of Action

The working hypothesis I am proposing here is that motor representations for acting automatically or consciously are one and the same thing, and that the two modes of representations are only distinguishable by the circumstances in which they are implemented into an overt action. The first theory to be considered is that of a monitoring of central and peripheral signals arising as a consequence of the execution of an action. This theory holds that the (central) efferent signals at the origin of an action are matched with those which result from its execution (the reafferent signals) and that this comparison provides cues about where and when the action originated. Its basic principle, inherited from the cybernetic era, and deeply rooted in physiological thinking, is that each time the motor centers generate an command signal for producing a movement, a "copy" of this command (the "efference copy") is retained. The reafference inflow signals (e.g., visual, proprioceptive) generated by the movement are compared with the copy so that, if a mismatch is recorded between the two types of signals, the state of the motor centers can be updated (Sperry 1950; von Holst and Mittelstaedt 1950).

More recent descriptions of this mechanism assume the existence of "internal models" in which the desired state of the system is represented. Internal models can predict the sensory consequences that should result from the execution of the motor command. In a self-generated movement, the predicted consequences are compared with the actual sensory feedback (Jeannerod 1995, Wolpert et al. 1995). This model of the control of action has been applied to the problem of action identification and self-identification. Identifying oneself as the agent of an action (the sense of agency) would rely on the degree of concordance between the predicted effects of that action and its actual sensory consequences. If perceived sensory changes correlate with the self-generated output signals, they are registered as consequences of one's own action. If not, on the contrary, they are registered as originating from an external origin. The correlation between efferent signals and the resultant incoming signals is thus an unambiguous feature of self-generated changes (Frith et al. 2000).

The introspective observations reported earlier in this section suggest that the same model could also account for some of the aspects of consciousness of action that have been described here. The situations where an action is delayed, incompletely executed, or blocked are typical examples of a mismatch between the desired output and an its observed result. Although we are still far from understanding why such a mismatch can create the conditions for consciousness of the action, recent experiments using neuroimaging techniques provide a tentative answer. In these experiments, a relatively limited cortical area, the posterior parietal cortex on the right side, has been found to be activated when a mismatch is created between an action and its sensory consequences (Fink et al. 1999). The activity of this area increases as a function of the degree of the mismatch (Farrer et al. 2003). Furthermore, lesions of this same area in the right posterior parietal cortex are associated with striking neuropsychological symptoms that testify to an alteration of self-consciousness and consciousness of action: neglect of contralateral space, neglect of the corresponding half of the body (denial of ownership), or even denial of the disease (anosognosia) (e.g., Daprati et al. 2000).

Keeping this model in mind, we may now ask further questions about the detailed mechanisms that may underlie the subjective experience of being conscious of a movement. One of these questions, addressed in the next section, concerns the respective roles of efferent and afferent mechanisms.

3 Is Consciousness of Action an Afferent or an Efferent Phenomenon?

According to the above model, several sources of information are potentially available to make a conscious judgment about one's own motor performance. Among the sensory sources are visual cues (directly derived from vision of the moving segment or indirectly from the effects of the movement on external objects) and proprioceptive cues (derived from movement-related mechanical deformations of the limb, through receptors located in the skin, joints, and muscles). Non-sensory sources are mainly represented by central signals originating from various levels of the action generation system. Note that, unlike visual cues, the proprioceptive and the central cues are unambiguously related to the self-generated movement: they are "first-person" cues in the sense that they can only conceivably arise from the self.

The Two Williams Debate

There is a long-standing controversy about the respective roles of the two main first-person cues in conscious knowledge about one's actions. This issue was the topic of the classical Two Williams Debate, in which Wilhelm Wundt held that our knowledge is based a priori on efferent information of a central origin and William James defended the opposite opinion that all that we know about our movements is based a posteriori on information from sensory organs. (See Jeannerod 1985 for historical references.) Experimenters have consistently failed to resolve this issue, mainly because of the methodological difficulty of isolating the two sources of information from one another. There are no reliable methods for suppressing proprioceptive information arising during the execution of a movement. Alternatively, it is possible to prevent muscular contractions in a subject who is attempting to move, e.g., by complete curarization of one limb: if the subject reports sensations from his attempts to move his paralyzed limb, these sensations should arise from outflow motor commands, not from proprioceptive inflow. The available evidence shows that no perception of movement arises in this condition. However, experiments where an arm is only partially curarized suggest a more balanced conclusion: subjects requested to estimate the heaviness of weights that they attempted to lift with their weakened arm report an increased perceived heaviness (McCloskey et al. 1974). This illusion was interpreted as reflecting the increase in motor outflow needed to lift the weights (Gandevia and McCloskey 1977). This result provides an indirect evidence as to the possibility for central signals to influence conscious experience.

A more direct solution to this problem is to examine patients with complete haptic deafferentation of pathological origin (e.g., following a sensory neuropathy). One such patient is GL, who has been extensively studied by several experimenters (Cole and Paillard 1995).

Exploring Consciousness of Action in Patient GL

Patient GL has no haptic information about the movements she performs. Thus, when visual feedback from her movements is either systematically distorted or suppressed, the only information on which she can rely to form a phenomenal experience about her own action should be derived from the action generation processes. An experimental study was performed to examine this point, using the apparatus already described. GL had to draw a line with her unseen hand while an angular bias to the right, increasing from 1° to 20° over successive trials, was introduced. Like a normal subject, GL performed the task without difficulty and was able to compensate for the bias. When asked, at the end of each trial, to estimate verbally the angle by which she thought her hand had deviated to the left for bringing the line to the target, GL never explicitly reported a feeling of discordance between what she had seen and the movement that she thought she had made. Remember that, in this task, normal subjects become clearly aware—although by underestimating it—of a displacement of their hand toward the left to compensate for the disturbance, when the discordance exceeds a certain value. Instead, GL gave responses indicating that she thought she had drawn the line in the sagittal direction. In spite of expressing perplexity at the end of some trials, GL never became aware of the discordance and, consequently, of any strategy of correction she had to apply to correct for the bias. When asked to describe her feelings, she only mentioned that she found the task "difficult" and requiring an "effort of concentration." Conversely, as I have mentioned, control subjects examined in this task were able to report their conscious strategy (Fourneret et al. 2001).

Another experiment with the same patient addressed the same question of a possible role of the efferent processes in motor consciousness by exploring the production and the perception of muscular force. When muscular force is applied isometrically (with no change in muscle length), e.g. on an ergometer, proprioceptive input is limited: thus, this condition should maximize the role of the central commands in the conscious appreciation of the exerted force. When instructed, first to apply a certain degree of force with one hand, and then to match this degree of force with the other hand, GL performed with a close to normal accuracy (Lafargue et al. 2003): this result indicates that GL was able to produce accurate central commands. Yet, she was unable to report any conscious feeling from her effort, neither did she experience fatigue when a high degree of muscular contraction had to be maintained.

The main point revealed by these observations is that the lack of proprioceptive input from movement execution or isometric force generation severely impairs the possibility of consciously monitoring the efferent process. The central, non-sensory cues, which are still available in patient GL, appear to be of no use for consciously monitoring one's movements, except for the vague feelings of effort and difficulty that GL reported in one of the tasks. However, the mere opposition between peripheral and central sources of information in providing cues for consciousness (which was the core of the Two Williams Debate) does not take into account the complete set of events arising during the voluntary execution of a movement. The model of action monitoring proposed above postulates that central signals are used as a reference for the desired action, and that reafferent sensory signals from the executed movement are compared with this reference. In GL, because no reafference from the executed movement was present, this comparison process could not take place. In normal subjects, the conscious information would be derived, not directly from the reafferent (proprioceptive) signals themselves, but from the output of the comparison process, for which the presence of both central and peripheral signals is required. The lack of conscious feelings during attempted movements in completely paralyzed subjects (produced by curarization, for example, a situation I have mentioned briefly) in spite of the generation of intense motor commands, can also be explained by the lack of corresponding proprioceptive reafferent signals. Conversely, when reafferent signals are present, but do not match the central signals, the comparison process generates signals proportional to the degree of mismatch between the two. This would account for the sensations of effort reported by subjects with a paresis of pathological origin (but with preserved proprioceptive input) (Brodal 1973) and in normal subjects during lifting weights with incompletely paralyzed arms (see above), as well as for the rise of consciousness in situations where a movement cannot reach its goal.

The above hypothesis is not incompatible with the fact that GL knew that she had attempted to perform the task at each trial, neither with the fact that she was aware of her intention to move, if not of her actual movements. In other words, awareness of one's actions is only one aspect of the general problem of action consciousness. Our present results suggest that the cues for accessing awareness of action-related mental states (like intending or imagining an action, for example) should be distinct from those that are generated at the time of execution.

Conclusion: Consciousness of Action as a Post Hoc Phenomenon

The picture of consciousness that arises when it is studied in its relation to action is that of a post hoc phenomenon. First, consciousness of action (and probably other forms of consciousness as well) is a lengthy process that can appear only if adequate time constraints are fulfilled. Second, given that the Two Williams Debate apparently turned in favor of William James, consciousness appears to be bound to a posteriori signals arising from the completion of the action itself, not to central signals that precede the action. As such, consciousness could not play a causal role in triggering the action, simply because it comes too late.

The type of consciousness (in fact, of non-consciousness) that is linked to the experience of the embodied self, like consciousness of action, is discontinuous. It operates on a moment-to-moment basis, as it is bound to particular bodily events. The embodied self mostly carries an implicit mode of action consciousness, where consciousness becomes manifest only when required by the situation. The related information has a short life span and usually does not survive the bodily event for very long. In contrast, the conscious sense of will that we may experience when we execute an action, which is at the origin of our narrative continuity, arises from the belief that our thoughts can have a causal influence on our behavior. (See Sperry 1980 for discussion.) While we tend to perceive ourselves as causal, we actually ignore the cause from which our actions originate. Conscious free choice, like conscious will, is not a direct perception of a causal relation between a thought and an action, but rather a feeling based on the causal inference one makes about the data that do become available to consciousness. This dissociation between the two levels of the self (an embodied self and a "narrative" self) has been considered by some authors as the origin of an illusion (e.g., Wegner 2002). Because the conscious thought and the observed action are consistently associated, even though they may not be causally related, the narrative self tends to build a cause-and-effect story. The embodied self, in contrast, by avoiding conscious introspection, reaches simpler (and perhaps more secure) conclusions about an action, its goal and its agent by monitoring on-line the degree of congruence between central and peripheral signals generated by the action.

The role of consciousness should rather be to ensure the continuity of subjective experience across actions which are—by necessity—executed automatically. Because it reads behavior rather than starting it, consciousness represents a background mechanism for the cognitive rearrangement after the action is completed, e.g., for justifying its results, or modifying the factors that have been at the origin of the movement if the latter turned out to be unsuccessful. In line with the idea proposed by Nisbett and Wilson (1977) that we tend to "tell more than we can know," this mechanism could have the role of establishing a declarative cognitive content about one's own preferences, beliefs, or desires.

References

Brodal, A. 1973. Self-observations and neuroanatomical considerations after a stroke. *Brain* 96: 675–694.

Castiello, U., Paulignan, Y., and Jeannerod, M. 1991. Temporal dissociation of motor responses and subjective awareness: A study in normal subjects. *Brain* 114: 2639–2655.

Cole, J., and Paillard J. 1995. In *The Body and the Self*, ed. J. Bermudez et al. MIT Press.

Daprati, E., Sirigu, A., Pradat-Diehl, P., Franck, N., and Jeannerod, M. 2000. Recognition of self produced movement in a case of severe neglect. *Neurocase* 6: 477–486.

de Vignemont, F., and Fourneret, P. 2004. The sense of agency: A philosophical and empirical review of the "Who" system. *Consciousness and Cognition* 13: 1–19.

Farrer, C., Franck, N., Georgieff, N., Frith, C. D., Decety, J., and Jeannerod, M. 2003. Modulating the experience of agency: A PET study. *Neuroimage* 18: 324–333.

Fink, G. R, Marshall, J. C., Halligan, P. W., Frith, C. D., Driver, J., Frackowiack, R. S. J., and Dolan, R. J. 1999. The neural consequences of conflict between intention and the senses. *Brain* 122: 497–512.

Fourneret, P., and Jeannerod, M. 1998. Limited conscious monitoring of motor performance in normal subjects. *Neuropsychologia* 36: 1133–1140.

Fourneret, P., Franck, N., Slachevsky, A., and Jeannerod, M. 2001. Self-monitoring in schizophrenia revisited. *NeuroReport* 12: 1203–1208.

Frith, C. D., Blakemore, S. J., and Wolpert, D. M. 2000. Abnormalities in the awareness and control of action. *Philosophical Transactions of the Royal Society London B* 355: 1771–1788.

Gandevia, S. G., and McCloskey, D. I. 1977. Changes in motor commands, as shown by changes in perceived heaviness, during partial curarization and peripheral anesthesia in man. *Journal of Physiology* 272: 673–689.

Jacob, P., and Jeannerod, M. 2003. *Ways of Seeing: The Scope and Limits of Visual Cognition.* Oxford University Press.

Jakobson, L. S., and Goodale, M. A. 1991. Factors affecting higher order movement planning: A kinematic analysis of human prehension. *Experimental Brain Research* 86: 199–208.

Jeannerod, M. 1985. *The Brain-Machine: The Development Of Neurophysiological Thought.* Harvard University Press.

Jeannerod, M. 1995. Mental imagery in the motor context. *Neuropsychologia* 33: 1419–1432.

Jeannerod, M. 1997. *The Cognitive Neuroscience of Action.* Blackwell.

Jeannerod, M. 2003a. The mechanisms of self-recognition in humans. *Behavioral Brain Research* 142: 1–15.

Jeannerod, M. 2003b. Consciousness of action and self-consciousness: A cognitive neuroscience approach. In *Agency and Self-Awareness*, ed. J. Roessler and N. Eilan. Oxford University Press.

Knoblich, G., and Kircher, T. T. J. 2004. Deceiving oneself about being in control: conscious detection of changes in visuomotor coupling. *Journal of Experimental Psychology: Human Perception and Performance* 30: 657–666.

Lafargue, G., Paillard, J., Lamarre, Y., and Sirigu, A. 2003. Production and perception of grip force without proprioception: Is there a sense of effort in deafferented subjects. *European Journal of Neuroscience* 17: 2741–2749.

Libet, B. 1992. The neural time-factor in perception, volition and free will. *Revue de Métaphysique et de Morale* 2: 255–272.

McCloskey, D. I., Ebeling, P., and Goodwin, G. M. 1974. Estimation of weights and tensions and apparent involvement of a "sense of effort." *Experimental Neurology* 42: 220–232.

Milner, A. D., and Goodale, M. A. 1993. Visual pathways to perception and action. In *Progress in Brain Research*, ed. T. Hicks et al. Elsevier.

Nielsen, T. I. 1963. Volition: A new experimental approach. *Scandinavian Journal of Psychology* 4: 225–230.

Nisbett, R., and Wilson, T. 1977. Telling more than we can know: Verbal reports on mental processes. *Psychological Review* 84: 231–259.

Perenin, M. T., and Rossetti, Y. 1996. Grasping without form discrimination in a hemianopic field. *Neuroreport* 7: 793–797.

Shoemaker, S. 1963. *Self-Knowledge and Self-Identity.* Cornell University Press.

Slachewsky, A., Pillon, B., Fourneret, P. Pradat-Diehl, Jeannerod, M., and Dubois, B. 2001. Preserved adjustment but impaired awareness in a sensory-motor conflict following prefrontal lesions. *Journal of Cognitive Neuroscience* 13: 332–340.

Sperry, R. W. 1950. Neural basis of the spontaneous optokinetic response produced by visual inversion. *Journal of Comparative and Physiological Psychology* 43: 482–489.

Sperry, R. W. 1980. Mind-brain interaction: Mentalism, yes; dualism, no. *Neuroscience* 5: 195–206.

von Holst, E., and Mittelstaedt, H. 1950. Das Reafferenzprinzip. Wechselwirkungen zwischen Zentralnervensystem und Peripherie. *Naturwissenschaften* 37: 464–476.

Wegner, D. 2002. *The Illusion of Conscious Will.* MIT Press.

Weiskrantz, L. 1986. *Blindsight: A Case Study and Implications.* Oxford University Press.

Wolpert, D. M., Ghahramani, Z., and Jordan, M. I. 1995. An internal model for sensorimotor integration. *Science* 269: 1880–1882.

3 Intentions, Actions, and the Self

Suparna Choudhury and Sarah-Jayne Blakemore

What gives me the right to speak of an 'I,' and indeed of an 'I' as a cause. . . . ?
—Nietzsche (1914)

The human subjective experience of freely willed action requires that the actor feels a sense of agency. In other words, willed action is one that the agent can own, "bearing [one's] signature" (Pettit 2001). In this chapter we discuss how a sense of self might emerge from action. How do we feel in control of our actions? The ability to attribute one's own actions to the self is crucial to feeling that the experience is "mine." We describe studies that have investigated how we recognize the consequences of our actions and how this "self-monitoring" system distinguishes between self and other. We review psychological studies of the conscious experience of willed action and neurophysiological studies that shed light on its possible underlying processes. In addition, studies of patients with disorders of volition will be discussed as evidence that a breakdown in the self-monitoring system may account for a disturbance to the normal experiential link between intention and the awareness of volitional control.

1 Distinguishing between Self and Other through Prediction

Being aware of one's own actions and distinguishing them from the actions of others is critical for feeling a sense of self and for communication with other agents. Usually, when we carry out an action, we *feel* a sense of agency—that is, we feel that we are both the author and the owner of our own action. How is this feeling of ownership possible? This is particularly problematic given the well-established mirror in the brain: the same parts of the brain fire both when I watch someone else make an action and when I make the action myself. This suggests that there is a shared representational system that codes our own actions and our perceptions of other people's actions (Decety et al. 1997; Umilta et al. 2001; Gallese 2003; Rizzolatti and Craighero 2004). If my brain "mirrors" observed actions, how do I know that it is someone else, and not me, who is moving when I observe an action? How does the brain distinguish between moving an arm and observing someone else moving their arm? Evidence from studies of motor control suggests that the brain solves the problem of agency through prediction.

Forward Models

It has been proposed that internal motor representations, also known as forward models, serve as predictors in the brain (Wolpert et al. 1995; Miall and Wolpert 1996; Wolpert and Flanagan 2001). Prediction is a necessary step in motor planning and can be used in many ways—for example, for fine motor adjustments, action planning, and motor learning. Several studies have suggested that, through the anticipation of future outcomes of actions, the brain links the consequences of a movement to the prior intention to confer a sense of agency.

For every intended action, the brain must issue a motor command to the muscles in order to execute the action. It is proposed that a duplicate of the motor command—an "efference copy"—is generated in parallel and used to make predictions about the sensory consequences of one's own action. The *forward dynamic model* predicts the sensory consequences of the movement and compares them with the desired effects—for example, the intended position of a hand. Discrepancies between predicted states and desired states result in error signals that can be used to fine-tune actions. A controller, also called an *inverse model*, gauges this relationship to provide the motor instructions required by the muscles to achieve the desired effect, such as a particular grip force for a given object. The *forward output model* predicts the sensory consequences of the motor act and compares them with the actual effect of the movement. Discrepancies between predicted states and actual states can be used for self-monitoring—that is, to distinguish between self-produced or externally produced actions, and in doing so to maintain a distinct sense of self.

Recognizing the Consequences of Action

This predictive control model may account for why self-produced touch differs from our experience of a touch stimulus produced by an external agent or object. For instance, it is well known that you cannot tickle yourself. Why do we react differently (or not at all) to a self-produced tickle and an externally produced tickle? A series of studies provide evidence that self-produced stimuli are perceptually attenuated whereas externally produced stimuli are not. In one experiment, a device was used to deliver a touch stimulus to the subject's right palm. In the first condition, subjects produced the stimulus themselves, using the left hand; in the second condition, the experimenter delivered the stimulus. Subjects consistently rated the self-produced touch less tickly and intense than the externally produced touch (Blakemore, Wolpert, and Frith 1999). This may be explained in terms of the framework of motor control outlined above. The forward output model can be used to make accurate predictions of the sensory outcome (in this case, the tickly sensation of the stimulus) of a self-produced action, using the motor command and efference copy. This results in attenuation or cancellation of the sensory outcome. In contrast, for an externally generated sensation, there is no efference copy available upon which to base a prediction, and hence, no attenuation. As a result, externally produced sensations are effectively perceptually enhanced.

Another study, in which the correspondence between self-generated movements and their sensory effects was manipulated, showed that attenuation of sensations is due to the accuracy of the sensory predictions (Blakemore, Frith, and Wolpert 1999). In this experiment, subjects held an object attached to a robot. This was connected to a second robot attached to which was a piece of foam that delivered a touch stimulus to the palm of the right hand. Movement of the participant's left hand therefore caused movement of the foam, as if by remote control. The robotic interface was used to introduce time delays of 100, 200, and 300 milliseconds, and trajectory rotations of 30°, 60°, and 90° between the movement of the participant's left hand and the tactile stimulus on the right palm, and subjects were asked to rate the "tickliness." As the delay and rotation increased, subjects reported a subsequent increase in the tickliness rating. Increasing the discrepancy between the initiation of action and the ensuing sensation temporally or spatially, therefore, results in the enhancement of the self-generated sensation, because the delayed or rotated sensory stimulus no longer matches the prediction based on the efference copy. In a sense, then, manipulating the correspondence between causes and effects of our actions deludes the motor system into treating the self as another. The study suggests that attenuation of sensations, as judged by subjects' experiential accounts, is correlated with the accuracy of sensory predictions. Since the forward model can make more accurate predictions of the consequences of our own actions relative to other people's actions, the system is used to attribute actions to the proper agent and in this way to distinguish between the self and others. Importantly, subjects reported that they were not aware of the perturbations between the movement and the consequences, which suggests that the signals for sensory discrepancies are not available to our conscious awareness.

This predictive process is also likely to be at the root of why physical fights always seem to escalate. Notice how tit-for-tat tussles between children tend to intensify, each child claiming that the other hit him or her harder. In a recent study (Shergill et al. 2003), a motor was used to apply a brief force to the tip of each participant's left index finger. Subjects were then asked to match the force they felt using their right index finger by pushing down on a force transducer attached to the motor. Results showed that subjects consistently applied a stronger force than had been applied to them. The authors suggest that, just as happens when we try to tickle ourselves, the brain predicts the sensory consequences of the self-generated force and then reduces the sensory feedback. Since the forward model can only predict the outcome of our own actions and not of those of someone else, sensations that are externally caused are enhanced relative to self-produced sensations. As a result, if you were to deliver a vengeful punch to match the force of your opponent's blow, it is likely that you would overestimate the strength of the opponent's punch and strike back harder.

Brain Areas Involved in Maintaining Awareness and Making Predictions

There is accumulating evidence that a cerebellar-parietal network is involved in predicting and attenuating self-produced actions relative to externally produced sensations (Blakemore, Wolpert, and Frith 1998; Blakemore, Rees, and Frith 1998; Blakemore, Frith, and Wolpert 2001). In an fMRI experiment that employed the tickling paradigm described above, during externally produced touch, activity in the bilateral parietal operculum (the secondary somatosensory cortex) and anterior cingulate cortex was higher than during the self-touch condition (Blakemore, Wolpert, and Frith 1998). In addition, there was less activity in the right cerebellar cortex during a self-generated movement with a tactile consequence compared to an identical movement with no tactile consequence. A positron emission tomography (PET) study revealed that activity in the right lateral cerebellar cortex increased as time delays between the onset of a self-generated movement and its sensory effect were increased. This suggests that this region is involved in signaling sensory discrepancies between predicted and actual sensory outcomes of motor acts (Blakemore, Rees, and Frith 1998).

These data support other studies that implicate the cerebellum and the parietal cortex in sensorimotor prediction. Electrophysiological studies show that neurons in the cerebellum are involved in reaching and grasping movements, firing before the onset of the action. They may therefore be involved in the rapid detection of errors during motor preparation and producing error signals at a subconscious level (Blakemore and Sirigu 2003). Electrophysiological studies have also demonstrated that neurons in the parietal cortex are activated during planning of eye movements (Duhamel et al. 1992) as well as during reaching and grasping movements (Buneo et al. 2002).

Neuroimaging studies have revealed differential activation of the inferior parietal cortex for tasks involving action of the self versus action of another. For instance, this region is activated more when an external agent controls a movement compared with when the subject controls a movement themselves (Farrer and Frith 2002). The inferior parietal cortex is activated when subjects mentally simulate actions from someone else's perspective compared with when they imagine performing the action themselves (Ruby and Decety 2001), answer conceptual questions from a third-person perspective compared with from their own perspective (Ruby and Decety 2003), and think about how another person would feel in certain situations relative to how they would feel (Ruby and Decety 2004). It has been argued that the cerebellum is involved in the rapid detection of discrepancies between actual and predicted sensory effects of movements, signaling errors below the level of awareness, while the parietal cortex is concerned with higher-level prediction, such as the maintenance of goals, the monitoring of intentions, and the distinction between the self and others. This information may be available to conscious awareness (Buneo et al. 2002; Blakemore and Sirigu 2003; Sirigu et al. 2004).

2   Losing the Sense of One's Own Volition

People diagnosed with schizophrenia who have delusions of control often report that their movements, thoughts, and emotions feel as if they are under the control of some other agent rather than caused by their own volition. The sense of agency and intentionality itself is not lost in these cases. In fact, patients often interpret other people's non-intentional actions as intentional (Blakemore, Sarfati, et al. 2003; Corcoran 2003). Self-produced action is, however, assigned to an external agent, rather than to the self, such that the movement feels involuntary. Studies of such patients have led several groups to interpret the cause of this experience as a failure in the self-monitoring system (Frith 1987; Frith, Blakemore, and Wolpert 2000; Johns et al. 2001). Indeed, patients with delusions of control or auditory hallucinations have different experiences of self-tickling than healthy controls or other patient controls who do not exhibit the symptoms (Blakemore, Smith, et al. 2000). There appears to be a failure in attenuation in the self-touch condition, such that the self-touch feels as intense and tickly as external touch. This suggests that something may have gone awry in the predictive mechanism that usually serves to reduce the sensory consequences of self-generated actions. A breakdown in the forward model might, therefore, account for the feeling that active movements are passive, and for the attribution of such sensations to alien sources.

Experience and Brain Activity during Delusions of Alien Control

The role of the parietal cortex and cerebellum in anticipating future states of the body and distinguishing between self and other has already been discussed. Neuroimaging studies of patients with delusions of control corroborate the suggested roles of these brain areas. In one study, subjects known to experience delusions of control were required to perform a simple "willed action" task using a joystick (Spence et al. 1997). Subjects were asked to move the joystick in one of four freely chosen directions. Subjects were scanned using positron emission tomography (PET), and brain activity was compared to a contrasting condition in which the movements of the joystick were paced and the subjects did not choose the directions with their own will. Higher activity in parietal cortex is characteristic of passive movements relative to active movements (Weiller et al. 1996). In the Spence et al. study, patients showed overactivity in the superior parietal cortex and in the cerebellum during the willed action condition relative to subjects who did not have delusions of control and to the patients themselves a few months later when these experiences had subsided. This suggests that in patients with delusions of control active movements are processed in the brain as passive movements. Many of these patients reported feelings of alien control while performing the willed action task, demonstrating a correspondence between the brain activation patterns and the phenomenology of passivity experiences.

Distinguishing our own movements from other people's movements is not always straightforward. In one experiment, normal healthy control subjects were instructed to execute various specified hand movements without directly watching their actions (Daprati et al. 1997). They were then presented with video-recorded images of their own moving hand as well as images of the experimenter's moving hand on a screen and asked to determine when the hand was theirs and when it belonged to the experimenter. Subjects tended to distinguish easily between their own hand and the experimenter's hand when the movements were distinct. However, when they were shown images of the experimenter's hand making the same movements they had made, they misjudged the ownership of the hand in about a third of the trials. When patients experiencing delusions of control and hallucinations performed this task, they gave mostly correct responses when distinguishing between images of their own hand movements and images of different actions performed by the experimenter's hand. However, the error rate rose to about 80 percent in the condition where they watched the experimenter's hand make movements identical to those they had made. Schizophrenic patients with delusions of control more readily attributed the experimenter's actions to themselves. It has been suggested that this could be due to an impairment in the forward model. In the condition in which all subjects were more error prone, the subject's (invisible) executed movement and the (visible) image of the experimenter's movement were identical. There was therefore no mismatch between the perceived consequence and the anticipated consequence (that is, the final hand position); hence the errors in both sets of subjects. Daprati et al. suggested, however, that whereas normal control subjects are able to use detailed timing and kinesthetic aspects of the movements to make correct agency judgments in most cases, schizophrenic patients fail to monitor these signals sufficiently, which leads to an inaccurate comparison between representations of self-produced and other-produced actions.

There are two issues that remain with this finding. First, the patients in this study tended to misattribute externally produced actions to themselves, whereas delusions of control are characterized by a misattribution of self-produced actions to an external source. Second, if delusions of control are caused by an impairment in the forward model, it must be at the level of the forward output model rather that the forward dynamic model. Patients with delusions of control show predictive grip-force modulation (Delevoye et al. 2003), which relies on a forward dynamic model comparison between predicted and intended states. Such patients also compensate for gain changes in a tracking task (Knoblich et al. 2004), which suggests that, at some level, the predictive mechanism is still intact.

3 Being Aware of Actions

Of What Aspects of Action Are We Aware?

Being aware of initiating and controlling actions is a major component of conscious experience, but many aspects of action occur without awareness. Evidence that sensations associated with actual movements are unavailable to awareness comes from a study in which the sensory consequences of movement were made to deviate from subjects' expectations (Pourneret and Jeannerod 1998). In this study the subjects' task was to draw a straight line on a computer screen. Subjects could not see their arm or hand and were given false feedback about the trajectory of their arm movement. They therefore had to make considerable deviations from a straight movement in order to achieve their goal. However, verbal reports indicated that subjects were not aware that they were making deviant movements—they claimed to have made straight movements. These results suggest that we are aware of the movements we intend rather than the movements we actually make. There is some evidence to suggest that the exact threshold above which the discrepancy between the intended and actual movement becomes available to awareness depends to some extent on the task at hand. When the task is to detect the mismatch, subjects seem to become aware that the movement is not their own when their movement and its sensory (visual) consequences are discrepant spatially by 15° or temporally by 150 ms (Franck et al. 2001). However, if subjects are not asked to detect a mismatch, they appear not to notice any discrepancy even when the sensory (tactile) consequences of their movements are delayed by 300 ms (Blakemore, Frith, and Wolpert 1999).

In his studies of motor consciousness, Benjamin Libet investigated the time at which awareness emerges during the generation of an action. Libet et al. (1983) asked normal volunteers to estimate retrospectively the time at which they initiated a finger movement (the time at which their finger started to move; the "M" judgment). This consistently anticipated the actual starting time of the movement by 50–80 ms. Recently, Patrick Haggard and his colleagues have carried out a series of experiments based on the Libet paradigm. They have shown that the perceived time of movement onset is slightly delayed (by about 75 ms) if the motor cortex is stimulated using transcranial magnetic stimulation (TMS), whereas this causes a far greater delay (of around 200 ms) in the initiation of the actual movement (Haggard and Magno 1999). These observations support the idea that our awareness of initiating a movement is not derived from sensory signals arising in the moving limb (which are not available until after the limb has started moving). Instead our awareness appears to be linked to a signal that precedes the movement, what Libet called an "unconscious cerebral initiative." One signal that is available before a movement is initiated is the prediction of the sensory consequences of the movement. Perhaps it is this prediction which we are aware of when making a movement.

Action in the Imagination

We often run a mental simulation, or a motor image, of ourself in action before making, or while watching, an action. For example, while a student watches her music teacher playing the flute or a football player kicking a ball, she will imagine the observed action, although she remains still. The imagined action can be vivid enough to produce physiological reactions—for example, an increase in heart rate that corresponds to the mental effort. Sensory prediction might underlie the ability to prepare and imagine movements. It is well established that imagining moving and preparing to move activate a subset of the brain regions activated by executing a movement (Decety et al. 1994; Stephan et al. 1995; Nyberg et al. 2001; Naito et al. 2002). Normal people can confuse actions performed in the imagination and actions performed in reality when they are asked to recall such actions two weeks later (Thomas and Loftus 2002). A recent fMRI study that directly compared movement execution with movement imagination demonstrated that imagining movements activates the left posterior and inferior parietal lobe to a greater extent than executing the same movement (Gerardin et al. 2000).

Typically, people show a speed-accuracy tradeoff for imaginary movements as well as for real movements. Several studies have demonstrated that it takes the same time to execute a real action as it does to imagine performing the same action, and that as the action becomes more difficult more time is needed to accomplish it. Walking blindfolded to a target takes progressively more time as the distance to the target increases, both in reality and in the imagination (Decety and Michel 1989). In addition, the times taken to walk to each of the targets in the walking condition were strikingly similar to the times taken to imagine the corresponding actions. This speed-accuracy tradeoff effect is lost in the imaginary movements of patients with parietal damage (Sirigu et al. 1996; Danckert et al. 2002). Taken together, these data suggest that the parietal lobe plays an important role in the generation of motor images, and that it may store motor representations that are necessary for motor imagery. The same lack of speed-accuracy tradeoff is seen in imagined movements made by schizophrenic patients with delusions of control (Maruff et al. 2003). This is in line with the proposal that delusions of control are associated with a faulty internal representation of action.

Awareness of Intentions

Are we aware of our *intentions* to move? In a second task, Libet asked volunteers to indicate the time at which they are aware of having the "urge" to make a movement (their subjective will, or intention, to move; the "W" judgment) (Libet et al. 1983). Subjects' W judgments consistently precede the production of the movement by about 200 ms. Interestingly, this is well after the onset of the readiness potential, the negative potential arising from the supplementary motor area (SMA), which precedes the movement by one second or more. On the basis of these results, Libet concluded that "the brain . . . decides to initiate . . . or prepares to initiate the act at a time before there is any reportable subjective awareness that such a decision has taken place." Data from several experiments, therefore, suggest that not all processes involved in action are available to our conscious awareness.

Indeed, in everyday life we often react automatically to situations and only later become aware of the stimulus that provoked us to move. For example, while driving, we might suddenly need to swerve the car to steer clear of an obstacle, and we might see the obstacle only after moving to avoid it. A series of experiments have shown that subjects can correctly track shifting targets without being aware of the shifts (Castiello et al. 1991). These experiments were designed to investigate subjects' awareness of motor corrections during a task that required them to reach for an object that changed position in front of them. In addition to reaching for the object, subjects were asked to signal vocally ("Tah!") as soon as they noticed that the target had shifted. Interestingly, the verbal responses, which Castiello et al. assumed reflected the onset of conscious awareness, occurred some 300 ms after the motor correction began. Similarly, a study that required subjects to change aspects (leg force or stride length and frequency) of their walking action on a treadmill in response to resistance changes of the treadmill showed that conscious awareness of the increased resistance lagged as long as 6 seconds behind the kinematic changes, in line with the notion of a temporal dissociation between (low-level) motor performance and (high-level) subjective awareness (Varraine et al. 2002). It was suggested that awareness of movement modifications was delayed as long as the goal feedback informed the subject of the success of their desired state. The awareness of the resistance change in the treadmill became available to consciousness only after a certain threshold in the discrepancy between the actual sensory consequences of the action and the desired effect. Clearly, this shows that we make motor adjustments before we are aware of them—that we react first and realize later.

A Sense of Agency

An important aspect of awareness of action is the sense of agency—the feeling of causing our movements and their consequences. Haggard et al. (2002) investigated the consequences of a sensory event's being causally linked to a subject's action. Subjects made a key-press, which on some trials was followed 250 ms later by an auditory tone. The subject's task was to judge the timing of either the key-press or the tone. When their key-press caused a tone, subjects judged the timing of their key-press as occurring about 15 ms later and the tone as occurring 46 ms earlier than if the two events occurred alone. This "temporal attraction" seems to depend on the perceived causal relationship between an action and its sensory consequence. In a second experiment, a varying delay (250, 450, or 650 ms) was introduced between the key-press and the tone. The further apart the key-press and tone, the more the temporal attraction of the tone to the key-press was diminished. Furthermore, the temporal attraction between the perception of actions and their sensory consequences did not occur when an involuntary movement (caused by stimulating the motor cortex using TMS) was followed 250 ms later by a tone, or when subjects judged the timing of two causally related external sensory events. The temporal attraction between self-generated actions and their sensory consequences binds together these events and enhances our experience of agency.

If an explicit goal is formed just before the action that achieves that goal, then the action will be perceived as intended. Wegner and Wheatley (1999) have shown that this can lead to errors in the perception of intention. A naive subject and a confederate simultaneously used a single mouse to control the position of a pointer on a screen. If the attention of the subject was drawn to an object on the screen and the pointer stopped near that object shortly afterwards, the subject frequently believed that she had intentionally moved toward the object even though in reality her arm had been moved passively by the confederate. As long as the action did not conflict with some explicitly formed goal, the action was perceived as intended.

Conclusion

The research discussed in this chapter investigated how we normally recognize our actions as our own. We have also described studies with people experiencing delusions of control, who lose the feeling of agency, which, in Western culture at least, is a mark of selfhood. In these cases, the boundary between self and other becomes permeable, such that one no longer feels like the executor but rather the vehicle of an action. It has been proposed that a self-monitoring system, which relies on a cerebellar-parietal network in the brain, is necessary for attributing actions to their veridical sources. This system provides a framework for understanding how we distinguish between self and other at the motor level, to maintain a sense of agency and ownership, and how this goes awry during abnormalities in the control and awareness of action. Finally, studies of willed action have been discussed to demonstrate that, although the intention to act precedes an action, the conscious awareness of an action can occur after the action. Philosophers have long argued that the sense of self is grounded in action (Merleau-Ponty 1962; Sartre 1995) and that "the person exists only in the performance of intentional acts" (Heidegger 1962). The experimental studies outlined above suggest that the *conscious awareness* of *unconsciously monitored* actions is the means by which our actions are experienced as subjectively real (Velmans 2004), willed, and owned. Consciousness is thus embodied: it is through action that we become conscious of ourselves as distinct selves.

References

Blakemore, S.-J., Frith, C. D., and Wolpert, D. W. 1999. Spatiotemporal prediction modulates the perception of self-produced stimuli. *Journal of Cognitive Neuroscience* 11: 551–559.

Blakemore, S.-J., Rees, G., and Frith, C. D. 1998. How do we predict the consequences of our actions? A functional imaging study. *Neuropsychologia* 36, no. 6: 521–529.

Blakemore, S.-J., Wolpert, D. M., and Frith, C. D. 1998. Central cancellation of self-produced tickle sensation. *Nature Neuroscience* 1, no. 7: 635–640.

Blakemore, S.-J., Wolpert, D. M., and Frith, C. D. 1999. The cerebellum contributes to somatosensory cortical activity during self-produced tactile stimulation. *Neuroimage* 10: 448–459.

Blakemore, S.-J., Smith, J., Steel, R., Johnstone, E., and Frith, C. D. 2000. The perception of self-produced sensory stimuli in patients with auditory hallucinations and passivity experiences: Evidence for a breakdown in self-monitoring. *Psychological Medicine* 30: 1131–1139.

Blakemore, S.-J., Frith, C. D., and Wolpert, D. W. 2001. The cerebellum is involved in predicting the sensory consequences of action. *NeuroReport* 12, no. 9: 1879–1885.

Blakemore, S.-J., Sarfati, Y., Bazin, N., and Decety, J. 2003. The detection of intentional contingencies in simple animations in patients with delusions of persecution. *Psychological Medicine* 33: 1433–1441.

Blakemore, S.-J., and Sirigu, A. 2003. Prediction in the cerebellum and parietal cortex. *Experimental Brain Research* 153, no. 2: 239–245.

Buneo, C. A., Jarvis, M. R., Batista, A. P., and Andersen, R. A. 2002. Direct visuomotor transformations for reaching. *Nature* 416, no. 6881: 632–636.

Castiello, U., Paulignan, Y., and Jeannerod, M. 1991. Temporal dissociation of motor responses and subjective awareness: A study in normal subjects. *Brain* 114: 2639–2655.

Corcoran, R. 2003. Inductive reasoning and the understanding of intention in schizophrenia. *Cognitive Neuropsychiatry* 8, no. 3: 223–235.

Danckert, J., Ferber, S., Doherty, T., Steinmetz, H., Nicolle, D., and Goodale, M. A. 2002. Selective, non-lateralized impairment of motor imagery following right parietal damage. *Neurocase* 8, no. 3: 194–204.

Daprati, E., Franck, N., Georgieff, N., Proust, J., Pacherie, E., Dalery, J., and Jeannerod, M. 1997. Looking for the agent: An investigation into consciousness of action and self-consciousness in schizophrenic patients. *Cognition* 65: 71–86.

Decety, J., and Michel, F. 1989. Comparative analysis of actual and mental movement times in two graphic tasks. *Brain and Cognition* 11: 87–97.

Decety, J., Perani, D., Jeannerod, M., Bettinardi, V., Tadary, B., Woods, R., Mazziotta, J. C., and Fazio, F. 1994. Mapping motor representations with positron emission tomography. *Nature* 371: 600–602.

Decety, J., Grezes, J., Costes, N., Perani, D., Jeannerod, M., Procyk, E., Grassi, F., and Fazio, F. 1997. Brain activity during observation of actions: Influence of action content and subject's strategy. *Brain* 120: 1763–1777.

Delevoye-Turrell, Y., Giersch, A., and Danion, J. M. 2003. Abnormal sequencing of motor actions in patients with schizophrenia: Evidence from grip force adjustments during object manipulation. *American Journal of Psychiatry* 160, no. 1: 134–141.

Duhamel, J., Colby, C. L., and Goldberg, M. E. 1992. The updating of the representation of visual space in parietal cortex by intended eye movements. *Science* 255: 90–92.

Farrer, C., and Frith, C. D. 2002. Experiencing oneself vs. another person as being the cause of an action: The neural correlates of the experience of agency. *Neuroimage* 15: 596–603.

Fourneret, P., and Jeannerod, M. 1998. Limited conscious monitoring of motor performance in normal subjects. *Neuropsychologia* 36: 1133–1140.

Franck, N., Farrer, C., Georgieff, N., Marie-Cardine, M., Dalery, J., d'Amato, T., and Jeannerod, M. 2001. Defective recognition of one's own actions in patients with schizophrenia. *American Journal of Psychiatry* 158, no. 3: 454–459.

Frith, C. D. 1987. The positive and negative symptoms of schizophrenia reflect impairment in the perception and initiation of action. *Psychological Medicine* 17: 631–648.

Frith, C. D., Blakemore, S.-J., and Wolpert, D. M. 2000. Abnormalities in the awareness and control of action. *Philosophical Transactions of the Royal Society London: Biological Sciences* 355: 1771–1778.

Gallese, V. 2003. The roots of empathy: The shared manifold hypothesis and the neural basis of intersubjectivity. *Psychopathology* 36: 171–180.

Gerardin, E., Sirigu, A., Lehericy, S., Poline, J. B, Gaymard, B., Marsault, C., Agid, Y., and Le Bihan, D. 2000. Partially overlapping neural networks for real and imagined hand movements. *Cerebral Cortex* 10: 1093–104.

Haggard, P., and Magno, E. 1999. Localising awareness of action with transcranial magnetic stimulation. *Experimental Brain Research* 127: 102–107.

Haggard, P., Clark, S., and Kalogeras, J. 2002. Voluntary action and conscious awareness. *Nature Neuroscience* 5: 382–385.

Heidegger, M. 1962. *Being and Time.* Harper and Row.

Jeannerod, M., and Frak, V. 1999. Mental imaging of motor activity in humans. *Current Opinions in Neurobiology* 9: 735–739.

Johns, L. C., Rossell, S., Frith, C., Ahmad, F., Hemsley, D., Kuipers, E., and McGuire, P. K. 2001. Verbal self-monitoring and auditory verbal hallucinations in patients with schizophrenia. *Psychological Medicine* 31: 705–715.

Knoblich, G., Stottmeister, F., and Kircher, T. 2004. Self-monitoring in schizophrenia. *Psychological Medicine* 34: 1–9.

Libet, B., Gleason, C. A., Wright, E. W., and Pearl, D. K. 1983. Time of conscious intention to act in relation to onset of cerebral activity (readiness potential): the unconscious initiation of a freely voluntary act. *Brain* 106: 623–642.

Maruff, P., Wilson, P. H., and Currie, J. 2003. Abnormalities of motor imagery associated with somatic passivity phenomena in schizophrenia. *Schizophrenia Research* 60: 229–238.

Merleau-Ponty, M. 1962. *Phenomenology of Perception.* Routledge and Kegan Paul.

Miall, R. C., and Wolpert, D. M. 1996. Forward models for physiological motor control. *Neural Net* 9: 1265–1279.

Naito, E., Kochiyama, T., Kitada, R., Nakamura, S., Matsumura, M., Yonekura, Y., and Sadato, N. 2002. Internally simulated movement sensations during motor imagery activate cortical motor areas and the cerebellum. *Journal of Neuroscience* 22: 3683–3691.

Nietzsche, F. W. 1914. *Beyond Good and Evil: Prelude to a Philosophy of the Future.* T. N. Foulis.

Nyberg, L., Petersson, K. M., Nilsson, L. G., Sandblom, J., Aberg, C., and Ingvar, M. 2001. Reactivation of motor brain areas during explicit memory for actions. *Neuroimage* 14: 521–528.

Pettit, P. 2001. *A Theory of Freedom: From the Psychology to the Politics of Agency*, Polity Press.

Rizzolatti, G., and Craighero, L. 2004. The Mirror-Neuron System. *Annual Review of Neuroscience* 27: 169–192.

Ruby, P., and Decety, J. 2001. Effect of subjective perspective taking during simulation of action: A PET investigation of agency. *Nature-Neuroscience* 4, no. 5: 546–555.

Ruby, P., and Decety, J. 2003. What you believe versus what you think they believe: A neuroimaging study of conceptual perspective-taking. *European Journal of Neuroscience* 17: 2475–248••.

Ruby, P., and Decety, J. 2004. How would *you* feel versus how do you think *she* would feel? A neuroimaging study of perspective-taking with social emotions. *Journal of Cognitive Neuroscience* 16: 988–999.

Sartre, J.-P. 1995. *Being and Nothingness: An Essay on Phenomenological Ontology*. Routledge.

Sirigu, A., Duhamel, J. R., Cohen, L., Pillon, B., Dubois, B., and Agid, Y. 1996. The mental representation of hand movements after parietal cortex damage. *Science* 273, no. 5281: 1564–1568.

Sirigu, A., Daprati, E., Ciancia, S., Giraux, P., Nighoghossian, N., Posada, A., and Haggard, P. 2004. Altered awareness of voluntary action after damage to the parietal cortex. Nature Neuroscience. 7: 80–84.

Shergill, S. S., Bays, P., Frith, C. D., and Wolpert, D. M. 2003. Two eyes for an eye: the neuroscience of force escalation. *Science* 301, no. 5630: 187.

Spence, S. A., Brooks, D. J., Hirsch, S. R., Liddle, P. F., Meehan, J., and Grasby, P. M. 1997. A PET study of voluntary movement in schizophrenic patients experiencing passivity phenomena (delusions of alien control). *Brain* 120, no. 11: 1997–2011.

Stephan, K. M., Fink, G. R., Passingham, R. E., Silbersweig, D., Ceballos-Baumann, A. O., Frith, C. D., and Frackowiak, R. S. 1995. Functional anatomy of the mental representation of upper extremity movements in healthy subjects. *Journal of Neurophysiology* 73, no. 1: 373–386.

Thomas, A. K., and Loftus, E. F. 2002. Creating bizarre false memories through imagination. *Memory and Cognition* 30, no. 3: 423–431.

Umilta, M. A., Kohler, E, Gallese, V., Fogassi, L., Fadiga, L., Keysers, C., and Rizzolatti, G. 2001. I know what you are doing: a neurophysiological study. *Neuron* 31, no. 1: 155–165.

Varraine, E., Bonnard, M., and Pailhous, J. 2002. The top down and bottom up mechanisms involved in the sudden awareness of low level sensorimotor behavior. *Cognitive Brain Research* 13, no. 3: 357–361.

Velmans, M. 2004. Self-realization, meaning and scientific studies of consciousness. Lecture at BPS CEP Conference, University of Oxford, September 18.

Wegner, D. M., and Wheatley, T. 1999. Apparent mental causation: Sources of the experience of will. *American Psychologist* 54: 480–492.

Weiller, C., Juptner, M., Fellows, S., Rijntjes, M., Leonhardt, G., Kiebel, S., Muller, S., Diener, H. C., and Thilmann, A. F. 1996. Brain representation of active and passive movement. *NeuroImage* 4: 105–110.

Wolpert, D. M., Ghahramani, Z., and Jordan, M. I. 1995. An internal model for sensorimotor integration. *Science* 269: 1880–1882.

Wolpert, D. M., and Flanagan, J. R. 2001. Motor prediction. *Current Biology* 11: R729–R732.

4 Free Choice and the Human Brain

Richard E. Passingham and Hakwan C. Lau

The term 'free choice' is used in this chapter to refer to choices that are not imposed on the subject by an external agent. In a psychological experiment subjects can be asked to choose between alternatives without there being any external cue to instruct the subjects as to which to choose. Alternatively they can be asked to act spontaneously, for example pressing their forefinger whenever they want. The distinction drawn is between actions that are the result of changes within the individual and actions that are prompted from outside. The use of the term 'free' in this context carries no implication about whether one can reconcile the impression that the subjects have that their choice is undetermined with a causal account of the brain events leading up to that choice.

What we can contribute is an account of the brain mechanisms underlying spontaneous choices—that is, choices that are not specified by external cues. It has long been known that in the human brain, about 1 to $1^1/_2$ second before a spontaneous finger movement, it is possible to detect a slow negative going potential, the Bereitschaftspotential or Readiness Potential (Kornhuber and Deecke 1965). This is measured by using electroencephalography (EEG), with an array of electrodes on the surface of the scalp. This potential is present when the subjects move their finger whenever they want, but not when they move it in response to an unpredictable tone (Jahanshahi et al. 1995). The early part of the potential can be shown to come from the supplementary motor area (SMA). This lies at the midline on the medial surface of the hemisphere. This has been shown by recording with magnetoencephalography (MEG), which allows a more precise localization than EEG of the source of the signal (Erdler et al. 2001). The localization has also been checked by carrying out both an MEG study and a functional brain imaging study on the same subjects, since the latter method has the best spatial resolution of all these methods (Pedersen et al. 1998).

Before a spontaneous movement, activity in the SMA occurs earlier than activity in the motor cortex itself. This has been demonstrated in two ways. First, functional magnetic resonance imaging (fMRI) has been used to study the temporal order of events. The signal rises earlier in the Pre-SMA and SMA than in motor cortex (Weilke et al. 2001; Cunnington et al. 2002; Hunter et al. 2003). However, the signal measured by fMRI reflects cerebral blood flow to the active region, and has a poor temporal resolution. The more convincing evidence comes from studies using MEG which has a millisecond temporal resolution, and these show that when subjects perform spontaneous finger movements activity occurs earlier in the SMA than in motor cortex (Pedersen et al. 1998; Erdler et al. 2001).

Two questions arise. The first is whether activity in the SMA carries specific information or simply reflects general preparation. To find out it is necessary to record directly from the cells themselves and to determine whether the activity of single cells specifies or codes for particular movements. This has been done in animals. It could be argued that free choice is unique to the human brain, and thus that such experiments are invalid. However, in the sense in which 'free choice' is used in this chapter, one can also distinguish movements that animals perform in response to external cues and movements that are spontaneous. For example, Okano and Tanji (1987) showed that more cells in the SMA of monkeys fire early before spontaneous movements than before movements that are cued. The critical observation is that if monkeys perform different sequences of movements, where there are no external cues to specify which movements to make, there are cells in the SMA that fire before one sequence but not before the others (Tanji and Shima 1994; Shima and Tanji 2000). In other words, the activity does not reflect general preparation for performing sequences but specifies particular movements.

The second question is whether activity in the SMA is necessary for spontaneous action. One way to find out is to interfere with activity in this area and to measure the behavioral effect. Thus, Thaler et al. (1995) made lesions that included both the supplementary motor cortex (SMA) and the area in front of it, the pre-supplementary motor cortex (Pre-SMA); the lesions were made in both hemispheres. The monkeys were tested in the dark so as to exclude any possible visual cues. The animals were trained to raise their arm whenever they wanted a peanut; however, they were not directly reaching toward anything, since the peanut was delivered to a food well below. After the lesion the monkeys failed to initiate these movements, though they would still raise their arm if trained to do so when a tone sounded.

A similar effect was found with lesions in the cingulate motor areas that lie below the SMA and the Pre-SMA. Like the SMA, the cingulate motor areas send anatomical connections to the motor cortex (Dum and Strick 2002). A large lesion that includes the SMA, the Pre-SMA, and the cingulate cortex can lead to a syndrome in which the patients fail to initiate movements (akinesia) or to speak of their own accord (Laplane et al. 1977; Masdeu et al. 1978; Damasio and van Hoesen 1983; Jonas 1987). The symptoms tend to recover, but this may be because the lesions are incomplete and only involve one hemisphere.

Lesions of the SMA prevent activity in this area at any point before movement. It could therefore be argued that the critical period might be late in the evolution of the movement. However, patients with Parkinson's disease also suffer from akinesia (lack of spontaneous movement), and they show a reduction in the potentials recorded at the midline early before movement (Filipovic et al. 1997; Ikeda et al. 1997). It is true that this reduction does not correlate with their reaction times to external stimuli (Filipovic et al. 1997), but the SMA is primarily involved in self-generated movements rather than movements that are externally initiated (Okano and Tanji 1987; Mushiake et al. 1991; Passingham 1993).

1   Intention

Given the evidence that there are events in the brain that occur at least one second before a spontaneous movement, the question arises as to when subjects make the decision to move. Libet et al. (1983) introduced a method by which subjects could report the earliest moment at which they were aware of the intention to move. They did so by viewing a clock with a spot revolving around the outside, and later reporting at what time they first "wanted or intended" to act. This judgment (W) could also be compared with the time at which they timed their actual movement (M). The finding was that the subjects judged W to occur earlier than M, as one might expect, but roughly 350 milliseconds after the start of the readiness potential. Even if trials were only included in which the subjects were sure that they had genuinely acted spontaneously and had not prepared in any way, the difference was still 150 milliseconds. The finding that it is possible to measure brain activity before W judgments has been confirmed by Haggard and Eimer (1999). These authors showed that this was true whether the subjects simply decided when to move a finger, as in the experiment of Libet et al. (1983), or decided whether to move their left or right finger.

The Libet task requires subjects to attend to their internal states. Lau et al. (2004b) therefore used fMRI to scan subjects while they attended either to the urge to move (W) or to their movement (M). The subjects reported the time at which they were aware of W or M after a variable delay period, and did so by using a game pad to move a cursor to the appropriate point on the clock's face. In both W and M the subjects judged timing by using the clock, and therefore activity related to the use of the clock is subtracted out by the comparison of W with M. This comparison therefore reveals activity associated with attention to intention (W). The result of the experiment was that there was more activity in the Pre-SMA for the W than for the M judgment (figure 4.1). The diagram shows the anatomical location of the activity in the Pre-SMA, and the graph shows that activity was greater

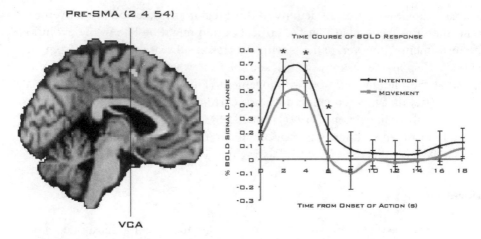

PRE-SMA (2 4 54)

VCA

Figure 4.1
The diagram at left shows the activation in the pre-supplementary motor cortex when subjects attend to their intention (W) compared with attending to their movement (M). The plot at right shows the enhanced haemodynamic response for the two conditions. Adapted from Lau et al. 2004a.

at this location for the W than for the M judgment. As already described, activity in the SMA and the Pre-SMA is associated with the early part of the readiness potential (Jahanshahi et al. 1995; Erdler et al. 2001). Functional magnetic resonance imaging (fMRI) has also been used to record activity in the Pre-SMA and the SMA when subjects decide when to move a finger (Jenkins et al. 2000; Weilke et al. 2001; Cunnington et al. 2002) or decide which finger to move and when to do so (Hunter et al. 2003).

However, the activity reported by Lau et al. (2004b) in the Pre-SMA when subjects judge their intention cannot be accounted for simply by pointing to the fact that the subjects were making spontaneous finger movements. In this experiment they did this in both conditions, W and M, and therefore activity due simply to the generation of movement would be subtracted out in the comparison of W and M. What the experiment shows is that activity in the Pre-SMA is enhanced when subjects attend to their intention compared with attending to the execution of the movement. (See figure 4.1.)

Subjects differ in the degree of this enhancement. In a follow-up study (Lau et al., submitted), we re-analyzed the data from the earlier study (Lau et al. 2004b) and plotted for each subject the degree of enhancement for activity in the Pre-SMA when comparing W with M. These values were then related to the times at which each subject judged W to occur. There was a significant negative correlation (−0.576), that is, the greater the degree of enhancement the earlier the subject judged W to occur (figure 4.2a).

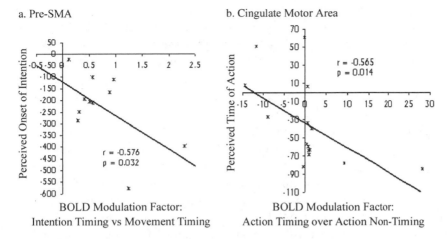

a. Pre-SMA

b. Cingulate Motor Area

BOLD Modulation Factor:
Intention Timing vs Movement Timing

BOLD Modulation Factor:
Action Timing over Action Non-Timing

Figure 4.2
a: Correlation between enhancement of activity (timing W vs. non-timing control) in the pre-SMA and the time at which W was reported. b: Correlation between enhancement of activity (timing M vs. non-timing control) in the cingulate motor area and the time at which M was reported.

It could be argued that this means that the more subjects attend, the more accurate they are in judging the time of W. The conclusion would then be that the true time of W may be earlier than many subjects report it to be. However, we have no independent measure of W, and therefore no way of estimating the accuracy of W judgments. On the other hand, we do have an independent measure of M, and that is the actual time at which the subjects perform the movement. Lau et al. (submitted) scanned subjects while they judged the time of their movement (M). When subjects judged M, compared with a matched condition in which they also made spontaneous movements but did not judge the time of M, there was activity in the cingulate motor area. Again the degree of enhancement differed between subjects, and there was a significant negative correlation (−0.565) between the degree of enhancement and the time at which the subjects reported that their movement occurred; the greater the enhancement, the earlier before the actual movement subjects reported it to occur (figure 4.2b).

It could again be argued that the more that subjects attended the more sensitive they were to early signs of movement. The argument would be that we know from electrophysiological recordings in monkeys that there is activity in motor cortex immediately before the actual movement (Halsband et al. 1994; Tanji and Shima 1994). Perhaps subjects use this activity to judge the time of the actual movement rather than waiting for kinesthetic feedback from the finger. However, the instruction given to the subjects was to judge the actual time of the movement, and thus judgments of M that occurred before the actual movement were objectively inaccurate. Three subjects did not judge M to occur earlier than the actual time of the button press, and in these subjects there was no significant enhancement of activity in the cingulate motor cortex. Putting these results together with those for W, we conclude that the demand to attend may bias the temporal judgments to be too early.

Under normal circumstances subjects make spontaneous movements without being required to attend to what they are doing, but the Libet task makes the unusual demand that subjects attend to their internal states. We know from other imaging studies that when either the demands of the task or the instructions given to the subjects require or allow attention to external stimuli there is enhancement of activity in the relevant sensory areas (Rees et al. 1997; Brefczynski and De Yoe 1999). There may be a link between visual awareness and this enhancement. Moutoussis and Zeki (2002) used fMRI to show that there is enhanced activity in higher visual areas when subjects are aware of a visual stimulus rather than unaware. The problem with the Libet task is that the demand to attend to the intention may influence the time at which subjects report awareness.

2 Ideo-Motor Theory of Action

The ideo-motor theory of action, as described by William James (1890), proposes that voluntary actions are preceded by the idea of the action, and that subjects are aware of this intention. James argues that even when movements have become automatic, as in well-rehearsed piano playing, the idea or representation of the action is still present in consciousness, however briefly. The assumption is that the representation causes the action. This assumption has been questioned by Wegner (2002, 2003), who argues that subjects wrongly conclude that it is their intentions that cause their actions because they are correlated with them in time. The way to test whether correlations genuinely reflect causes is to intervene: if A and B are correlated in time, one can test whether preventing A has the effect of preventing B.

This suggests an experiment in which one prevents awareness of W and tests the effect on spontaneous actions. This could be done by using transcranial magnetic brain stimulation (TMS) to interfere with activity in the Pre-SMA. In TMS, a coil is placed over the skull, and magnetic pulses are imposed through the skull on the underlying brain tissue, causing a temporary disruption in the normal pattern of electrical activity (Walsh and Cowey 2000). Thus, TMS can be thought of as a tool for introducing neural noise.

However, such an experiment poses a technical challenge because we have no way of knowing in advance when W will occur, and thus no way of acting to prevent it. On the other hand, we do know when the movement itself occurs. If TMS after

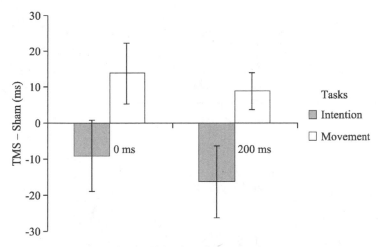

Figure 4.3
The effect of TMS at 0 and 200 ms on the time at which intention (W) and movement (M) were reported. The data are plotted against the baseline for sham TMS trials.

the time of the movement were to influence W, this might have implications for the hypothesis that W causes the action. Therefore, we used TMS to interfere with activity in the Pre-SMA either at the time at which the movement occurs or 200 milliseconds afterward (Lau et al., submitted).

In our experiment the subjects were required to judge W on some trials and M on other trials. As in our earlier experiment (Lau et al. 2004b) the subjects reported the time at which they were aware of W and M after a variable delay period by moving a cursor to the appropriate point on the clock's face. On TMS trials, whether a single pulse was imposed at 0 second (the time of the movement) or 200 milliseconds afterward, the subjects judged W to occur significantly earlier than on control trials in which a sham coil was used (figure 4.3). On the other hand, TMS also caused judgments of M to be delayed (figure 4.3). There was a significant difference between the effect on W and M (figure 4.4, first histogram). Yet, there was no effect if TMS was applied 500 milliseconds later, or at the time at which the subjects moved the cursor to make their report (figure 4.4, second histogram). This shows that the effect is not simply to disrupt the memory of W. It is crucial in interpreting this result to show that TMS over the Pre-SMA does not have a similar effect on the timing of other events. For this reason we included a condition in which the subjects judged the time of tactile stimulation. The tactile stimulus was vibration applied to the fingertip. The stimulus started at low amplitude and gradually increased in strength. It was set up this way so as to mimic the slow change in the

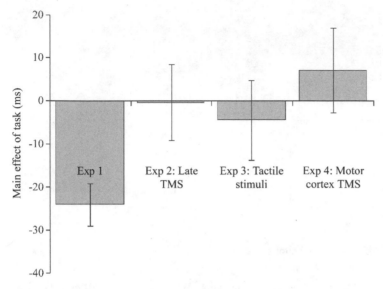

Figure 4.4
The effect of TMS for the comparison of the difference in the times for W – M. The data are plotted against the baseline for sham TMS trials. The first histogram give the data for W – M with TMS over the pre-SMA at 0 and 200 ms combined. The second histogram the data for W – M for TMS over the pre-SMA at 500 ms and the time of report combined. The third histogram gives the data for judgments of the onset of the tactile stimulus minus the peak for TMS over the pre-SMA at 0 and 200 ms combined. The fourth histogram gives the data for W – M with TMS over the motor cortex at 0 and 200 ms combined.

readiness potential. This allowed us to distinguish two judgments, the time of onset and the peak. The subjects judged the time of onset to be 133 milliseconds earlier than the time of the peak; this figure was similar to the difference of 98 milliseconds between judgments of W and M on trials in which no TMS was applied. The third histogram in figure 4.4 shows that TMS over the Pre-SMA at 0 and 200 milliseconds did not change the difference between the times at which onset and peak were reported. TMS over motor cortex had no effect (figure 4.4, fourth histogram). Thus, the effect was spatially and temporally specific.

The first conclusion from this experiment is that temporarily inactivating the Pre-SMA has a different effect on judgments of W and M. This fits with our earlier finding (Lau et al. 2004b) that there is more activity in the Pre-SMA when subjects judge W than M. However, the results also suggest that the neural activity underlying the experience of W continues for at least 200 milliseconds after the actual movement. It is true that this in itself does not prove that W could not cause the movement as supposed by the ideo-motor theory. However, it does show that causing the action cannot be the only function of W, since the activity that continues after the action cannot in principal be viewed as its cause.

3   Willed Actions

The debate so far has centered on spontaneous finger movements. But it could be argued that performing such movements is normally a relatively automatic process. We do not usually need to attend to them. William James (1890) suggested that the key to will was the holding in mind and attention to an idea in the face of competing alternatives. Frith et al. (1991) therefore used the term 'willed action' to refer to choices to which we must attend. The task they gave subjects was to make a series of movements, moving either the forefinger or the second finger as they chose, but avoiding a stereotyped sequence. Similar instructions were given in a study conducted at the same time by Deiber et al. (1991) in which the subjects chose in which of four directions to move a joystick. In both studies there was activity in the dorsal prefrontal cortex when comparing such movements with movements instructed by external cues. This finding has since been replicated (Spence et al. 1998; Rowe et al. 2004).

There are two ways in which this activity could be explained. The first is that it reflects the need to hold items in working memory. The instructions stress that the subjects should not engage in stereotyped sequences, and subjects may try to achieve this by holding the last few moves in mind so as to avoid repeating them (Spence and Frith 1999). We have investigated this possibility by trying to eliminate the requirement for working memory. In the first study, Hadland et al. (2001) instructed subjects to move each of their eight fingers in any order but without repeating a finger movement. Each time they moved a finger, lights appeared on the screen to indicate the fingers that had been moved, and these lights remained on throughout the sequence. Thus, the subjects could always see which fingers they had moved. Yet, when repetitive TMS (rTMS) was applied over the dorsal prefrontal cortex, there was a disruption in their movements as measured by inter-response times; this did not occur when the movements were made in response to visual cues.

This study does not eliminate the possibility that the subjects were preparing sequences of moves and holding these in working memory. So Lau et al. (2004a) gave subjects the choice between colored pictures; these were computer-generated "fractals." The instruction was to choose the fractal that the subject "preferred," and new fractals were presented on every trial. Thus, the subjects made new choices each time, they could not prepare their choice for the next trial, and past choices were irrelevant. Again there was activity in the dorsal prefrontal cortex. This activity cannot be explained in terms of working memory or response preparation.

It is important, however, not to draw a stronger conclusion than is warranted. What these results show is that when working memory has been minimized or excluded it is still possible to demonstrate activity in the dorsal prefrontal cortex. What the results do not show is that none of the activity reported in this area on free selection tasks (Deiber et al. 1991; Frith et al. 1991; Spence et al. 1998; Rowe et al. 2004) can be accounted for by working memory. It is certainly the case that when subjects are asked to produce a random series of finger movements, responding every three seconds or so, they remember the last few moves, and this almost certainly contributes to the activity seen in the dorsal prefrontal cortex. It is well established that this area is activated when subjects must hold a series of recent items in mind and must select between them on the basis of some rule (Cohen et al. 1997; Owen et al. 1998).

There is a second way in which activity in the dorsal prefrontal cortex might be explained when subjects choose between alternatives. This is that the task requires attention to the selection of action. It was this that led Frith et al. (1991) to use the term 'willed action'. Psychologists assess the degree to which a task demands attention by studying the extent to which performance of a secondary task at the same time interferes with the primary task. If the primary task is to generate a series of finger movements, the movements become less random (that is, more stereotyped) if the subjects have to generate digits at the same time (Baddeley et al. 1998). If on the other hand the secondary task is not attentionally demanding, for example simple counting, there is no such interference effect.

There is evidence that activation occurs in the dorsal prefrontal cortex when subjects have to attend to the selection of their actions. Rowe et al. (2002b) taught subjects a simple motor sequence which they could perform automatically. In a separate condition the subjects were then instructed to attend to their performance. There was no significant activity in the dorsal prefrontal cortex when the subjects performed the sequence without attention, but considerable activity when the task was performed under attentional control (figure 4.5). Thus, even though the moves were the same and could be performed automatically, the simple requirement to attend to the upcoming response was enough to activate the dorsal prefrontal cortex. This raises the question of whether prefrontal activation when subjects are given a free choice reflects the fact that the subjects attend to the selection of their actions or the fact that the choice is free. Lau et al. (2004a) investigated this by varying the attentional load by presenting two, three or five fractals from which to choose. As already described, in one condition the subjects freely chose the fractal that they preferred. However, in another condition a smaller central fractal was presented which matched one of the others, and the task was to choose the match. As expected, in both conditions response times increased with the number of fractals. However, there was activity in the dorsal prefrontal cortex not only when the subjects freely chose between the fractals but also when they performed the task of matching. Lau et al. interpreted these results to imply that the crucial factor for activation of the dorsal prefrontal cortex is not freedom of choice but the attentional demands of the task.

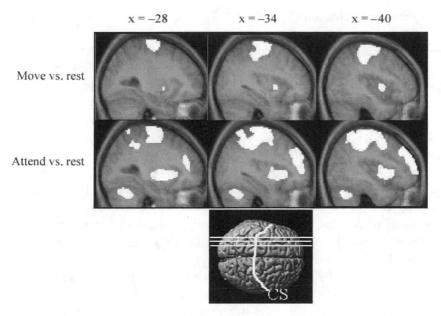

Figure 4.5
Parasaggital slices showing the activations for automatic performance of the sequence (Move – Rest) and for performance of the sequence under attentional control (Attend – Rest). The brain at the bottom shows the planes at which the sections were taken, and marks the central sulcus. The sections are oriented with the frontal lobes to the right.

Frith (2000) has suggested an alternative explanation for the activation of the dorsal prefrontal cortex when subjects select between actions. He points out that when subjects are required to generate a series of actions in the laboratory they must select the set of responses that are appropriate given the instructions. He calls this "sculpting the response space." He argues that holding the set of potential responses in mind continues throughout a series of trials, and that it is this that accounts for the activation in the dorsal prefrontal cortex. He supports this argument by pointing to data from Jahanshahi et al. (2000) showing that the activity in the dorsal prefrontal cortex did not increase the more frequently the responses were generated, as might be expected if the activity was time-locked to the response.

However, in the study by Lau et al. (2004a) the fMRI data were specifically analyzed so as to reveal activity at the time of the action. The "event related" analysis looked for activity that was time-locked to a particular event, and in these studies the event was the response. The fact that the analysis revealed prefrontal activity in these studies suggests at the least that there was a change in that activity when the subjects selected the action. These results are consistent with the view that the prefrontal cortex is involved in the selection of the particular action.

4   Relation between Prefrontal Cortex and Pre-SMA

If this is the case, the question arises as to the relative contributions of the prefrontal cortex and the Pre-SMA and SMA when subjects decide on action. It is known that in macaque monkeys the dorsal prefrontal cortex is interconnected with the Pre-SMA as well as the premotor cortex on the lateral surface (Lu et al. 1994). When subjects perform spontaneous finger movements, the earliest signal that can be picked up by MEG is in the dorsal prefrontal cortex, followed by activity in the Pre-SMA/SMA and premotor cortex (Pedersen et al. 1998). Though spontaneous finger movements could be performed without attention, in the laboratory the subjects are required to perform a series of such movements and instructed not to move their finger at stereotyped intervals, and this may encourage attention to the task.

It is possible to analyze the covariance in activity between the dorsal prefrontal cortex and Pre-SMA in imaging data. Rowe et al. (2002b) used structural equation modeling to do this. The covariance in activity between two areas is accounted for in part by the connections between them. By setting up an anatomical model that includes these, as well as other connections, one can work out the functional strengths of the paths that minimize the difference between the observed covariance and that implied by the model. Rowe et al. (2002b) were able to show in this way that when subjects attended to the selection of their actions there was an increase in the functional path strengths between the dorsal prefrontal cortex and the SMA, and also between the dorsal prefrontal cortex and the lateral premotor cortex. These changes were specific to the connections with the prefrontal cortex, since they were not found for the path between the parietal cortex and the premotor cortex (Rowe et al. 2002a).

In these studies attention was manipulated by instructing the subjects to attend in one condition, and this is inelegant. It is more usual for psychologists to manipulate attention by comparing different tasks that make different demands on attention. As already described above, Lau et al. (2004a) manipulated the object of attention by requiring subjects to time either their intention or their actual movement. When subjects attended to their intention, there was an enhancement of activity in the Pre-SMA, but there were similar enhancements in the dorsal prefrontal cortex and the parietal cortex. But, whereas there was an increase in the effectiveness of the interconnections between the prefrontal cortex and the Pre-SMA, this was not found for the parietal cortex and the Pre-SMA.

The fact that the dorsal prefrontal cortex and the Pre-SMA are connected does not mean that their functions are identical. Lau et al. (2004a) specifically compared activity in these two areas when subjects chose between pictures. As already mentioned above, there was activity in the dorsal prefrontal cortex irrespective of whether the choice was determined by the subject or specified by the match between two of the pictures. However, there was only activity in the Pre-SMA in the first of these conditions—that is, when the subjects made the choice on the basis of their own preference. This fits with other data suggesting a specialization of the Pre-SMA and the SMA for self-generated actions (Passingham 1993). For example, Mushiake et al. (1991) compared cell activity in the SMA and in the lateral premotor cortex, and found that there was a bias for cells in the SMA to fire when movements were not specified by visual cues, but for cells in the lateral premotor cortex to fire when movements were so specified. Monkeys with lesions of the Pre-SMA and SMA fail to produce self-initiated actions, though they still respond when the actions are triggered by tones (Thaler et al. 1995). By comparison, monkeys with lateral premotor lesions still produced self-initiated actions (ibid.).

5 Attention, Awareness, and the Global Workspace

We have argued above for a role for the dorsal prefrontal cortex in attention to the selection of action, and have demonstrated activity in the prefrontal cortex and the Pre-SMA that is associated with attention to intention. It has been suggested that the prefrontal cortex forms part of a "global workspace" (Dehaene et al. 1998; Dehaene and Naccache 2001). This concept bears some relation to the "central executive" of Baddeley (2003). The crucial difference is that both Dehaene and colleagues (Dehaene et al. 1998; Dehaene and Naccache 2001) and Baars and Franklin (2003) have produced computational models that permit testable predictions.

The critical notion is that there is a stage at which information processing becomes integrated and serial (Baars 2002; Baars and Franklin 2003). The suggestion is that at earlier stages the processing is carried out by distributed specialized processors which can operate in parallel, but that where the response is not automatic information must be integrated so as to determine the appropriate response. At this stage, processing is serial in the sense that it is not possible to handle two tasks simultaneously—that is, only one consistent content can be dominant at any one moment (Baars 2002).

There is evidence that processing in the prefrontal cortex fits both criteria. First, the prefrontal cortex receives inputs from all posterior regions of association cortex (Barbas 2000; Miller and Cohen 2001). It is the only area that receives information from all sense modalities, and the information that it receives is already highly processed. Thus, it can be regarded as sitting at the top of the hierarchy of information processing (Fuster 1997; Passingham et al. 2005).

To demonstrate that information is integrated at this stage, one can record the activity from cells in macaque monkeys. In this way it has been shown that the same cells can become active, for example, to both taste inputs and smell inputs (Rolls and Baylis 1994). Many cells in the prefrontal cortex fire both when monkeys remember spatial locations and when they remember objects (Rolls and Baylis 1994; Rao et al. 1997), even though the inputs for spatial and object information enter the prefrontal cortex by different routes (Wilson et al. 1993). Finally, there is cell activity in the dorsal prefrontal cortex that reflects the integration of information about spatial location and information about rewards (Kobayashi et al. 2002; Wallis and Miller 2003). Information about rewards is first processed by cells in the orbito-frontal cortex, but can be integrated with information about location through connections between the orbito-frontal and lateral frontal cortex (Barbas 1988; Wallis and Miller 2003).

Processing in the prefrontal cortex also fits the second criterion: that it be serial. This can be demonstrated by studying the interference with performance of a primary task by the requirement to carry out a secondary task at the same time. We have taught subjects a motor sequence by trial and error (Passingham 1998). Early in learning, performance of the sequence was considerably disrupted if the subjects were required to generate verbs from nouns at the same time. However, we also gave the subjects long practice on the task until it became automatic, and at that stage there was minimal interference in the dual task condition.

An explanation of these results is provided by the activity that can be recorded in the prefrontal cortex during performance of these tasks. There is activity in the prefrontal cortex both when subjects learn a motor sequence (Jueptner et al. 1997; Toni et al. 1998) and when they generate verbs (Raichle et al. 1994). However, as learning progresses the activity in the prefrontal cortex falls to near baseline levels at the time when the task is becoming automatic (Toni et al. 1998). Thus, early in learning the prefrontal cortex is engaged both by motor sequence learning and by verb generation, and decisions concerning both responses cannot be carried out at exactly the same time. Late in motor learning, the prefrontal cortex is no longer engaged in motor learning, and thus there is no interference (Passingham 1998).

It is a critical observation that the prefrontal cortex is not engaged once the task has become automatic. Dehaene and Naccache (2001) suggest that the global workspace is needed when responses are not automatic—for example, when the situation is novel. This is also a feature of the "supervisory attentional system" that was modeled by Norman and Shallice (1980). Novel situations require consideration of the current context and reference to current goals. Dehaene and Naccache (2001) specifically cite the spontaneous generation of intentional behavior as making demands on the global workspace, since there is no stereotyped response.

Evidence that the prefrontal cortex might form part of a global workspace can be derived from its anatomical connections and the properties of cells in this area, and we can collect data on these from macaque monkeys, as outlined above. However, both Dehaene and Naccache (2001) and Baars (2002) further suggest that the contents of the global workspace are conscious, and this cannot be tested on animal models. The reason is that the operational index of consciousness is the ability to report (Weiskrantz 1997).

There are at least two approaches to studying the neural correlates of consciousness. The first approach proposes that information must reach particular brain areas to be conscious (Weiskrantz 1997). For example, Crick and Koch (1998) and Jack and Shallice (2001) stress processing in the prefrontal cortex. The second approach suggests differences in the type of processing, involving, for example, synchronous high-frequency oscillations (Engel and Singer 2001) or enhanced activity under conditions of awareness (Moutoussis and Zeki 2002). For example, if a stimulus such as a word is immediately followed by another stimulus, the subject can be unaware of the first one; this is "backward masking." There is roughly a tenfold increase in activity in the temporal cortex when human subjects view unmasked words of which they are aware compared with masked words of which they are unaware (Dehaene et al. 2001). The cell activity continues significantly longer for unmasked stimuli (Rolls et al. 1999).

We make no claims to solve here the issue of the neural basis of consciousness. We claim only that the prefrontal cortex is part of the global workspace and that there is more activity in the prefrontal cortex under conditions of attentional control. We hesitate to say that the presence of activity in the prefrontal cortex guarantees awareness, for two reasons. First, activity can be recorded in the prefrontal cortex even when subjects are unaware, for example during implicit motor learning, though it is much more extensive during explicit learning when subjects are aware that there is a task to be learned (Aizenstein et al. 2004). Second, enhanced activity in parietal and visual areas also correlates with conscious awareness (Rees et al. 2002a,b).

6 Conscious Decisions and Deliberation

We started with the Libet task and the ideo-motor theory. It is the results on this task that have much exercised philosophers as well as psychologists. They appear to challenge the view that the action is first represented in awareness before the mechanisms for the preparation of action are engaged.

However, it may be that the problem is misconceived. When subjects perform the Libet task they are well aware of the aim of the task. This was set up by the verbal instructions they were given beforehand. Since a series of spontaneous movements is required, the instructions stress that the subject should act randomly, not repeating a stereotyped sequence of intervals. The activity recorded in this situation in the prefrontal cortex (Jahanshahi et al. 1995; Pedersen et al. 1998; Jenkins et al. 2000) represents in part the attentional control of performance according to this instruction. Furthermore, Sakai, and Passingham (2003) have suggested that the prefrontal cortex establishes a task set by interacting with posterior areas. Even if subjects only become aware of their specific intention just before action, they are aware of what they are supposed to be doing well before this.

Whereas the goals of action are set in the laboratory by the instructions given, in the everyday world they are set by the goals that people set for themselves. The sorts of decisions over which they deliberate are not when to make a random finger movement. The decisions are ones that have consequences. These decisions require the integration of all the relevant information about the current context, the alternative possibilities and the costs and values associated with them. It is for such decisions that the global workspace model has been proposed. Evidence that the prefrontal cortex plays a role comes from imaging studies in which subjects choose, for example, between menus (Arana et al. 2003) or between gambles (Rogers et al. 2004). Furthermore, it has been shown that there is an integration of information about goals and action in the human anterior prefrontal cortex (Ramnani and Miall 2003). It is not the purpose of this chapter to say whether the fact that we are aware of these decisions implies a causal role for awareness. It is true both that decisions of this sort demand the neural integration of highly processed information and that we report awareness of our deliberations. It is for the philosophers contributing to this volume to comment on the relation between the brain events and awareness.

References

Aizenstein, H. J., Stenger, V. A., Cochran, J., Clark, K., Johnson, M., Nebes, R. D., and Carter, C. S. 2004. Regional brain activation during concurrent implicit and explicit sequence learning. *Cerebral Cortex* 14: 199–208.

Arana, F. S., Parkinson, J. A., Hinton, E., Holland, A. J., Owen, A. M., and Roberts, A. C. 2003. Dissociable contributions of the human amygdala and orbitofrontal cortex to incentive motivation and goal selection. *Journal of Neuroscience* 23: 9632–9638.

Baars, B. J. 2002. The conscious access hypothesis: origins and recent evidence. *Trends in Cognitive Science* 6: 47–52.

Baars, B. J., and Franklin, S. 2003. How conscious experience and working memory interact. *Trends in Cognitive Science* 7: 166–172.

Baddeley, A. 2003. Working memory: Looking back and looking forward. *Nature Reviews Neuroscience* 4: 829–839.

Baddeley, A., Emslie, H., Kolodny, J., and Duncan, J. 1998. Random generation and the executive control of working memory. *Quarterly Journal of Experimental Psychology A* 51: 819–852.

Barbas, H. 1988. Anatomical organization of basoventral and mediodorsal visual recipient prefrontal region in the rhesus monkey. *Journal of Comparative Neurology* 276: 313–342.

Barbas, H. 2000. Connections underlying the synthesis of cognition, memory, and emotion in primate prefrontal cortices. *Brain Research Bulletin* 52: 319–330.

Brefczynski, J. A., and DeYoe, E. A. 1999. A physiological correlate of the 'spotlight' of visual attention. *Nature Neuroscience* 2: 370–374.

Cohen, J. D, Perlstein, W. M, Braver, T. S, Nystrom, L. E, Noll, D. C, Jonides, J., and Smith, E. E. 1997. Temporal dynamics of brain activation during a working memory task. *Nature* 386: 604–607.

Crick, F., and Koch, C. 1998. Consciousness and neuroscience. *Cerebral Cortex* 8: 97–107.

Cunnington, R., Windischberger, C., Deecke, L., and Moser, E. 2002. The preparation and execution of self-initiated and externally-triggered movement: a study of event-related fMRI. *Neuroimage* 15: 373–385.

Damasio, A. R., and van Hoesen, G. W. 1983. Emotional disturbances associated with focal lesions of the limbic frontal lobe. In *Neuropsychology of Human Emotion*, ed. K. Heilman and P. Satz. Guilford.

Dehaene, S., and Naccache, L. 2001. Towards a cognitive neuroscience of consciousness: basic evidence and a workspace framework. *Cognition* 79: 1–37.

Dehaene, S., Kerszberg, M., and Changeux, J.-P. 1998. A neuronal model of a global workspace in effortful cognitive tasks. *Proceedings of the National Academy of Sciences* 95: 14529–14534.

Dehaene, S., Naccache, L., Cohen, L., Bihan, D. L., Mangin, J. F., Poline, J. B., and Riviere, D. 2001. Cerebral mechanisms of word masking and unconscious repetition priming. *Nature Neuroscience* 4: 752–758.

Deiber, M.-P., Passingham, R. E., Colebatch, J. G., Friston, K. J., Nixon, P. D., and Frackowiak, R. S. J. 1991. Cortical areas and the selection of movement: a study with positron emission tomography. *Experimental Brain Research* 84: 393–402.

Dum, R. P., and Strick, P. L. 2002. Motor areas in the frontal lobe of the primate. *Physiology and Behavior* 77: 677–682.

Engel, A. K., and Singer, W. 2001. Temporal binding and the neural correlates of sensory awareness. *Trends in Cognitive Science* 5: 16–25.

Erdler, M., Beisteiner, R., Mayer, D., Kaindl, T., Edward, V., Windischberger, C., Lindiger, G., and Deecke, L. 2001. Supplementary motor area activating preceding voluntary movement is detectable with a whole-scalp magnetoencephalography system. *Neuroimage* 11: 697–707.

Filipovic, S. R., Covickovic-Sternic, N., Radovic, V. M., Dragasevic, N., Stojanovic-Svetel, M., and Kostic, V. S. 1997. Correlation between Bereitschaftspotential and reaction time measurements in patients with Parkinson's disease. Measuring the impaired supplementary motor area function? *Journal of Neurological Science* 147: 177–183.

Frith, C. D. 2000. The role of dorsolateral prefrontal cortex in the selection of action. In: *Control of Cognitive Processes: Attention and Performance XVIII*, ed. S. Monsell and J. Driver. MIT Press.

Frith, C. D., Friston, K., Liddle, P. F., and Frackowiak, R. S. J. 1991. Willed action and the prefrontal cortex in man: a study with PET. *Proceedings of the Royal Society of London, series B* 244: 241–246.

Fuster, J. 1997. *The Prefrontal Cortex*. Lippincott-Raven.

Hadland, K. A., Rushworth, M. F., Passingham, R. E., Jahanshahi, M., and Rothwell, J. C. 2001. Interference with performance of a response selection task that has no working memory component: An rTMS comparison of the dorsolateral prefrontal and medial frontal cortex. *Journal of Cognitive Neuroscience* 13: 1097–1108.

Haggard, P., and Eimer, M. 1999. On the relation between brain potentials and the awareness of voluntary movements. *Experimental Brain Research* 126: 128–133.

Halsband, U., Matsuzaka, Y., and Tanji, J. 1994. Neuronal activity in the primate supplementary, presupplementary and premotor cortex during externally- and internally instructed sequential movements. *Neuroscience Research* 20: 149–155.

Hunter, M. D., Griffiths, T. D., Farrow, T. F., Zheng, Y., Wilkinson, I. D., Hegde, N., Woods, W., Spence, S. A., and Woodruff, P. W. 2003. A neural basis for the perception of voices in external auditory space. *Brain* 126: 161–169.

Ikeda, A., Shibasaki, H., Kaji, R., Terada, K., Nagamine, T., Honda, M, and Kimura, J. 1997. Dissociation between contingent negative variation (CNV) and Bereitschaftspotential (BP) in patients with parkinsonism. *Electroencephalography and Clinical Neurophysiology* 102: 142–151.

Jack, A. I., and Shallice, T. 2001. Introspective physicalism as an approach to the science of consciousness. *Cognition* 79: 161–196.

Jahanshahi, M., Dirnberger, G., Fuller, R., and Frith, C. D. 2000. The role of the dorsolateral prefrontal cortex in random number generation: A study with positron emission tomography. *Neuroimage* 12: 713–725.

Jahanshahi, M., Jenkins, I. H., Brown, R. G., Marsden, C. D., Passingham, R. E., and Brooks, D. J. 1995. Self-initiated versus externally triggered movements. I. An investigation using regional cerebral blood flow and movement-related potentials in normals and Parkinson's disease. *Brain* 118: 913–934.

James, W. 1890. *The Principles of Psychology*. Holt.

Jenkins, I. H., Jahanshahi, M., Jueptner, M., Passingham, R. E., and Brooks, D. J. 2000. Self-initiated versus externally triggered movements. II. The effect of movement predictability on regional cerebral blood flow. *Brain* 123: 1216–1228.

Jonas, S. 1987. The supplementary motor region and speech. In *The Frontal Lobes Revisited*, ed. E. Perecman. IRBN Press.

Jueptner, M., Stephan, K. M., Frith, C. D, Brooks, D. J., Frackowiak, R. S. J., and Passingham, R. E. 1997. Anatomy of motor learning. I. Frontal cortex and attention to action. *Journal of Neurophysiology* 77: 1313–1324.

Kobayashi, S., Lauwereyns, J., Koizumi, M., Sakagami, M., and Hikosaka, O. 2002. Influence of reward expectation on visuospatial processing in macaque lateral prefrontal cortex. *Journal of Neurophysiology* 87: 1488–1498.

Kornhuber, H. H., and Deecke, L. 1965. Hirnpotentialanderungen bei willkurbewegungen und passiven bewegungen des Menschen: bereitschaftspotential und reafferente potentiale. *Pflügers Archiv* 284: 1–17.

Laplane, D, Tailarach, J, Meininger, V, Bancaud, J., and Orgogozo, J. M. 1977. Clinical consequences of corticectomies involving the supplementary motor area in man. *Journal of Neurological Science* 34: 301–314.

Lau, H. C., Rogers, R. D., Ramnani, N., and Passingham, R. E. 2004a. Willed action and attention to the selection of action. *Neuroimage* 21: 1407–1415.

Lau, H. C., Rogers, R. D., Haggard, P., and Passingham, R. E. 2004b. Attention to intention. *Science* 303: 1208–1210.

Libet, B., Gleason, C. A., Wright, E. W., and Pearl, D. K. 1983. Time of conscious intention to act in relation to onset of cerebral activity (readiness-potential). The unconscious initiation of a freely voluntary act. *Brain* 106: 623–642.

Lu, M.-T., Preston, J. B., and Strick, P. L. 1994. Interconnections between the prefrontal cortex and the premotor areas in the frontal lobe. *Journal of Comparative Neurology* 341: 375–392.

Masdeu, J. C, Schoene, W. C., and Funkenstein, A. 1978. Aphasia following infarction of the left supplementary motor area. *Neurology* 28: 1220–1223.

Miller, E. K., and Cohen, J. D. 2001. An integrative theory of prefrontal cortex function. *Annual Review of Neuroscience* 24: 167–202.

Moutoussis, K., and Zeki, S. 2002. The relationship between cortical activation and perception investigated with invisible stimuli. *Proceedings of the National Academy of Sciences* 99: 9527–9532.

Mushiake, H., Inase, M., and Tanji, J. 1991. Neuronal activity in the primate premotor, supplementary, and precentral motor cortex during visually guided and internally determined sequential movements. *Journal of Neurophysiology* 66: 705–718.

Norman, D. A., and Shallice, T. 1980. Attention to Action: Willed and Automatic Control of Behavior. Technical Report 99, Center for Human Information Processing.

Okano, K., and Tanji, J. 1987. Neuronal activity in the primate motor fields of the agranular frontal cortex preceding visually triggered and self-paced movements. *Experimental Brain Research* 66: 155–166.

Owen, A. M., Stern, C. E., Look, R. B., Tracey, I., Rosen, B. R., and Petrides, M. 1998. Functional organization of spatial and nonspatial working memory processing within the human lateral frontal cortex. *Proceedings of the National Academy of Sciences* 95: 7721–7726.

Passingham, R. E. 1993. *The Frontal Lobes and Voluntary Action*. Oxford University Press.

Passingham, R. E. 1998. Attention to action. In *The Prefrontal Cortex*, ed. A. Roberts et al. Oxford University Press.

Passingham, R. E., Rowe, J. B., and Sakai, K. 2005. Prefrontal cortex and attention to action. In *Attention in Action*, ed. G. Humphreys and M. Riddoch. Psychology Press.

Pedersen, J. R., Johansoen, P., Bak, C. K., Kofoed, B., Saermark, K., and Gjedde, A. 1998. Origin of human readiness field linked to left middle frontal gyrus by MEG and PET. *Neuroimage* 8: 214–220.

Raichle, M. E., Fiez, J. A., Videen, T. O., MacLeod, A. K., Pardo, J. V., Fox, P. T., and Petersen, S. E. 1994. Practice-related changes in human brain functional anatomy during non-motor learning. *Cerebral Cortex* 4: 8–26.

Ramnani, N., and Miall, R. C. 2003. Instructed delay activity in the human prefrontal cortex is modulated by monetary reward expectation. *Cerebral Cortex* 13: 318–327.

Rao, S. C., Rainer, G., and Miller, E. K. 1997. Integration of what and where in the primate prefrontal cortex. *Science* 276: 821–824.

Rees, G., Frith, C. D., and Lavie, N. 1997. Modulating irrelevant motion perception by varying attentional load in an unrelated task. *Science* 278: 1616–1619.

Rees, G., Kreiman, G., and Koch, C. 2002a. Neural correlates of consciousness in humans. *Nature Neuroscience Reviews* 3: 261–270.

Rees, G., Wojciulik, E., Clarke, K., Husain, M., Frith, C., and Driver, J. 2002b. Neural correlates of conscious and unconscious vision in parietal extinction. *Neurocase* 8: 387–393.

Rogers, R. D., Ramnani, N., Mackay, C., Wilson, J. L., Jezzard, P., Carter, C. S., and Smith, S. M. 2004. Distinct portions of anterior cingulate cortex and medial prefrontal cortex are activated by reward processing in separable phases of decision-making cognition. *Biological Psychiatry* 55: 594–602.

Rolls, E., and Baylis, G. C. 1994. Gustatory, olfactory and visual convergence within the primate orbitofrontal cortex. *Journal of Neuroscience* 14: 5432–5452.

Rolls, E. T., Tovee, M. J., and Panzeri, S. 1999. The neurophysiology of backward visual masking: information analysis. *Journal of Cognitive Neuroscience* 11: 300–311.

Rowe, J., Friston, K., Frackowiak, R., and Passingham, R. 2002a. Attention to action: Specific modulation of corticocortical interactions in humans. *Neuroimage* 17: 988–998.

Rowe, J., Stephan, K. E., Friston, K., Frackowiak, R., Lees, A., and Passingham, R. 2002b. Attention to action in Parkinson's disease: Impaired effective connectivity among frontal cortical regions. *Brain* 125: 276–289.

Rowe, J. B., Stephan, K. E., Friston, K., Frackowiak, R. S. J., and Passingham, R. E. 2005. The prefrontal cortex shows context-specific changes in effective connectivity to motor or visual cortex during the selection of action or colour. *Cerebral Cortex* 15: 85–95.

Sakai, K., and Passingham, R. E. 2003. Prefrontal interactions reflect future task operations. *Nature Neuroscience* 6: 75–81.

Shima, K., and Tanji, J. 2000. Neuronal activity in the supplementary and presupplementary motor areas for temporal organization of multiple movements. *Journal of Neurophysiology* 84: 2148–2160.

Spence, S. A., and Frith, C. 1999. Towards a functional anatomy of volition. In *The Volitional Brain*, ed. B. Libet et al. Imprint Academic.

Spence, S. A., Hirsch, S. R., Brooks, D. J., and Grasby, P. M. 1998. Prefrontal cortex activity in people with schizophrenia and control subjects. *Journal of Psychiatry* 172: 1–8.

Tanji, J., and Shima, K. 1994. Role for supplementary motor area cells in planning several moves ahead. *Nature* 371: 413–416.

Thaler, D., Chen, Y.-C., Nixon, P. D., Stern, C., and Passingham, R. E. 1995. The functions of the medial premotor cortex (SMA). I. Simple learned movements. *Experimental Brain Research* 102: 445–460.

Toni, I., Krams, M., Turner, R., and Passingham, R. E. 1998. The time-course of changes during motor sequence learning: A whole-brain fMRI study. *Neuroimage* 8: 50–61.

Wallis, J. D., and Miller, E. K. 2003. Neuronal activity in primate dorsolateral and orbital prefrontal cortex during performance of a reward preference task. *European Journal of Neuroscience* 18: 2069–2081.

Walsh, V., and Cowey, A. 2000. Transcranial magnetic stimulation and cognitive neuroscience. *Nature Reviews Neuroscience* 1: 73–79.

Wegner, D. M. 2002. *The Illusion of Conscious Will*. MIT Press.

Wegner, D. M. 2003. The mind's best trick: How we experience conscious will. *Trends in Cognitive Science* 7: 65–69.

Weilke, F., Spiegel, S, Boecker, H., von Einsiedel, H. G., Conrad, B., Schwaiger, M., and Erhard, P. 2001. Time-resolved fMRI of activation patterns in MI and SMA during complex voluntary movement. *Journal of Neurophysiology* 85: 1858–1863.

Weiskrantz, L. 1997. *Consciousness Lost and Found.* Oxford University Press.

Wilson, F. A. W., Schalaidhe, S. P., and Goldman-Rakic, P. S. 1993. Dissociation of object and spatial processing domains in primate prefrontal cortex. *Science* 260: 1955–1958.

5 Consciousness, Intentionality, and Causality

Walter J. Freeman

What is consciousness? It is known through experience of the activities of one's own body and observation of the bodies of others. In this respect, the question whether it arises from the soul (Eccles 1994), or from panpsychic properties of matter (Whitehead 1938; Penrose 1994; Chalmers 1996), or as a function of brain operations (Searle 1992; Dennett 1991; Crick 1994) is not relevant. The pertinent questions are—however it arises and is experienced—how and in what senses does it cause the functions of brains and bodies, and how do brain and body functions cause it? How do actions cause perceptions; how do perceptions cause awareness; how do states of awareness cause actions? Analysis of causality is a necessary step toward a comprehension of consciousness, because the forms of answers depend on the choice among meanings that are assigned to "cause": (a) to make, move and modulate (an agency in linear causality); (b) to explain, rationalize and blame (cognition in circular causality without agency but with top-down-bottom-up interaction); or (c) to flow in parallel as a meaningful experience, by-product, or epiphenomenon (noncausal interrelation).

The elements of linear causality (a) are shown in figure 5.1 in terms of stimulus-response determinism. A stimulus initiates a chain of events that includes activation of receptors, transmission by serial synapses to cortex, integration with memory, selection of a motor pattern, descending transmission to motor neurons, and activation of muscles. At one or more nodes along the chain awareness occurs, and meaning and emotion are attached to the response. Temporal sequencing is crucial; no effect can precede or occur simultaneously with its cause. At some instant each effect becomes a cause. The demonstration of causal invariance must be based on repetition of trials. The time line is reinitiated at zero in observer time, and S-R pairs are collected. Some form of generalization is used, in the illustration it is by time ensemble averaging. Events with small variance in time of onset close to stimulus arrival are retained. Later events with varying latencies are lost. The double dot indicates a point in real time; it is artificial in observer time. This conceptualization is inherently limited, because awareness cannot be defined at a point in time.

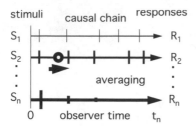

Figure 5.1
Linear causality of the observer. Linear causality is the view of connected events by which causal chains are constructed. The weaknesses lie in requirements to assign points in time to the beginning and the end of each chain, and to intervening events in the chain in strict order, and to repeat pairs of observations in varying circumstances in order to connect pairs of classes of events. As Davidson (1980) remarked, events have causes; classes have relations. In the example, analysis of stimulus-dependent events such as evoked potentials is done by time ensemble averaging, which degrades nonsynchronized events, and which leads to further attempts at segmentation in terms of the successive peaks, thus losing sight of an event extended in time. The notion of 'agency' is implicit in each event in the chain acting to produce an effect, which then becomes the next cause.

The elements of circular causality (b) are shown in figure 5.2. The double dot shows a point moving counterclockwise on a trajectory idealized as a circle, in order to show that an event exists irresolvably as a state through a period of inner time, which we reduce to a point in real time. Stimuli from the world impinge on this state. So also do stimuli arising from the self-organizing dynamics within the brain. Most stimuli are ineffective, but occasionally one succeeds as a "hit" on the brain state, and a response occurs. The impact and motor action are followed by a change in brain structure that begins a new orbit.

Noncausal relations (c) are described by statistical models, differential equations, phase portraits, and so on, in which time may be implicit or reversible. Once the constructions are completed by the calculation of risk factors and degrees of certainty from distributions of observed events and objects, the assignment of causation is optional. In describing brain functions awareness is treated as irrelevant or epiphenomenal.

These concepts are applied to animal consciousness on the premise that the structures and activities of brains and bodies are comparable over a broad variety of animals including humans. The hypothesis is that the elementary properties of consciousness are manifested in even the simplest of extant vertebrates, and that structural and functional complexity increases with the evolution of brains into higher mammals. The dynamics of simpler brains is described in terms of neural operations that provide goal-oriented behavior.

In sections 1–5 I describe the neural mechanisms of intention, reafference, and learning, as I see them. I compare explanations of neural mechanisms using linear and circular causality at three levels of hierarchical function. In the remaining

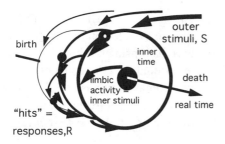

Figure 5.2
Circular causality of the self. Circular causality expresses the interrelations between levels in a hierarchy: a top-down macroscopic state simultaneously influences microscopic particles that bottom-up create
and sustain the macroscopic state. The state exists over a span of inner time in the system that can be
collapsed to a point in external time. Events in real time are marked by changes in the state of the system,
which are discrete. This conceptualization is widely used in the social and physical sciences. In an example
used by Haken (1983), the excited atoms in a laser cause coherent light emission, and the light imposes
order on the atoms. The laser was also used by Cartwright (1989) to exemplify levels of causality, by
which she contrasted simple, direct cause-effect relations not having significant interactions or second-
order perturbations with higher order "capacities" (according to her, closely related to Mill's "tendencies," but differing by "material abstraction," p. 226), which by virtue of abstraction have an enlarged
scope of forward action, but which lack the circular relation between microscopic and macroscopic entities that is essential for explaining lasers—and brains. The notion of an 'agency' does not enter, and multiple scales of time and space are required for the different levels. A succession of orbits can be conceived
as a cylinder with its axis in real time, extending from birth to death of an individual and its brain. Events
are intrinsically not reproducible. Trajectories in inner time may be viewed as fusing past and future into
an extended present by state transitions. The circle is a candidate for representing a state of awareness.

sections I describe some applications of this view in the fields of natural sciences.
The materials I use to answer the question "What is causality?" come from several
disciplines, including heavy reliance on neurobiology and nonlinear dynamics. In the
words of computer technologists, these two disciplines make up God's own firewall,
which keeps hackers from burning in to access and crack the brain codes. For
reviews on neuroflaming I recommend as introductory texts *Brain, Mind, and
Behavior* (Bloom and Lazerson 1988) and *A Visual Introduction to Dynamical
Systems Theory for Psychology* (Abraham et al. 1990).

1   Level 1: The Circular Causality of Intentionality

An elementary process requiring the dynamic interaction between brain, body,
and world in all animals is an act of observation. This is not a passive receipt of
information from the world, as expressed implicitly in figure 5.1. It is the culmina-
tion of purposive action by which an animal directs its sense organs toward a
selected aspect of the world and abstracts, interprets, and learns from the resulting
sensory stimuli (figure 5.2). The act requires a prior state of readiness that
expresses the existence of a goal, a preparation for motor action to position

the sense organs, and selective sensitization of the sensory cortices. Their excitability has already been shaped by the past experience that is relevant to the goal and the expectancy of stimuli. A concept that can serve as a principle by which to assemble and interrelate these multiple facets is intentionality. This concept has been used in different contexts since its synthesis by Thomas Aquinas (1272) 700 years ago. The properties of intentionality as it is developed here are its intent or directedness toward some future state or goal, its unity, and its wholeness (Freeman 1995).

Intent comprises the endogenous initiation, construction, and direction of behavior into the world, combined with changing the self by learning in accordance with the perceived consequences of the behavior. Its origin lies within brains. Humans and other animals select their own goals, plan their own tactics, and choose when to begin, modify, and stop sequences of action. Humans at least are subjectively aware of themselves acting. This facet is commonly given the meaning of purpose and motivation by psychologists, because, unlike lawyers, they usually do not distinguish between intent and motive. Intent is a forthcoming action, and motive is the reason.

Unity appears in the combining of input from all sensory modalities into Gestalten; in the coordination of all parts of the body, both musculoskeletal and autonomic, into adaptive, flexible, yet focused movements; and in the full weight of all past experience in the directing of each action. Subjectively, unity may appear in the awareness of self. Unity and intent find expression in modern analytic philosophy as "aboutness," meaning the way in which beliefs and thoughts symbolized by mental representations refer to objects and events in the world, whether real or imaginary. The distinction between inner image and outer object calls up a dichotomy between subject and object that was not part of the originating Thomistic view.

Wholeness is revealed by the orderly changes in the self and its behavior that constitute the development and maturation of the self through learning, within the constraints of its genes and its material, social, and cultural environments. Subjectively, wholeness is revealed in the striving for the fulfillment of the potential of the self through its lifetime of change. Its root meaning is "tending," the Aristotelian view that biology is destiny. It is also seen in the process of healing of the brain and body from damage and disruption. The concept appears in the description by a fourteenth-century surgeon, LaFranchi of Milan, of two forms of healing, by first intention with a clean scar, and by second intention with suppuration. It is implicit in the epitaph of the sixteenth-century French surgeon Ambroise Paré: Je le pansay, Dieu le guarit [I bound his wounds, God healed him]. Pain is intentional in that it directs behavior toward facilitation of healing, and that it mediates learning when actions have gone wrong with deleterious, unintended consequences. Pain serves to exemplify the differences between volition, desire, and intent; it is willed by sadists, desired by masochists, and essential for normal living.

Intentionality cannot be explained by linear causality, because actions under that concept must be attributed to environmental (Skinner 1969) and genetic (Herrnstein and Murray 1994) determinants, leaving no opening for self-determination. Acausal theories (Hull 1943; Grossberg 1982) describe statistical and mathematical regularities of behavior without reference to intentionality. Circular causality explains intentionality in terms of "action-perception cycles" (Merleau-Ponty 1945) and "affordances" (Gibson 1979), in which each perception concomitantly is the outcome of a preceding action and the condition for a following action. Dewey (1914) phrased the same idea in different words: an organism does not react to a stimulus but acts into it and incorporates it. That which is perceived already exists in the perceiver, because it is posited by the action of search and is actualized in the fulfillment of expectation. The unity of the cycle is reflected in the impossibility of defining a moving instant of "now" in subjective time, as an object is conceived under linear causality. The Cartesian distinction between subject and object does not appear, because they are joined by assimilation in a seamless flow.

2   Level 2: The Circular Causality of Reafference

Brain scientists have known for over a century that the necessary and sufficient part of the vertebrate brain to sustain minimal intentional action, a component of intentionality, is the ventral forebrain, including those parts that comprise the external shell of the phylogenetically oldest part of the forebrain, the paleocortex, and the underlying nuclei such as the amygdala with which the cortex is interconnected. These components suffice to support identifiable patterns of intentional behavior in animals, when all of the newer parts of the forebrain have been surgically removed (Goltz 1892) or chemically inactivated by spreading depression (Bures et al. 1974). Intentional behavior is severely altered or lost following major damage to these parts. Phylogenetic evidence comes from observing intentional behavior in salamanders, which have the simplest of the existing vertebrate forebrains (Herrick 1948; Roth 1987) comprising only the limbic system. Its three cortical areas are sensory (which is predominantly the olfactory bulb), motor (the pyriform cortex), and associational (figure 5.3). The latter has the primordial hippocampus connected to the septal, amygdaloid, and striatal nuclei. It is identified in higher vertebrates as the locus of the functions of spatial orientation (the "cognitive map") and temporal orientation in learning ("short-term memory"). These integrative frameworks are essential for intentional action into the world. Even the simplest actions, such as observation, searching for food, and evading predators, require an animal to

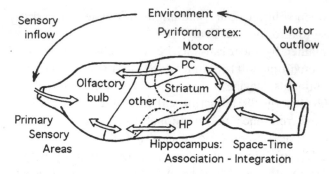

Figure 5.3
Schematic diagram of the dorsal view of the right cerebral hemisphere of the salamander (adapted from Herrick 1948). The unbroken sheet of superficial neuropil sustains bidirectional interactions between all of its parts, which are demarcated by their axonal connections with sensory receptors (olfactory bulb and 'Transitional zone' for all other senses, descending connections to the corpus striatum, amygdaloid and septum from the pyriform area, and the intrinsic connections between these areas and the primordial hippocampus posteromedially. This primitive forebrain suffices as an organ of intentionality, comprising the limbic system with little else besides.

coordinate its position in the world with that of its prey or refuge, and to evaluate its progress during evaluation, attack, or escape.

The crucial question for neuroscientists is "How are the patterns of neural activity that sustain intentional behavior constructed in brains?" A route to an answer is provided by studies of the electrical activity of the primary sensory cortices of animals that have been trained to identify and respond to conditioned stimuli. An answer appears in the capacity of the cortices to construct novel patterns of neural activity by virtue of their self-organizing dynamics.

Two approaches to the study of sensory cortical dynamics are in contrast. One is based in linear causality (figure 5.1). An experimenter identifies a neuron in sensory cortex by recording its action potential with a microelectrode, and then determines the sensory stimulus to which that neuron is most sensitive. The pulse train of the neuron is treated as a symbol to "represent" that stimulus as the "feature" of an object—for example, the color, contour, or motion of an eye or a nose. The pathway of activation from the sensory receptor through relay nuclei to the primary sensory cortex and then beyond is described as a series of maps, in which successive representations of the stimulus are activated. The firings of the feature detector neurons must then be synchronized or "bound" together to represent the object, such as a moving colored ball, as it is conceived by the experimenter. This representation is thought to be transmitted to a higher cortex, where it is compared with representations of previous objects that are retrieved from memory storage. A solution to the "binding problem" is still being sought (Gray 1994; Hardcastle 1994; Singer and Gray 1995).

The other approach is based in circular causality (figure 5.2). In this view, the experimenter trains a subject to cooperate through the use of positive or negative reinforcement, thereby inducing a state of expectancy and search for a stimulus, as it is conceived by the subject. When the expected stimulus arrives, the activated receptors transmit pulses to the sensory cortex, where they elicit the construction by nonlinear dynamics of a macroscopic, spatially coherent oscillatory pattern that covers the entire cortex (Freeman 1975, 1991). It is observed by means of the electroencephalogram (EEG) from electrode arrays on all the sensory cortices (Freeman 1975, 1992, 1995; Barrie et al. 1996; Kay and Freeman 1998). It is not seen in recordings from single neuronal action potentials, because the fraction of the variance in the single neuronal pulse train that is covariant with the neural mass is far too small, on the order of 0.1 percent.

The emergent pattern is not a representation of a stimulus, nor a ringing as when a bell is struck, nor a resonance as when one string of a guitar vibrates when another string does so at its natural frequency. It is a phase transition that is induced by a stimulus, followed by a construction of a pattern that is shaped by the synaptic modifications among cortical neurons from prior learning. It is also dependent on the brain-stem nuclei that bathe the forebrain in neuromodulatory chemicals. It is a dynamic action pattern that creates and carries the meaning of the stimulus for the subject. It reflects the individual history, present context, and expectancy, corresponding to the unity and the wholeness of intentionality. Owing to dependence on history, the patterns created in each cortex are unique to each subject.

The visual, auditory, somesthetic, and olfactory cortices serving the distance receptors all converge their constructions through the entorhinal cortex into the limbic system, where they are integrated with each other over time. Clearly they must have similar dynamics, in order that the messages be combined into Gestalten. The resultant integrated meaning is transmitted back to the cortices in the processes of selective attending, expectancy, and the prediction of future inputs (Freeman 1995; Kay and Freeman 1998).

The same wave forms of EEG activity as those found in the sensory cortices are found in various parts of the limbic system. This similarity indicates that the limbic system also has the capacity to create its own spatiotemporal patterns of neural activity. They are embedded in past experience and convergent multisensory input, but they are self-organized. The limbic system provides interconnected populations of neurons that, according to the hypothesis being proposed, generate continually the patterns of neural activity that form goals and direct behavior toward them.

EEG evidence shows that the process in the various parts occurs in discontinuous steps (figure 5.2), like frames in a motion picture (Freeman 1975; Barrie, Freeman, and Lenhart 1996). Being intrinsically unstable, the limbic system continually transits across states that emerge, transmit to other parts of the brain, and then

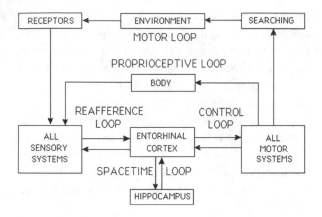

Figure 5.4
The dynamic architecture of the limbic system. In the view of dynamics the limbic architecture is formed by multiple loops. The mammalian entorhinal cortex is the target of convergence of all sensory input, the chief source of input for the hippocampus, its principal target for its output, and a source of centrifugal input to all of the primary sensory cortices. The hypothesis is proposed that intentional action is engendered by counterclockwise flow of activity around the loops into the body and the world, comprising implicit cognition, and that awareness and consciousness are engendered by clockwise flow within the brain, comprising explicit cognition. The intentional flow consists in the microscopic activity of brain subsystems, and the back flow is the macroscopic order parameter that by circular causality regulates and holds or releases the activity of the subsystems.

dissolve to give place to new ones. Its output controls the brain-stem nuclei that serve to regulate its excitability levels, implying that it regulates its own neurohumoral context, enabling it to respond with equal facility to changes, both in the body and in the environment, that call for arousal and adaptation or rest and recreation. Again by inference it is the neurodynamics of the limbic system, with contributions from other parts of the forebrain such as the frontal lobes and basal ganglia, that initiates the novel and creative behavior seen in search by trial and error.

The limbic activity patterns of directed arousal and search are sent into the motor systems of the brain stem and the spinal cord (figure 5.4). Simultaneously, patterns are transmitted to the primary sensory cortices, preparing them for the consequences of motor actions. This process has been called "reafference" (von Holst and Mittelstädt 1950; Freeman 1995), "corollary discharge" (Sperry 1950), "focused arousal," and "preafference" (Kay and Freeman 1998). It compensates for the self-induced changes in sensory input that accompany the actions organized by the limbic system, and it sensitizes sensory systems to anticipated stimuli prior to their expected times of arrival.

The concept of preafference began with an observation by Helmholtz (1872) on patients with paralysis of lateral gaze, who, on trying and being unable to move an eye, reported that the visual field appeared to move in the opposite direction. Helmholtz concluded that "an impulse of the will" that accompanied voluntary behavior was unmasked by the paralysis: "These phenomena place it beyond doubt that we judge the direction of the visual axis only by the volitional act by means of which we seek to alter the position of the eyes." J. Hughlings Jackson (1931) repeated the observation, but postulated alternatively that the phenomenon was caused by "an in-going current," which was a signal from the non-paralyzed eye that moved too far in the attempt to fixate an object, and which was not a recursive signal from a "motor centre." He was joined in this interpretation by William James (1893) and Edward Titchener (1907). Thus was deployment of the concept of neural feedback in re-entrant cognitive processes delayed until late in the twentieth century.

The sensory cortical constructions consist of brief staccato messages to the limbic system, which convey what is sought and the result of the search. After multisensory convergence, the spatiotemporal activity pattern in the limbic system is updated through temporal integration in the hippocampus. Accompanying sensory messages there are return updates from the limbic system to the sensory cortices, whereby each cortex receives input that has been integrated with the input from all others, reflecting the unity of intentionality. Everything that a human or an animal knows comes from the circular causality of action, preafference, perception, and updating. It is done by successive frames of self-organized activity patterns in the sensory and limbic cortices.

3 Level 3: Circular Causality among Neurons and Neural Masses

The "state" of the brain is a description of what it is doing in some specified time period. A phase transition occurs when the brain changes and does something else. For example, locomotion is a state within which walking is a rhythmic pattern of activity that involves large parts of the brain, spinal cord, muscles, and bones. The entire neuromuscular system changes almost instantly with the transition to a pattern of jogging or running. Similarly, a sleeping state can be taken as a whole or divided into a sequence of slow wave and REM stages. Transit to a waking state can occur in a fraction of a second, whereby the entire brain and body "shift gears." The state of a neuron can be described as active and firing or as silent, with sudden changes in patterns of firing constituting phase transitions. Populations of neurons also have a range of states, such as slow wave, fast activity, seizure, or silence. The science of dynamics describes states and their phase transitions.

The most critical question to ask about a state concerns its degree of stability or resistance to change. Stability is evaluated by perturbing an object or a system (Freeman 1975). For example, an egg on a flat surface is unstable, but a coffee mug is stable. A person standing on a moving bus and holding on to a railing is stable, but someone walking in the aisle is not. If a person regains his chosen posture after each perturbation, no matter in which direction the displacement occurred, that state is regarded as stable, and it is said to be governed by an attractor. This is a metaphor to say that the system goes ("is attracted to") the state through interim transiency. The range of displacement from which recovery can occur defines the basin of attraction, in analogy to a ball rolling to the bottom of a bowl. If a perturbation is so strong that it causes concussion or a broken leg, and the person cannot stand up again, then the system has been placed outside the basin of attraction, and a new state supervenes, with its own attractor and basin of attraction.

Stability is always relative to the time duration of observation and to the criteria for what is chosen to be observed. In the perspective of a lifetime, brains appear to be highly stable in their numbers of neurons, in their architectures and major patterns of connection, and in the patterns of behavior they produce (including the character and identity of the individual, which can be recognized and followed for many years). A brain undergoes repeated transitions from waking to sleeping and back again, coming up refreshed with a good night or irritable with insomnia but still giving arguably the same person as the night before. But in the perspective of the short term, brains are highly unstable. Thoughts go fleeting through awareness, and the face and the body twitch with the passing of emotions. Glimpses of the internal states of neural activity reveal patterns that are more like hurricanes than the orderly march of symbols in a computer, with the difference that hurricanes don't learn. Brain states and the states of populations of neurons that interact to give brain function are highly irregular in spatial form and time course. They emerge, persist for a small fraction of a second, then disappear and are replaced by other states. We neuroscientists aim to describe and measure these states and to tell what they mean both to observations of behavior and to experiences with awareness. We approach the dynamics by defining three kinds of stable state, each with its type of attractor. The simplest is the point attractor. The system is at rest unless perturbed, and it returns to rest when allowed to do so. As it relaxes to rest, it has a brief history, but loses it on convergence to rest. Examples of point attractors are neurons or neural populations that have been isolated from the brain, and also the brain that is depressed into inactivity by injury or a strong anesthetic to the point where the EEG has gone flat. A special case of a point attractor is noise. This state is observed in populations of neurons in the brain of a subject at rest, with no evidence of overt behavior or awareness. The neurons fire continually but not in concert with each other. Their pulses occur in long trains at irregular times. Knowledge about the prior pulse trains from each neuron and those of its neighbors up to the present fails to support the prediction of when the next pulse will occur. The state of noise has continual activity with no history of how it started, and it gives only the expectation that its average amplitude and other statistical properties will persist unchanged.

A system that gives periodic behavior is said to have a limit cycle attractor. The classic example is the clock. When it is viewed in terms of its ceaseless motion, it is regarded as unstable until it winds down, runs out of power, and goes to a point attractor. If it resumes its regular beat after it is re-set or otherwise perturbed, it is stable as long as its power lasts. Its history is limited to one cycle, after which there is no retention of its transient approach in its basin to its attractor. Neurons and populations rarely fire periodically, and when they appear to do so, close inspection shows that the activities are in fact irregular and unpredictable in detail, and when periodic activity does occur, it is either intentional, as in rhythmic drumming, or pathological, as in nystagmus and Parkinsonian tremor.

The third type of attractor gives aperiodic oscillation of the kind that is observed in recordings of EEGs and of physiological tremors. There is no frequency or small number of frequencies at which the system oscillates. The system's behavior is therefore unpredictable, because performance can only be projected far into the future for periodic behavior. This type was first called "strange"; it is now widely known as "chaotic." The existence of this type of oscillation was known to mathematicians a century ago, but systematic study was possible only recently after the full development of digital computers. The best-known simple systems with chaotic attractors have a small number of components and a few degrees of freedom—for example, the double-hinged pendulum and the dripping faucet. Large and complex systems such as neurons and neural populations are thought to be capable of chaotic behavior, but proof is not yet possible at the present level of developments in mathematics.

The discovery of chaos has profound implications for the study of brain function (Skarda and Freeman 1987). A dynamic system has a collection of attractors, each with its basin, which forms an "attractor landscape" with all three types. The system can jump from one state to another in an itinerant trajectory (Tsuda 1991). Capture by a point or limit cycle attractor wipes the history of the system clean upon asymptotic convergence, but capture in a chaotic basin engenders continual aperiodic activity, thereby creating novel, unpredictable patterns that retain the system's history.

Although the trajectory is not predictable, the statistical properties such as the mean and the standard deviation of the state variables of the system serve as measures of its steady state. Chaotic fluctuations carry the system endlessly around in the basin. However, if energy is fed into the system so that the fluctuations increase in amplitude, or if the landscape of the system is changed so that the basin shrinks or flattens, a microscopic fluctuation can carry the trajectory across the boundary between basins to another attractor. This crossing constitutes a first-order phase transition.

In each sensory cortex there are multiple chaotic attractors with basins corresponding to previously learned classes of stimuli, including that for the learned background stimulus configuration, which constitutes an attractor landscape. This chaotic prestimulus state of expectancy establishes the sensitivity of the cortex by warping the landscape, so that a very small number of sensory action potentials driven by an expected stimulus can carry the cortical trajectory into the basin of an appropriate attractor. Circular causality enters in the following way. The state of a neural population in an area of cortex is a macroscopic event that arises through the interactions of the microscopic activity of the neurons comprising the neuropil. The global state is upwardly generated by the microscopic neurons, and simultaneously the global state downwardly organizes the activities of the individual neurons.

Each cortical phase transition requires this circularity. It is preceded by a conjunction of antecedents. A stimulus is sought by the limbic brain through orientation of the sensory receptors in sniffing, looking, and listening. The landscape of the basins of attraction is shaped by limbic preafference, which facilitates access to an attractor by expanding its basin for the reception of a desired class of stimuli. Preafference provides the ambient context by multisensory divergence. The web of synaptic connections modified by prior learning maintains the basins and attractors. Pre-existing chaotic fluctuations are enhanced by input, forcing the selection of a new macroscopic state that then engulfs the stimulus-driven microscopic activity.

The first proposed reason that all the sensory systems (visual, auditory, somatic, and olfactory) operate this way is the finite capacity of the brain faced with the infinite complexity of the environment. In olfaction, for example, a significant odorant may consist of a few molecules mixed in a rich and powerful background of undefined substances, and it may be continually changing in age, temperature, and concentration. Each sniff in a succession with the same chemical activates a different subset of equivalent olfactory receptors, so the microscopic input is unpredictable and unknowable in detail. Detection and tracking require an invariant pattern over trials. This is provided by the attractor, and the generalization over equivalent receptors is provided by the basin. The attractor determines the response, not the particular stimulus. Unlike the view proposed by stimulus-response reflex determinism, the dynamics give no linear chain of cause and effect from stimulus to response that can lead to the necessity of environmental determinism. The second proposed reason is the requirement that all sensory patterns have the same basic form, so that they can be combined into Gestalten once they are converged to be integrated over time.

4   Circular Causality in Awareness

Circular causality, then, occurs with each phase transition in sensory cortices and the olfactory bulb, when fluctuations in microscopic activity exceed a certain threshold, such that a new macroscopic oscillation emerges to force cooperation on the very neurons that have brought the pattern into being. EEG measurements show that multiple patterns self-organize independently in overlapping time frames in the several sensory and limbic cortices, coexisting with stimulus-driven activity in different areas of the neocortex, which structurally is an undivided sheet of neuropil in each hemisphere receiving the projections of sensory pathways in separated areas.

Circular causality can serve as the framework for explaining the operation of awareness in the following way. The multimodal macroscopic patterns converge simultaneously into the limbic system, and the results of integration over time and space are simultaneously returned to all of the sensory systems. Here I propose that another level of hierarchy exists in brain function as a hemispheric attractor, for which the local macroscopic activity patterns are the components. The forward limb of the circle provides the bursts of oscillations converging into the limbic system that destabilize it to form new patterns. The feedback limb incorporates the limbic and sensory cortical patterns into a global activity pattern or order parameter that enslaves all of the components. The enslavement enhances the coherence among all of them, which dampens the chaotic fluctuation instead of enhancing it, as the receptor input does in the sensory cortices.

A global operator of this kind must exist, for the following reason. The synthesis of sense data first into cortical wave packets and then into a multimodal packet takes time. After a Gestalt has been achieved through embedding in past experience, a decision is required as to what the organism is to do next. This also takes time for an evolutionary trajectory through a sequence of attractors constituting the attractor landscape of possible goals and actions (Tsuda 1991). The triggering of a phase transition in the motor system may occur at any time, if the fluctuations in its multiple inputs are large enough, thereby terminating the search trajectory. In some emergent behavioral situations an early response is most effective: action without reflection. In complex situations with unclear ramifications into the future, precipitate action may lead to disastrous consequences. More generally, the forebrain appears to have developed in phylogenetic evolution as an organ taking advantage of the time provided by distance receptors for the interpretation of raw sense data. The quenching function of a global operator to delay decision and action can be seen as a necessary complement on the motor side, to prevent premature closure of the process of constructing and evaluating possible courses of action. This view is comparable to that of William James (1879), who wrote that "the study *a posteriori* of the *distribution* of consciousness shows it to be exactly such as we might expect in an organ added for the sake of steering a nervous system grown too complex to regulate itself," except that consciousness is provided not by another "organ" (an add-on part of the human brain) but by a new hierarchical level of organization of brain dynamics.

Action without the deferral that is implicit in awareness can be found in "automatic" sequences of action in the performance of familiar complex routines. Actions "flow" without awareness. Implicit cognition is continuous, and it is simply unmasked in the conditions that lead to "blindsight." In this view, emotion is defined as the impetus for action—more specifically, as impending action. Its degree is proportional to the amplitude of the chaotic fluctuations in the limbic system, which appears as the modulation depth of the carrier waves of limbic neural activity patterns. In accordance with the James-Lange theory of emotion (James 1893), it is experienced through awareness of the activation of the autonomic nervous system in preparation for and support of overt action, as described by Cannon (1939). It is observed in the patterns of behavior that social animals have acquired through evolution (Darwin 1872). Emotion is not in opposition to reason. Behaviors that are seen as irrational and "incontinent" (Davidson 1980) result from premature escape of the chaotic fluctuations from the leavening and smoothing of the awareness operator. The most intensely emotional behavior, experienced in artistic creation, in scientific discovery, and in religious awe, occurs as the intensity of awareness rises in concert with the strength of the fluctuations (Freeman 1995). As with all other difficult human endeavors, self-control is achieved through long and arduous practice.

Evidence for the existence of the postulated global operator is found in the high level of covariance in the EEGs simultaneously recorded from the bulb and the visual, auditory, somatic, and limbic (entorhinal) cortices of animals and from the scalp of humans (Lehmann and Michel 1990). The magnitude of the shared activity can be measured in limited circumstances by the largest component in principal-components analysis (PCA). Even though the wave forms of the several sites vary independently and unpredictably, the first component has 50–70 percent of the total variance (Smart et al. 1997; Gaál and Freeman 1997). These levels are lower than those found within each area of 90–98 percent (Barrie, Freeman, and Lenhart 1996), but they are far greater than can be accounted for by any of a variety of statistical artefacts or sources of correlation, such as volume conduction, pacemaker driving, or contamination by the reference lead in monopolar recording. The high level of coherence holds for all parts of the EEG spectrum and for aperiodic as well as near-periodic waves.

The maximal coherence appears to have zero phase lag over distances up to several centimeters between recording sites and even between hemispheres (Singer and Gray 1995). Attempts are being made to model the observed zero time lag among the structures by cancellation of delays in bidirectional feedback transmission (König and Schillen 1991; Traub et al. 1996; Roelfsma et al. 1997).

5   Consciousness Viewed as a System Parameter Controlling Chaos

A clear choice can be made now between the three meanings of causality proposed in the introduction. Awareness and neural activity are not acausal parallel processes, nor does either make or move the other as an agency in temporal sequence. Circular causality is a form of explanation that can be applied at several hierarchical levels without recourse to agency. This formulation provides the sense or feeling of necessity that is essential for human comprehension, by addressing the elemental experience of cause and effect in acts of observation, even though logically it is very different from linear causality in all aspects of temporal order, spatial contiguity, and invariant reproducibility. The phrase is a cognitive metaphor. It lacks the attribute of agency, unless and until the loop is broken into the forward (microscopic) limb and the recurrent (macroscopic) limb, in which case the agency that is so compelling in linear causality can be re-introduced. This move acquiesces to the needs of the human observers to use it in order to comprehend dynamic events and processes in the world.

I propose that the globally coherent activity, which is an order parameter, may be an objective correlate of awareness through preafference, comprising expectation and attention, which are based in prior proprioceptive and exteroceptive feedback of the sensory consequences of previous actions, after they have undergone limbic integration to form Gestalten, and in the goals that are emergent in the limbic system. In this view, awareness is basically akin to the intervening state variable in a homeostatic mechanism, which is both a physical quantity, a dynamic operator, and the carrier of influence from the past into the future that supports the relation between a desired set point and an existing state. The content of the awareness operator may be found in the spatial pattern of amplitude modulation of the shared wave form component, which is comparable to the amplitude modulation of the carrier waves in the primary sensory receiving areas.

What is most remarkable about this operator is that it appears to be antithetical to initiating action. It provides a pervasive neuronal bias that does not induce phase transitions, but defers them by quenching local fluctuations (Prigogine 1980). It alters the attractor landscapes of the lower-order interactive masses of neurons that it enslaves. In the dynamicist view, intervention by states of awareness in the process of consciousness organizes the attractor landscape of the motor systems, prior to the instant of its next phase transition, the moment of choosing in the limbo of indecision, when the global dynamic brain activity pattern is increasing its complexity and fine-tuning the guidance of overt action. This state of uncertainty and unreadiness to act may last a fraction of a second, a minute, a week, or a lifetime. Then when a contemplated act occurs, awareness follows the onset of the act and does not precede it.

In that hesitancy, between the last act and the next, comes the window of opportunity, when the breaking of symmetry in the next limbic phase transition will make apparent what has been chosen. The observer of the self intervenes by awareness that organizes the attractor landscape, just before the instant of the next transition:

Between the conception
And the creation
Between the emotion
And the response
Falls the Shadow
   Life is very long
—T. S. Eliot, "The Hollow Men" (1936)

The causal technology of self-control is familiar to everyone: hold off fear and anger; defer closure; avoid temptation; take time to study; read and reflect on the opportunity, the meaning, and the consequences; take the long view as it has been inculcated in the educational process. According to Mill (1843, p. 550): "We cannot, indeed, directly will to be different from what we are; but neither did those who are supposed to have formed our characters directly will that we should be what we are. Their will had no direct power except over their own actions. . . . We are exactly as capable of making our own character, *if we will*, as others are of making it for us."

There are numerous unsolved problems with this hypothesis. Although strong advances are being made in analyzing the dynamics of the limbic system and its centerpieces, the entorhinal cortex and the hippocampus (Boeijinga and Lopes da Silva 1988; O'Keefe and Nadel 1978; Rolls et al. 1989; McNaughton 1993; Wilson and McNaughton 1993; Buzsaki 1996; Eichenbaum 1997; Traub et al. 1996), their self-organized spatial patterns, their precise intentional contents, and their mechanisms of formation in relation to intentional action are still unknown. The pyriform cortex, to which the bulb transmits, is strongly driven by its input, and it lacks the phase cones that indicate self-organizing capabilities comparable to those of the sensory cortices. Whether the hippocampus has those capabilities or is likewise a driven structure is unknown. The neural mechanisms by which the entire neocortical neuropil in each hemisphere maintains spatially coherent activity over a broad spectrum with nearly zero time lag are unknown. The significance of this coherent activity for behavior is dependent on finding correlates with behaviors, but these are unknown. If those correlates are meanings, then the subjects must be asked to make representations of the meanings in order to communicate them, so that they are far removed from overt behavior. Knowledge of human brain function is beyond the present reach of neurodynamics because our brains are too complex, owing to their mechanisms for language and self-awareness.

6   Causality Belongs in Technology, Not in Science

The case has now been made on the grounds of neurodynamics that causality is a form of knowing through intentional action. Thus causality is inferred not to exist in material objects, but to be assigned to them by humans with the intent to predict and control them. The determinants of human actions include not only genetic and environmental factors but also self-organizing dynamics in brains, operating primarily through the dynamics of intentional action and secondarily through neural processes that support consciousness, which is commonly but mistakenly attached to free will. Though this inference is not new, it is given new cogency by recent developments in neuroscience. What, then, might be the consequences for natural science, philosophy, and medicine if this inference is accepted?

The concept of causality is fundamental in all aspects of human behavior and understanding, which includes our efforts in laboratory experiments and the analysis of data to comprehend the causal relations of world, brain and mind. In my own work I studied the impact on brain activity of stimuli that animals were trained to ignore or to respond to, seeking to determine how the stimuli might cause new patterns of brain activity to form, and how the new patterns might shape how the animals behaved in response to the stimuli. I attempted to interpret my findings and those of others in terms of chains of cause and effect, which I learned to identify as linear causality (Freeman 1975).

These attempts repeatedly foundered in the complexities of neural activity and in the incompatibility of self-organized, goal-directed behavior of my animals with behaviorist models based on input-output determinism. I found that I was adapting to the animals at least as much as they were being shaped by me. My resort to acausal correlation based in multivariate statistical prediction was unsatisfying. Through my readings in physics and philosophy I learned the concept of circular causality, which invokes hierarchical interactions of immense numbers of semiautonomous elements such as neurons, which form nonlinear systems. These exchanges lead to the formation of macroscopic population dynamics that shapes the patterns of activity of the contributing individuals. I found this concept to be applicable at several levels, including the interactions between neurons and neural masses, between component masses of the forebrain, and between the behaving animal and its environment, under the rubric of intentionality (Freeman 1995).

By adopting this alternative concept I changed my perspective (Freeman 1995). I now sought not to pin events at instants of time, but to conceive of intervals at differing time scales; not to fill the gaps in the linear chains, but to construct the feedback pathways from the surround; not to average the single responses to monotonously repeated stimuli, but to analyze each event in its uniqueness before generalizing; not to explain events exclusively in terms of external stimuli and context, but to allow for the contribution of self-organizing dynamics.

Circular causality departs so strongly from the classical tenets of necessity, invariance, and precise temporal order that the only reason to call it that is to satisfy the human habitual need for causes. The most subtle shift is the disappearance of agency, which is equivalent to loss of Aristotle's efficient cause. Agency is a powerful metaphor. For example, it is common sense to assert that an assassin causes a victim's death, that an undersea quake causes a tsunami, that a fallen tree causes a power failure by breaking a transmission line, that an acid-fast bacillus causes tuberculosis, that an action potential releases transmitter molecules at a synapse, and so forth. But interactions across hierarchical levels do not make sense in these terms. Molecules that cooperate in a hurricane cannot be regarded as the agents that cause the storm. Neurons cannot be viewed as the agents that make consciousness by their firing.

The very strong appeal of agency to explain events may come from the subjective experience of cause and effect that develops early in human life, before the acquisition of language, when as infants we go through the somatomotor phase (Piaget 1930; Thelen and Smith 1994) and learn to control our limbs and to focus our sensory receptors. "I act (cause); therefore I feel (effect)." Granted that causality can be experienced through the neurodynamics of acquiring knowledge by the use of the body, the question I raise here is whether brains share this property with other material objects in the world. The answer I propose is that assignment of cause and effect to one's self and to others having self-awareness is entirely appropriate, but that investing insensate objects with causation is comparable to investing them with teleology and soul.

The further question is: Does it matter whether or not causality is assigned to objects? The answer here is "Very much." Several examples are given of scientific errors attributable to thinking in terms of linear causality. The most important, with wide ramifications, is the assumption of universal determinacy, by which the causes of human behavior are limited to environmental and genetic factors, and the causal power of self-determination is excluded from scientific consideration. We know that linear extrapolation often fails in a nonlinear world. Proof of the failure of this inference is by reductio ad absurdum. It is absurd in the name of causal doctrine to deny our capacity as humans to make choices and decisions regarding our own futures, when we exercise the causal power that we experience as free will.

7 Anthropocentricity in Acts of Human Observation

Our ancestors have a history of interpreting phenomena in human terms appropriate to the scales and dynamics of our brains and bodies. An example of our limitations and our cognitive means for surmounting them is our spatial conception of the earth as flat. This belief is still quite valid for lengths of the size of the human body, such as pool tables, floors, and playing fields, where we use levels, transits, and gradometers, and even for distances that we can cover by walking and swimming. The subtleties of ships that were hull-down over the horizon were mere curiosities, until feats of intellect and exploration such as circumnavigation of the earth opened a new spatial scale. Inversely, at microscopic dimensions of molecules flatness has no meaning. Under an electron microscope the edge of a razor looks like a mountain range.

In respect to time scales, we tend to think of our neurons and brains as having static anatomies, despite the evidence of continual change from time lapse cinematography, as well as the cumulative changes that passing decades reveal to us in our bodies. An intellectual leap is required to understand that form and function are both dynamic, differing essentially in our time scales of measurements and experiences with them. The embryological and phylogenetic developments of brains are described by sequences of geometric forms and the spatiotemporal operations by which each stage emerges from the one preceding. The time scales are in days and eons, not in seconds as in behavior and its neurophysiological correlates.

The growth of structure and the formation of the proper internal axonal and dendritic connections is described by fields of attraction and repulsion, with gradient descents mediated by contact sensitivities and the diffusion of chemicals. Moreover, recent research shows that synapses undergo a process of continual dynamic formation, growth and deletion throughout life (Smythies 1997). The same and similar terms are used in mathematics and the physical sciences such as astronomy and cosmology, over a variety of temporal and spatial scales, many of which are far from the scales of kinesthesia to which we are accustomed. On the one hand, morphogenesis is the geometry of motion, which we can grasp intuitively through time lapse photography. On the other hand, the motions of speeding bullets and hummingbird wings are revealed to us by high-speed cinematography.

The attribution of intention as a property of material objects was common in earlier times by the assignment of spirits to trees, rocks, and the earth. An example is the rising sun. From the human perspective the sun seems to ascend above the horizon and move across the sky. In mythology this motion was assigned to an agency such as a chariot carrying the sun, or to motivation by the music of Orpheus, because music caused people to dance. In the Middle Ages the sun, moon, planets and stars were thought to be carried by spheres that encircled the earth and gave ineffable music as they rotated. The current geometric explanation is that an observer on the earth's surface shifts across the terminator with inertial rotation in an acausal space-time relation. Still, we watch the sun move.

Similarly, humans once thought that an object fell because it desired to be close to the earth, tending to its natural state. In Newtonian mechanics it was pulled down by gravity. In acausal, relativistic terms, it follows a geodesic to a minimal energy state. The Newtonian view required action at a distance, which was thought to be mediated by the postulated quintessence held over from Aristotle, the "ether." Physicists were misled by this fiction, which stemmed from the felt need for a medium to transmit a causal agent. The experimental proof by Michaelson and Morley that the ether did not exist opened the path to relativistic physics and an implicit renunciation of gravitational causality. But physicists failed to pursue this revolution to its completion, and instead persisted in the subject-object distinction by appealing to the dependence of the objective observation on the subjective reference frame of the observer.

In complex, multivariate systems interactive at several levels like brains, causal sequences are virtually impossible to specify unequivocally. Because it introduced indeterminacy, evidence for feedback in the nervous system was deliberately suppressed in the first third of the twentieth century. It was thought that a neuron in a feedback loop could not distinguish its external input from its own output. An example was the reaction of Ramón y Cajal to a 1929 report by his student Rafael Lorente de Nó, who presented Cajal with his Golgi study of neurons in the entorhinal cortex (Freeman 1984). He constructed diagrams of axodendritic connections among the neurons with arrows to indicate the direction of transmission, and he deduced that they formed feedback loops. Cajal told him that his inference was unacceptable, because brains were deterministic and could not work if they had feedback. He withdrew his report from publication until Cajal's death, in 1934. After he published it (Lorente de Nó 1934), it became an enduring classic, leading to the concept of the nerve cell assembly by its influence on Donald Hebb (1949), and to neural networks and digital computers by inspiring Warren McCulloch and through him John von Neumann (1958). The concept of linear causality similarly slowed recognition and acceptance of processes of self-organization in complex systems, by the maxim that "nothing can cause itself." The phrase "self-determination" was commonly regarded as an oxymoron. A similar exclusion delayed acceptance of the concept of reafference, also called corollary discharge (Freeman 1995).

8   Applications in Philosophy

Description of a linear causal connection is based on appeal to an invariant relationship between two events. If an effect follows, the cause is sufficient; if an effect is always preceded by it, then the cause is necessary. From the temporal order and its invariance, as attested by double-blind experimental controls to parcellate the antecedents, an appearance of necessity is derived. The search concludes with assignment of an agency, that has responsibility for production, direction, control or stimulation, and that has its own prior agency, since every cause must also be an effect.

According to David Hume (1739), causation does not arise in the events; it emerges in the minds of the observers. The temporal succession and spatial contiguity of events that are interpreted as causes and effects comprise the invariant connection. It is the felt force of conjoined impressions that constitutes the quale of causality. Since the repetition of these relations adds no new idea, the feeling of the necessity has to be explained psychologically. He came to this conclusion from an abstract premise in the doctrine of the nominalism, according to which there are no universal essences in reality, so the mind cannot frame a concept or image that corresponds to any universal or general term, such as causality. This was opposed, then as now, to the doctrine of scientific realism. Hume and his nominalist colleagues were anticipated 500 years earlier by the work of Thomas Aquinas (1272), who conceived that the individual forms of matter are abstracted by the imagination ("phantasia") to create universals that exist only in the intellect, not in matter. Early-twentieth-century physicists should have completed the Humean revolution in their development of quantum mechanics, but they lost their nerve and formulated instead the Copenhagen interpretations, which reaffirmed the subject-object distinction of Plato and Descartes, despite the force of their own discoveries staring them in the face. Phenomenologists before Heidegger maintained the error, and postmodern structuralists persist in it. For example, instead of saying "Causality is a form of knowing," they say "The attribution of causality is a form of knowing." That is, "Causality really does exist in matter, but it is a matter of choice by humans whether to believe it."

Conversely, Mill (1873, pp. 101–102)) accepted "the universal law of causation" but not necessity: ". . . the doctrine of what is called Philosophical Necessity" weighed on my existence like an incubus. . . . I pondered painfully on the subject, till gradually I saw light through it. I perceived, that the word Necessity, as a name for the doctrine of Cause and Effect applied to human action, carried with it a misleading association; and that this association was the operative force in the depressing and paralyzing influence which I had experienced." Mill developed his position fully in "A System of Logic" (1843).

Kant (1781) insisted that science could not exist without causality. Since causality was for him a category in mind, it follows that science is a body of knowledge about the world but is not in the world. Causality then becomes a basis for agreement among scientists regarding the validation of relationships between events, and the prediction of actions to be taken for control of events in the world. Since it could not be validated by inductive generalization from sense data, but was nevertheless essential to give wholeness and completion to experience [Apperzeption], Kant concluded that it must be "a priori" and "transcendental" over the sense data. This led him to designate causality as a category [Kategorie] in and of the mind, along with space and time as the forms of perception [Anschauungsformen] by which the sense data were irretrievably modified during assembly into perceptions, making the real world [das Ding an sich] inaccessible to direct observation.

Friedrich Nietzsche (1886, p. 48) placed causality in the mind as the expression of free will: "The question is in the end whether we really recognize the will as efficient, whether we believe in the causality of the will: if we do—and at bottom our faith in this is nothing less than our faith in causality itself—then we have to make the experiment of positing the causality of the will hypothetically as the only one . . . the will to power."

Hilary Putnam (1990, p. 81) assigned causality to the operation of brains in the process of observation: "Hume's account of causation . . . is anathema to most present-day philosophers. Nothing could be more contrary to the spirit of recent philosophical writing than the idea that there is nothing more to causality than regularity or the idea that, if there is something more, that something more is largely subjective." Putnam (ibid., p, 75) also wrote: "If we cannot give a single example of an ordinary observation report which does not, directly or indirectly, presuppose causal judgments, then the empirical distinction between the 'regularities' we 'observe' and the 'causality' we 'project onto' the objects and events involved in the regularities collapses. Perhaps the notion of causality is so primitive that the very notion of observation presupposes it?"

Davidson (1980, p. 19) made a case for "anomalous monism" to resolve the apparent contradiction between the deterministic laws of physics, the necessity for embodiment of mental processes in materials governed by those fixed laws, and the weakness of the "laws" governing psychophysical events as distinct from statistical classes of events: "Why on earth should a cause turn an action into a mere happening and a person into a helpless victim? Is it because we tend to assume, at least in the arena of action, that a cause demands a causer, agency and agent? So we press the question; if my action is caused, what caused it? If I did, then there is the absurdity of an infinite regress; if I did not, I am a victim. But of course the alternatives are not exhaustive. Some causes have no agents. Among these agentless causes are the states and changes of state in persons which, because they are reasons as well as causes, constitute certain events free and intentional actions."

Davidson's premises have been superseded in two respects. First, he postulated that brains are material systems, for which the laws of physics support accurate prediction. He described brains as "closed systems." In the past three decades numerous investigators have realized that brains are open systems, as are all organs and living systems, with an infinite sink in the venous return for waste heat and entropy, so that the 1st and 2nd laws of thermodynamics do not hold for brains, thus negating one of his two main premises. Second, he postulated that, with respect to meaning, minds are "open" systems, on the basis that they are continually acting into the world and learning about it. The analyses of electrophysiological data taken during the operations of sensory cortices during acts of perception indicate that meaning in each mind is a closed system, and that meaning is based in chaotic constructions, not in information processing, thus negating the other of his two main premises. In my view, neurons engage in complex biochemical operations that have no meaning or information in themselves, but inspire meaning in researchers who measure them. The degree of unpredictability of mental and behavioral events is in full accord with the extent of variations in the space-time patterns of the activity of chaotic systems, thus removing the requirement for the adjective, "anomalous," because it applies to both sets of laws for the material and mental aspects of living systems. Moreover, the adoption of the concept "circular causality" from physics and psychology removes agency. That which remains is "dynamical monism."

9 Applications of Causality in Medical Technology

Causality is properly attributed to intentional systems, whose mechanisms of exploring, learning, choosing, deciding, and acting constitute the actualization of the feeling of necessary connection, and of the cognitive metaphor of agency. It is properly used to describe technological intervention into processes of the material world after analysis of the interrelations of events. Surmounting linear causal thinking may enable neuroscientists to pursue studies in the dynamics of the limbic system to clarify the meanings of statistical regularities in chaotic, self-organizing systems and change their outcomes by experimental manipulation. Social scientists may take advantage of the discovery of a biological basis for choice and individual responsibility to strengthen our social and legal institutions by complementing environmental and genetic linear causation. The nature-nurture debate has neglected a third of the determinant triad: the self. People can and do make something of themselves. Neurophilosophers studying consciousness in brain function may find new answers to old questions by re-opening the debate on causality. What acausal relations arise among the still inadequately defined entities comprising brains? What is the global operator of consciousness? The mind-brain problem is not solved, but it can be transplanted to more fertile ground.

My proposal is not to deny or abandon causality, but to adapt it as an essential aspect of the human mind/brain by virtue of its attachment to intentionality. This can be done by using the term 'circular causality' divorced from agency in the sciences, and the term 'linear causality' in combination with agency in the technologies, including medical, social, legal, and engineering applications.

For example, medical research is widely conceived as the search for the causes of diseases and the means for intervention to prevent or cure them. A keystone in microbiology is expressed in the postulates Robert Koch formulated in 1881 to specify the conditions that must be met in order to assign a causal relation between a microorganism and a disease:

(1) the germ must always be found in the disease; (2) it must be isolated in pure culture from the diseased individual; (3) inoculation with the isolated culture must be followed by the same disease in a suitable test animal; and (4) the same germ must be isolated in pure culture from the diseased test animal.

These postulates have served well for understanding transmissible diseases and providing a biological foundation for developing chemotherapies, vaccines, and other preventatives. Public health measures addressing housing, nutrition, waste disposal, and water supplies had already been well advanced in the nineteenth century for the prevention of pandemics such as cholera, typhoid, tuberculosis, and dysentery, on the basis of associations and to a considerable extent on the basis of the maxim "Cleanliness is next to godliness." This was intentional behavior of a high order indeed. The new science brought an unequivocal set of targets for research on methods of prevention and treatment.

The most dramatic development in neuropsychiatry was the finding of spirochetes in the brains of patients with general paresis, for which the assigned causes had been lifestyles of dissolution and moral turpitude. The discovery of the "magic bullet" 606 (arsphenamine) established the medical model for management of neuropsychiatric illness, which was rapidly extended to viruses (rabies, polio, measles), environmental toxins (lead, mercury, ergot), vitamin and mineral deficiencies (cretinism, pellagra), hormonal deficits (hypothyroidism, diabetic coma, lack of dopamine in postencephalitic and other types of Parkinson's disease), and genetic abnormalities (phenylketonuria, Tourette's Syndrome, Huntington's chorea). Massive research programs are under way to find the unitary causes and the magic bullets of chemotherapies, replacement genes, and vaccines for Alzheimer's, neuroses, psychoses, and schizophrenias. The current explanations of the affective disorders—too much or too little dopamine, serotonin, etc. —resemble the Hippocratic doctrine of the four humors, imbalances of which were seen as the causes of diseases.

There are compelling examples of necessary connections. Who can doubt that *Vibrio* causes cholera, or that a now-eradicated virus caused smallpox? However, these examples come from medical technology, in which several specific conditions hold. First, the discoveries in bacteriology came through an extension of human perception through the microscope to a new spatial scale. This led to the development by Rudolf Virchow of the cellular basis of human pathology. The bacterial adversaries were then seen as having the same spatial dimensions as the cells with which they were at war. The bacterial invaders and the varieties of their modes of attack did not qualitatively differ from the macroscopic predators with which mankind had always been familiar, such as wolves and crocodiles, which humans eradicate, avoid, or maintain in laboratories and zoos. Second, the causal metaphor motivated the application of controlled experiments to the isolation and analysis of target bacterial and viral species, vitamins, toxic chemicals, hormones, and genes. It still does motivate researchers, with the peculiar potency of intermittent reinforcement by occasional success. The latest example is the recognition that pyloric ulcers are caused by a bacillus and not by psychic stress or a deleterious lifestyle, implying that the cause is "real" and not just "psychosomatic." Third, the research and therapies are directly addressed to humans, who take action by ingesting drugs and seeking vaccinations, and who perceive changes in their bodies thereafter. A feeling of causal efficacy is very powerful in these circumstances, and many patients commit themselves without reservation to treatments, well after FDA scientists by controlled studies have shown them to be ineffective. The urgency of conceptualizing causality to motivate beneficial human actions does not thereby establish the validity of that agency among the objects under study. Feeling is believing, but it is not knowing. The feeling of causal agency in medicine has led to victories, but also to mistakes with injury and death on a grand scale.

Koch's postulates approach a necessary connection of a bacillus to an infectious disease, but not the sufficient conditions. Pathogens are found in healthy individuals as well, and often not in the sick. Inoculation does not always succeed in producing the disease. These anomalies can be, and commonly are, ignored, if the preponderance of evidence justifies doing so, but the classical criteria for causality are violated, or are replaced with statistical judgments. A positive culture of a bacillus is sufficient reason to initiate treatment with an antibiotic, even if it is the wrong disease. Similarly, pathologists cannot tell the cause of death from their findings at autopsy. They are trained to state what the patient died "with" and not "of." It is the job of the coroner or a licensed physician to assign the cause of death. The causes of death are not scientific. They are social and technological, and they concern public health, economic well being, and the apprehension of criminals.

Another example of the social value of causality is the statement "Smoking causes cancer." This is a clear and valid warning that a particular form of behavior is likely to end in early and painful death. On the one hand, society has a legitimate interest in maintaining health and reducing monetary and emotional costs by investing the strong statistical connection with the motivating status of causality. On the other hand, the "causal chain" by which tobacco tars are connected to the unbridled proliferation of pulmonary epithelial tissue is still being explored, and a continuing weakness of evidence for the complete linear causal chain is being used by tobacco companies to claim that there is no proof that smoking causes cancer. Thus the causal argument has been turned against society's justifiable efforts to prevent tobacco-related illnesses.

10   The Technology of Mental Illness

The most complex and ambiguous field of medicine concerns the causes and treatments of mental disorders. Diagnosis and treatment for the past century have been polarized between the medical model of the causes of diseases, currently held in biological psychiatry, and psychoanalysis, the talking cure. Sigmund Freud was impressed with the phenomena of hysteria, in which patients suffered transient disabilities, such as blindness and paralysis, but presented no evidence of infection or anatomical degeneration in their brains. He drew on his background in clinical neurology to develop a biological hypothesis (1895) for behavior, based on the flow of nerve energy between neurons through "contact barriers" (named 'synapses' by Foster and Sherrington 3 years later). Some axonal pathways developed excessive resistance at these barriers, deflecting nerve energy into unusual channels by "neuronic inertia," giving rise to hysterical symptoms. Within a decade he had abandoned the biological approach as "premature," working instead with his symbolic model of the id, the ego, and the superego, but his ideas were generalized to distinguish "functional" from "organic" diseases. Traumatic childhood experiences warped the development of the contact barriers. Treatment was to explore the recesses of memory, bring the resistances to awareness, and reduce them by client and therapist reasoning together following transference and countertransference.

The bipolarization between the organic and the functional has been stable for a century. Patients and practitioners have been able to choose their positions in this spectrum of causes according to their beliefs and preferences. Some patients are delighted to be informed that their disorders are due to chemical imbalances, that are correctable by drugs and are not their fault or responsibility. Others bitterly resent the perceived betrayal by their bodies, and they seek healing through the exercise of mental discipline and the power of positive thinking. But the balance has become unstable with two new circumstances. One is the cost of medical care. Health maintenance organizations are pressuring psychiatrists to see more patients in shorter visits, to dispense with oral histories and the meanings of symptoms for the patients, and to get them quickly out the door with packets of pills. The power of biological causality is clearly in operation as a social, not a scientific, impetus, operating to the detriment of people with complex histories and concerns.

The other circumstance is the growing realization among mental health care specialists that chemical imbalances, poor genes, and unfortunate experiences of individuals are insufficient explanations to provide the foundations for treatment. Of particular importance for the onset, the course, and the resolution of an illness are the social relations of individuals, families, neighborhoods, and religious communities and the milieu of national policies and events. Conflicts rage over the assignment of the cause of chronic fatigue syndrome to neuroticism or to a virus, of "Gulf War Syndrome" to malingering or a neurotoxin, and of post-traumatic stress disorder to battle fatigue or a character deficit. The dependence of the debates on causality is fueled by technological questions of human action: What research is to be done? What treatments are to be given? Who is to pay for the treatments? Successful outcomes are known to depend less on pills and counseling than on mobilization of community support for distressed individuals (Frankl 1973). These complex relations, involving faith and meaning among family and friends, may be seriously violated by reduction to unidirectional causes. Patients may be restored to perfect chemical balance and then die anyway in despair. Families may disintegrate into endless recrimination and self-justification, from lack of tolerance of misdirected parental and filial intentions and honest mistakes. So it is with patient-doctor relations. To seek and find a cause is to lay the blame, opening the legal right to sue for compensation for psychological injury and distress. These, too, are legacies of linear causal thinking.

Abnormal behavior in states of trance or seizure was attributed in past centuries to the loss or willing surrender of self-control to possession by exotic spirits. In the West the failure of responsibility was codified as legal insanity in 1846 according to the McNaughton Rule: "[To] establish a defense on the grounds of insanity, it must be clearly proven that at the time of the committing of the act, the party accused was laboring under such a defect of reason, from disease of the mind, as not to know the nature and quality of the act he was doing, or, if he did know it, that he did not know he was doing what was wrong." In the terms of the present analysis, for behavior to be insane the neural components of the limbic system must have entered into basins of attraction that are sufficiently strange or unusually stable to escape control by the global state variable. This view encompasses the two facets of causality, microscopic and macroscopic, that compete for control of the self, but it is not an adequate statement of the problem. In fact the case on which the rule was based was decided on political grounds (Moran 1981). Daniel McNaughton was a Scotsman engaged in ideal-driven assassination, and his transfer by the British authorities from Newgate Prison to Bethlam Hospital was designed to prevent him from testifying in public. A similar move for similar reasons was made by the American government by sending the poet Ezra Pound, charged with treason in World War II, to St. Elizabeth's Hospital rather than to the federal prison at Leavenworth. The point is that judgments about which acts are intentional and which are not are made by society, in last resort by judges and juries in courts of law, not by doctors, scientists, or individuals in isolation. What biology can offer is a foundation on which to construct a social theory of self-control.

11   The Science versus the Technology of Self-Control

The role of causality in self-awareness is close to the essence of what it is to be human. Nowhere is this more poignant than in the feeling of the need for self-control. Materialists and psychoanalysts see the limbic self as a machine driven by metabolic needs and inherited instincts, the id, that carries the ego as a rational critic that struggles to maintain causal control, as befits the Cartesian metaphor of the soul as the pilot of a boat, by adjudicating blind forces. Structure and chemistry are genetically determined. Behaviorist psychologists confuse motivation with intention and view behavior as the sum of reflexes, caused by environmental inputs and sociobiological processes, while consciousness is epiphenomenal.

Functionalists see the mind as equivalent to software that can be adapted to run on any platform, once the algorithms and rules have been discovered. Logical operations on symbols as representations are the causes of rational behavior, and the unsolved problems for research concern the linkage of the symbols with activities of neurons and with whatever the symbols represent in the world. That research will be unnecessary, if the linkages can made instead to the components of intelligent machines resembling computers (Fodor 1981). Unfortunately the only existing intelligent beings have evolved from lower species, and our brains contain the limbic system as irrational baggage. Outputs from the logic circuits in the neocortex, before reaching the motor apparatus, are filtered through the limbic system, where emotions are attached that distort and degrade the rational output. Consciousness is a mystery to be explained by "new laws of physics" (Penrose 1994; Chalmers 1996).

Existentialists hold that humans choose what they become by their own actions. The cause of behavior is the self, which is here described as emerging through the dynamics in the limbic system. The ego constituting awareness of the self discovers its own nature by observing and analyzing its actions and creations, but cannot claim credit for them. In extreme claims advanced by Nietzsche and Sartre, the ego is unconstrained by reality. In more modest terms, because of the circularity of the relation of the self and its awareness, the future actions of the self are shaped in the context of its irrevocable past, its body, its given cultural and physical environment, and its present state of awareness, which is its own creation. The finite brain grapples with the infinity of the world and the uncertainty of the interlocked futures of world and brain, by continually seeking the invariances that will support reliable predictions. Those predictions exist as awareness of future possibilities, without which the self cannot prevail. They are expressed in the feeling of hope: the future need not merely happen; to some extent it can be caused.

Conclusion

The interactions between microscopic and macroscopic domains lie at the heart of self-organization. How do all those neurons simultaneously get together in a virtual instant, and switch from one harmonious pattern to another in an orderly dance, like the shuttle of lights on the "magic loom" of Sherrington (1940)? The same problem holds for the excitation of atoms in a laser, leading to the emergence of coherent light from the organization of the whole mass; for the coordinated motions of molecules of water and air in a hurricane; for the orchestration of the organelles of caterpillars in metamorphosing to butterflies; and for the inflammatory spread of behavioral fads, rebellions, and revolutions that sweep entire nations. All these kinds of events call for new laws such as those developed in physics by Haken (1983), in chemistry by Prigogine (1980), in biology by Eigen and Schuster (1979), in sociology by Foucault (1976), and in neurobiology by Edelman (1987), which can address new levels of complexity that have heretofore been inaccessible to human comprehension. Perhaps these will serve as the "new laws" called for by Penrose (1994) and Chalmers (1996), but they need not lead to dualism or panpsychism. They can arise as logical extensions from the bases of understanding we already have in these several realms of science, none of which can be fully reduced to the others.

Consciousness in the neurodynamic view is a global internal state variable composed of a sequence of momentary states of awareness. Its regulatory role is comparable to that of the operator in a thermostat, that instantiates the difference between the sensed temperature and a set point, and that initiates corrective action by turning a heater on or off. The machine state variable has little history and no capacities for learning or determining its own set point, but the principle is the same: the internal state is a form of energy, an operator, a predictor of the future, and a carrier of information that is available to the system as a whole. It is a prototype, an evolutionary precursor, not to be confused with awareness, any more than tropism in plants and bacteria is to be confused with intentionality. In humans, the operations and informational contents of the global state variable, which are sensations, images, feelings, thoughts, and beliefs, constitute the experience of causation.

To deny this comparability and assert that humans are not machines is to miss the point. Two things distinguish humans from all other beings. One is the form and function of the human body, including the brain, which has been given to us by 3 billion years of biological evolution. The other is the heritage given to us by 2 million years of cultural evolution. Our mental attributes have been characterized for millennia as the soul or spirit or consciousness that makes us not-machines. The uniqueness of the human condition is not thereby explained, but the concept of circular causality provides a tool for intervention, when something has gone wrong, because the circle can be broken into forward and feedback limbs. Each of them can be explained by linear causality, which tells us where and how to intervene. The only error would be to assign causal agency to the parts of the machine.

Science provides knowledge of relations among objects in the world, whereas technology provides tools for intervention into the relations by humans with intent to control the objects. The acausal science of understanding the self distinctively differs from the causal technology of self-control. "Circular causality" in self-organizing systems is a concept that is useful to describe interactions between microscopic neurons in assemblies and the macroscopic emergent state variable that organizes them. In this review intentional action is ascribed to the activities of the subsystems. Awareness (fleeting frames) and consciousness (continual operator) are ascribed to a hemisphere-wide order parameter constituting a global brain state. Linear causal inference is appropriate and essential for planning and interpreting human actions and personal relations, but it can be misleading when it is applied to microscopic-microscopic relations in brains. It is paradoxical to assign linear causality to brains, and thereby cast doubt on the validity of causal agency (free will) in choices in and by humans, just because they are materialized in phase transitions in their brains.

Acknowledgments

The author's research was supported by grants from the National Institutes of Health (MH-06686) and the Office of Naval Research (N00014-93-1-0938). This work originally appeared in the *Journal of Consciousness Studies* (6, 1999, no. 11: 143–172).

References

Abraham, F. D, Abraham, R. H., Shaw, C. D., and Garfinkel, A. 1990. *A Visual Introduction to Dynamical Systems Theory for Psychology*. Aerial.

Aquinas, St. Thomas. 1272. *The Summa Theologica* (Encyclopedia Britannica, Inc., 1952).

Barrie, J. M, Freeman, W. J., and Lenhart, M. 1996. Modulation by discriminative training of spatial patterns of gamma EEG amplitude and phase in neocortex of rabbits. *Journal of Neurophysiology* 76: 520–539.

Bloom, F. E., and Lazerson, A. 1988. *Brain, Mind, and Behavior*, second edition. Freeman.

Boeijinga, P. H., and Lopes da Silva, F. H. 1988. Differential distribution of beta and theta EEG activity in the entorhinal cortex of the cat. *Brain Research* 448: 272–286.

Bures, J., Buresová, O., and Krivánek, J. 1974. *The Mechanism and Applications of Leão's Spreading Depression of Electroencephalographic Activity*. Academic Press.

Buzsaki, G. 1996. The hippocampal-neocortical dialogue. *Cerebral Cortex* 6: 81–92.

Cannon, W. B. 1939. *The Wisdom of the Body*. Norton.

Cartwright, N. 1989. *Nature's Capacities and their Measurement*. Clarendon.

Chalmers, D. J. 1996. *The Conscious Mind: In Search of a Fundamental Theory*. Oxford University Press.

Crick, F. 1994. *The Astonishing Hypothesis: The Scientific Search for the Soul*. Scribner.

Darwin, C. 1872. *The Expression of the Emotions in Man and Animals*. J. Murray.

Davidson, D. 1980. Actions, reasons, and causes. In *Essays on Actions and Events*. Clarendon.

Dennett, D. H. 1991. *Consciousness Explained*. Little, Brown.

Dewey, J. 1914. Psychological doctrine in philosophical teaching. *Journal of Philosophy* 11: 505–512.

Eccles, J. C. 1994. *How the Self Controls Its Brain*. Springer-Verlag.

Edelman, G. M. 1987. *Neural Darwinism: The Theory of Neuronal Group Selection*. Basic Books.

Eichenbaum, H. 1997. How does the brain organize memories? *Science* 277: 330–332.

Eigen, M., and Schuster, P. 1979. *The Hypercycle. A Principle of Natural Self-Organization*. Springer-Verlag.

Eliot, T. S. 1936. "The Hollow Men." In *Collected Poems 1909–1935*. Harcourt Brace.

Fodor, J. A. 1981. *Representations: Philosophical Essays on the Foundations of Cognitive Science*. MIT Press.

Foucault, M. 1976. *The History of Sexuality*, volume 1 (Random House, 1980).

Frankl, V. 1973. *The Doctor and the Soul*. Random House.

Freeman, W. J. 1975. *Mass Action in the Nervous System*. Academic Press.

Freeman, W. J. 1984. Premises in neurophysiological studies of learning. In *Neurobiology of Learning and Memory*, ed. G. Lynch et al. Guilford.

Freeman, W. J. 1991. The physiology of perception. *Scientific American* 264: 78–85.

Freeman, W. J. 1992. Tutorial in Neurobiology: From Single Neurons to Brain Chaos. *International Journal of Bifurcation and Chaos* 2: 451–482.

Freeman, W. J. 1995. *Societies of Brains. A Study in the Neuroscience of Love and Hate*. Erlbaum.

Freud, S. 1895. The project of a scientific psychology. In *The Origins of Psychoanalysis*, ed. M. Bonaparte et al. Basic Books, 1954.

Gaál, G., and Freeman, W. J. 1997. Relations among EEGs from entorhinal cortex and olfactory bulb, somatomotor, auditory and visual cortices in trained cats. *Society of Neuroscience Abstracts* 407: 19.

Gibson, J. J. 1979. *The Ecological Approach to Visual Perception*. Houghton Mifflin.

Gloor, P. 1997. *The Temporal Lobe and the Limbic System*. Oxford University Press.

Goltz, F. L. 1892. Der Hund ohne Grosshirn. Siebente Abhandlung über die Verrichtungen des Grosshirns. *Pflügers Archiv* 51: 570–614.

Gray, C. M. 1994. Synchronous oscillations in neuronal systems: Mechanisms and functions. *Journal of Comparative Neuroscience* 1: 11–38.

Grossberg, S. 1982. *Studies of Mind and Brain: Neural Principles of Learning, Perception, Development, Cognition, and Motor Control*. Reidel.

Haken, H. 1983. *Synergetics: An Introduction*. Springer-Verlag.

Hardcastle, V. G. 1994. Psychology's binding problem and possible neurobiological solutions. *Journal of Consciousness Studies* 1: 66–90.

Hebb, D. O. 1949. *The Organization of Behavior*. Wiley.

Helmholtz, H. L. F. von. 1872. *Handbuch der physiologischen Optik*, volume 3 (L. Voss, 1909).

Herrnstein, R. J., and Murray, C. 1994. *The Bell Curve*. Free Press.

Herrick, C. J. 1948. *The Brain of the Tiger Salamander*. University of Chicago Press.

Hull, C. L. 1943, *Principles of Behavior, An Introduction to Behavior Theory*. Appleton-Century.

Hume, D. 1739. *Treatise on Human Nature*. J. Noon.

Jackson, J. H. 1931. *Selected Writings of John Hughlings Jackson*. Hodder and Stoughton.

James, W. 1879. Are we automata? *Mind* 4: 1–21.

James, W. 1893. *The Principles of Psychology.* Holt.

Kant, I. 1781. *Kritik der reinen Vernunft* (Suhrkamp, 1974).

Kay, L. M, and Freeman, W. J. 1998. Bidirectional processing in the olfactory-limbic axis during olfactory behavior. *Behavioral Neuroscience* 112: 541–553.

König, P., and Schillen, T. B. 1991. Stimulus-dependent assembly formation of oscillatory responses. I. synchronization. *Neural Computation* 3: 155–166.

Lehmann, D., and Michel, C. M. 1990. Intracerebral dipole source localization for FFT power maps. *Electroencephalography and Clinical Neurophysiology* 76: 271–276.

Lorente de Nó, R. 1934. Studies on the structure of the cerebral cortex. I The area entorhinalis. *Journal für Psychologie und Neurologie* 45: 381–438.

McNaughton, B. L. 1993. The mechanism of expression of long-term enhancement of hippocampal synapses: Current issues and theoretical implications. *Annual Review of Physiology* 55: 375–396.

Merleau-Ponty, M. 1942. *The Structure of Behavior* (Beacon, 1963).

Mill, J. S. 1843. *Of Liberty and Necessity* (Longmans, Green, 1965).

Mill, J. S. 1873. *Autobiography* (Columbia University Press. 1924).

Moran, R. 1981. *Knowing Right from Wrong: The Insanity Defense of Daniel McNaughtan.* Macmillan.

Nietzsche, F. 1886. *Beyond Good and Evil. A Prelude to a Philosophy of the Future* (Random House, 1966).

O'Keefe, J., and Nadel, L. 1978. *The Hippocampus as a Cognitive Map.* Clarendon.

Penrose, R. 1994. *Shadows of the Mind.* Oxford University Press.

Piaget, J. 1930. *The Child's Conception of Physical Causality.* Harcourt, Brace.

Prigogine, I. 1980. *From Being to Becoming: Time and Complexity in the Physical Sciences.* Freeman.

Putnam, H. 1990. *Realism with a Human Face.* Harvard University Press.

Roelfsema, P. R., Engel, A. K., König, P., and Singer, W. 1997. Visuomotor integration is associated with zero time-lag synchronization among cortical areas. *Nature* 385: 157–161.

Rolls, E. T., Miyashita, Y., Cahusac, P. B. M., Kesner, R. P., Niki, H., Feigenbaum, J. D., and Bach, L. 1989. Hippocampal neurons in the monkey with activity related to the place in which the stimulus is shown. *Journal of Neuroscience* 9: 1835–1845.

Roth, G. 1987. *Visual Behavior in Salamanders.* Springer-Verlag

Searle, J. R. 1992. *The Rediscovery of the Mind.* MIT Press.

Sherrington, C. S. 1940. *Man on His Nature.* Oxford University Press.

Singer, W., and Gray, C. M. 1995. Visual feature integration and the temporal correlation hypothesis. *Annual Review of Neuroscience* 18: 555–586.

Skarda, C. A., and Freeman, W. J. 1987. How brains make chaos in order to make sense of the world. *Behavioral and Brain Sciences* 10: 161–195.

Skinner, B. F. 1969. *Contingencies of Reinforcement; A Theoretical Analysis.* Appleton-Century-Crofts

Smart, A., German, P., Oshtory, S., Gaál, G., Barrie, J. M., and Freeman, W. J. 1997. Spatio-temporal analysis of multi-electrode cortical EEG of awake rabbit. *Society of Neuroscience Abstracts* 189. 13.

Smythies, J. 1997. The biochemical basis of synaptic plasticity and neural computation: A new theory. *Proceedings of the Royal Society London B* 264: 575–579.

Sperry, R. W. 1950. Neural basis of the spontaneous optokinetic response. *Journal of Comparative Physiology* 43: 482–489.

Thelen, E., and Smith, L. B. 1994. *A Dynamic Systems Approach to the Development of Cognition and Action.* MIT Press.

Titchener, E. B. 1907. *An Outline of Psychology.* Macmillan.

Traub, R. D., Whittington, M. A., Colling, S. B., Buzsaki, G., and Jefferys, J. G. R. 1996. A mechanism for generation of long-range synchronous fast oscillations in the cortex. *Nature* 383: 621–624.

Tsuda, I. 1991. Chaotic itinerancy as a dynamical basis of hermeneutics in brain and mind. *World Futures* 32: 167–184.

von Holst, E., and Mittelstädt, H. 1950. Das Reafferenzprinzip (Wechselwirkung zwischen Zentralnervensystem und Peripherie). *Naturwissenschaften* 37: 464–476.

von Neumann, J. 1958. *The Computer and the Brain.* Yale University Press.

Whitehead, A. N. 1938. *Modes of Thought.* Macmillan.

Wilson, M. A., and McNaughton, B. L. 1993. Dynamics of the hippocampal ensemble code for space. *Science* 261: 1055–1058.

II PHILOSOPHY

6 Where's the Action? Epiphenomenalism and the Problem of Free Will

Shaun Gallagher

Some philosophers argue that Descartes was wrong when he characterized animals as purely physical automata—robots devoid of consciousness. It seems to them obvious that animals (tigers, lions, and bears, as well as chimps, dogs, and dolphins, and so forth) are conscious. There are other philosophers who argue that it is not beyond the realm of possibility that robots and other artificial agents may someday be conscious—and it is certainly practical to take the intentional stance toward them (the robots as well as the philosophers) even now. I'm not sure that there are philosophers who would deny consciousness to animals but affirm the possibility of consciousness in robots. In any case, and in whatever way these various philosophers define consciousness, the majority of them do attribute consciousness to humans. Among this group, however, are philosophers and scientists who want to reaffirm the idea, explicated by Shadworth Holloway Hodgson in 1870, that in regard to action the presence of consciousness does not matter, since it plays no causal role. Hodgson's brain generated the following thought: Neural events form an autonomous causal chain that is independent of any accompanying conscious mental states. Consciousness is epiphenomenal, incapable of having any effect on the nervous system. James (1890, p. 130) summarizes the situation:

To Descartes belongs the credit of having first been bold enough to conceive of a completely self-sufficing nervous mechanism which should be able to perform complicated and apparently intelligent acts. By a singularly arbitrary restriction, however, Descartes stopped short at man, and while contending that in beasts the nervous machinery was all, he held that the higher acts of man were the result of the agency of his rational soul. The opinion that beasts have no consciousness at all was of course too paradoxical to maintain itself long as anything more than a curious item in the history of philosophy. And with its abandonment the very notion that the nervous system per se might work the work of intelligence, which was an integral, though detachable part of the whole theory, seemed also to slip out of men's conception, until, in this century, the elaboration of the doctrine of reflex action made it possible and natural that it should again arise. But it was not till 1870, I believe, that Mr. Hodgson made the decisive step, by saying that feelings, no matter how intensely they may be present, can have no causal efficacy whatever, and comparing them to the colors laid on the surface of a mosaic, of which the events in the nervous system are represented by the stones. Obviously the stones are held in place by each other and not by the several colors which they support.[1]

The question "Does consciousness cause behavior?" is thus answered in the negative by epiphenomenalists. It is often thought that (1) this question, *as it is commonly understood*,[2] is directly related to the question of free will, and (2) if one is an epiphenomenalist one cannot accept the idea of free will. Although it seems that the truth of the second statement would imply the truth of first one, I will argue that (1) is false, even if (2) is true (although, to be clear, I don't think that (2) is true). The reason for this has to do with what I am calling the common understanding of the question. This understanding can be stated succinctly as follows: when we ask whether consciousness causes behavior we are asking whether consciousness plays a role in the initiation of bodily movement and motor control. I do not want to claim that this understanding controls the entire discussion of free will. I suggest, however, that it does characterize a large part of the thinking that goes on in one corner of the discussion, specifically in the debates between epiphenomenalists and interactionists. I'll try to present evidence or examples for how pervasive this understanding is, at least in this one small corner of philosophical discussion.

1   The Question as Commonly Understood

The common understanding of the question can be seen in the epiphenomenalist answer where causal efficacy is attributed to neural mechanisms but not to consciousness. Neural events cause bodily movement and consciousness, but consciousness cannot cause neural events or bodily movement. The understanding of the question itself, however, had already been set by Descartes and involves the Cartesian concept of mind as a mental space in which I control my own thoughts and actions. Strictly speaking, for Descartes, only mental actions (volitions) are free; actions of the body are not free, but are governed by physical laws.[3] This concept of the mind, as an interior space that is accessible to reflection, frames the modern question. On the Cartesian view, the problem is to explain how the mind directs the body, since what makes a certain bodily movement an action is the contribution of these mental processes. Descartes suggested that the mental events somehow interact with the brain, which then activates the muscles.[4] Without such interaction we have mere behavior, the sort of thing possible for automata and animals. Unless the action is initiated in the mind—acted out, in some cases, explicitly in imagination—then the external behavior is not really an action. Action on this definition is always voluntary or intentional action. If my bodily movement is not intentional, then it is mere behavior, something like reflex behavior. If my bodily movement is determined by something other than my own reflective thought, then it is involuntary movement, but not action.

The epiphenomenalist adopts the same Cartesian framework and simply answers No to the question. Action is nothing more than motor behavior determined by processes other than conscious thought. The epiphenomenalist does not deny that there is conscious thought, or even necessarily that conscious thought appears to be something similar to that which Descartes describes. But consciousness simply does not have causal efficacy in regard to the organism's behavior.

On this reading, it is possible for a Cartesian and an epiphenomenalist to agree on the phenomenology, but disagree on the etiology of action. What is the phenomenology that they could agree on? Allegedly it is just this: when I act I reflectively experience having a desire or intention and then in some way experience the generation of bodily movement. My action appears to be formed in these mental processes, and insofar as I am conscious of these mental processes along with my bodily movements, my actions appear to be under my conscious control. The Cartesian will then say that what appears to be the case is the case; the epiphenomenalist will say that what appears to be the case is not the case. Both are answering the same question. Do these mental processes cause the bodily movements which constitute my behavior? The idea of free action emerges if the answer is Yes. The intention that we experience and the movement that follows is the result of our willing to do the action. If the answer is No, then the intention is nothing more than a feeling produced by brain processes that really control the action. My sense of agency is simply a by-product of neural happenings, and it lacks veracity.

The concept of free will, then, commonly gets understood in terms of this question. Does the conscious mental event operate as a cause that moves or directs the body? Is there some kind of direct transformation from conscious willing to moving muscles? Within this Cartesian frame of mind, Carpenter (1874) describes the mental state as closing a physical circuit in the "nerve-force" or as a translation between the psychical and the physical. For the epiphenomenalist, however, there is no interaction, no circuit to be closed, no translation. To say there is, is to say that physical causality is insufficient to explain physical events.

2 Reflective and Perceptual Theories

Within this debate different views of how consciousness relates to action are sometimes cast in terms of a reflective theory of how movements are under conscious control. On this kind of theory consciousness enters into the explanation of action just insofar as my action is controlled by my introspectively reflective choice-making, together with a self-monitoring of movement. The reflective theory, as Naomi Eilan characterizes it, "holds that it is some form of reflection on some aspect of the intention or the action that makes the action conscious" (2003, p. 189), and that puts me in control. That is, attentional consciousness is directed at my inner intention, and at how that intention is translated into bodily movement.[5] Perceptual theories, in contrast, state that "it is some form of consciousness of the environment that makes the action conscious" (ibid.). Eilan specifies this by explaining that perception plays two knowledge-yielding roles in regard to action. First, it delivers knowledge of the environmental objects or events that we target with the action. Second, perceptual feedback provides knowledge of whether the action was properly accomplished (see Eilan 2003, p. 190).

We can clarify the difference between the reflective and perceptual theories by considering a simple case of normal action such as getting a drink. I'm thirsty and decide to get a drink. I get up from my desk and walk to the fridge, open it and reach in for a drink. On the reflective theory, my action originates in (is caused by) my conscious decision to get a drink, and this conscious decision is usually described in terms of becoming aware of my desire for a drink motivated by thirst sensations, having a belief that there is something to drink in the fridge, and then, for just these reasons consciously moving my body in the direction of the drink. This may be an oversimplified version of the story, but it provides a clear indication of the kinds of conscious processes required to effect the action according to this theory. The basic idea is that I initiate and control my action by consciously deciding on what I want, and consciously moving my body to accomplish the goal. Consciousness, on this view, is self-attending or self-monitoring. On the perceptual theory, in contrast, consciousness is primarily directed toward the world. I'm conscious of the thing that I want to get, where I'm moving and what I'm looking for—the fridge, the drink. This perception-for-action is complemented by perceptual feedback—proprioceptive and visual—that tells me that I've accomplished (or failed to accomplish) my goal. Perceptual consciousness seems important for making the action successful, and so plays a necessary and causal role in moving the action along.

The perceptual theory of how consciousness causes behavior, however, fares no better than the reflective theory from the point of view of epiphenomenalism. All the perceptual aspects described above can be causally explained in terms of third-person physical mechanisms. The kind of perceptual information described by the perceptual theory is precisely the kind of perceptual input that is required for motor control. Indeed, most perceptual information of this sort is unconsciously processed, and, according to epiphenomenalism, it is that information processing that is running the show (see e.g., Jeannerod 2003; Pockett, this volume, for a summary of such accounts). It is clear that we can build a non-conscious robot that could retrieve a drink from the fridge, and it is also quite clear that the initial motivation—our thirst—is itself reducible to non-conscious processes that launch the larger action process. Consciousness may keep us informed about what is going on in broad and general terms, it can act as a "dormant monitor" (Jeannerod 2003, p. 162), and so allow us to know what we are doing, but it plays no role in the causal processes that move us. We, as conscious animals, are seemingly just along for the ride.

Differences between reflective and perceptual theories aside, what becomes clear about the way the question gets asked (and, as I will argue, what is problematic about this discourse when it is applied to the issue of free will), is summarized nicely by Joëlle Proust (2003, p. 202): "Standard philosophical approaches [to] action define action in terms of a particular psychological state causing a relevant bodily movement." She indicates that there is "now widespread convergence on this causal approach," even if there is some disagreement about the kind of psychological state involved. The familiar candidates, at least on the reflective approach, are desire and belief (Davidson 1980; Goldman 1970) or intentions (Searle 1983; Mele 1992), providing conceptual reasons for acting. The best arguments for giving causal efficacy to consciousness are posed in these terms, and these terms are precisely the ones rejected by epiphenomenalism. An epiphenomenalist might say that there is no necessary connection between the justification of action and the cause of action, since animals are capable of purposeful actions without having a worked out conceptual understanding of why they acted that way (Proust 2003, pp. 203–204). And we know that even humans who may have well-thought out reasons for acting in a particular way, may in fact be acting in that way due to different and unconscious reasons.

Proust's examination of "minimal" actions (Bach 1978), for example, postural shifts, pre-attentive movements such as the scratching of an itch or avoiding an object in the environment—even cast in terms of Searle's (1983) notion of "intention in action," which specifies the details of how intentions are to be realized, and even if it drops the quest for large or complex psychological states in favor of more perceptual models—retains the focus on causal control of relevant bodily movements. "An intention in action has to do with the routine, unplanned ways of coping with the environment . . . it also accounts for the specific dynamics of the bodily movements through which an action is being performed" (Proust 2003, p. 206). This brings us back to perceptual processes, and, as Proust notes, the difficulty (although not for epiphenomenalists) is that these minimal actions may be fully unconscious. For Proust, "what is pertinent is whether or not the bodily movements tend to be under the agent's guidance. . . . Whatever the causal antecedents of a specific goal-directed movement may be, what makes it an action is the contribution of the corresponding agent to actively maintain the orientation of his bodily effort towards achieving a target event." (p. 207) On this view, as on the "standard philosophical approaches," or on what I have called the common understanding of the question, which includes the epiphenomenal view, the agent performs its action by keeping its body under control. It does this either explicitly for reflective conscious reasons, or in an implicit (pre-reflective) perceptual way, or unconsciously.

In general terms I think that a good understanding of motor control and the performance of action can be worked out in terms of perceptual and non-conscious processes (Gallagher 1995). However, these issues get carried over into questions about whether action is free or not, and more generally into debates about free will, and this is where things start to go wrong.

3 Libetarian Experiments

A good example of how things can go wrong can be found in the debates that surround the experiments conducted by Benjamin Libet (1985; 1992; 1996; Libet et al. 1983). As Libet says, "the operational definition of free will in these experiments was in accord with common views" (1999, p. 47). Libet's experiments show that motor action and the sense of agency depend on neurological events that we do not consciously control, and that happen before our conscious awareness of deciding or moving. In one of Libet's experiments, subjects with their hands on a tabletop are asked to flick their wrists whenever they want to. Their brain activity is monitored, with special attention given to the time course of brain activity leading up to the movement, between 500 milliseconds and 1 second. Just before the flick, there is 50 ms of activity in the motor nerves descending from motor cortex to the wrist. But this is preceded by several hundred (up to 800) ms of brain activity known as the readiness potential (RP). Subjects report when they were first aware of their decision (or urge or intention) to move their wrists by referencing a large clock that allows them to report fractions of a second. On average, 350 ms before they are conscious of deciding (or of having an urge) to move, their brains are already working on the motor processes that will result in the movement. Thus, voluntary acts are "initiated by unconscious cerebral processes before conscious intention appears" (Libet 1985). The brain seemingly decides and then enacts its decisions in a nonconscious fashion, on a subpersonal level, but also inventively tricks us into thinking that we consciously decide matters and that our actions are personal events.

These results motivate a question, which Libet poses in precise terms: "The initiation of the freely voluntary act appears to begin in the brain unconsciously, well before the person consciously knows he wants to act. Is there, then, any role for conscious will in the performance of a voluntary act?" (1999, p. 51). The epiphenomenalist interpretation of these results is that what we call free will is nothing more than a false sense or impression, an illusion (Wegner 2002). Libet himself answers in the positive: Consciousness can have an effect on our action, and free will is possible, because there is still approximately 150 ms remaining after we become conscious of our intent to move, and before we move. So, he suggests, we have time to consciously veto the movement (1985, p. 2003).

Do these experiments actually address the question of free will? Only on the supposition that the question is correctly framed in terms of initiation and control
of bodily movement, which is, as I indicated, the common understanding of the
question. Patrick Haggard, who extends Libet's experiments to demonstrate
the importance of efferent binding, clearly makes this supposition, suggesting that
the experiments reframe the standard philosophical views: "A further consequence
of the efferent binding approach is to reorder the traditional philosophical priorities in this area. The central philosophical question about action has been whether
conscious free will exits. That is, how can 'I' control my body?" (Haggard 2003, p.
113).[6] Although Haggard maintains that the question of free will becomes unim-
portant, he does not attempt to make a clear distinction between the question of
motor control and the question of free will; indeed, for him, apparently, the question of free will is a question about motor control. Rather, his concern is to dismiss
reflective theories of free will and to focus on a more specific aspect of motor
control, namely, in Searle's terms, intention in action rather than prior intention. The
question becomes "*How* does my will or intention become associated with the
actions [i.e., the bodily movements] that it causes?" (ibid.) Will or intention, in
action, is captured, for Haggard, in the milliseconds of physiological signals of the
lateralized readiness potential, which is a more specific part of the RP. Approximately 500 ms prior to the onset of movement, the bilateral RP activity begins to
lateralize to the motor cortex contralateral to the hand that will move. It is this lateralized signal that generates not only the movement, but our awareness of initiating the movement. "This view places consciousness of intention much closer to the
detailed pattern of motor execution than some other accounts. [Awareness of
willing] thus looks rather like intention in action, and much less like prior intention." (ibid., p. 118) Thus, consciousness of an action is "intertwined with the internal models thought to underlie movement control" (119).

The common understanding in the standard reflective, perceptual, or epiphenomenal theories, as well as in the recent debates richly informed by neuroscience,
is that free will is either explained or explained away by what we have learned about
motor control—that is, about how "I" control my body. I propose, however, that
these are two different questions, in the same way that "Shall we go for a ride?" is
different from "How does this car work?" You should think it strange if in response
to your question "Shall we go for a ride today?" I start to tell you in precise terms
how the internal-combustion engine in my car turns the wheels. Developing a good
answer to one of these questions is not the same as answering the other.

The best answers we have to the question of motor control indicate that most
control processes happen at a sub-personal, unconscious level. As we move through
the world we do not normally monitor the specifics of our motor action in any
explicitly conscious way. As I walk out to the beach I am not normally conscious of

how I am activating my leg muscles. The object of my awareness is the beach, the ocean, the anticipated enjoyment of sitting in the sun and reading the latest volume on voluntary action, or perhaps a troubling discussion I've just had with my friend. Body schematic processes that involve proprioception, efference copy, forward comparators, and ecological information keep me moving in the right direction. Both phenomenology and neuropsychology support a combination of perceptual and non-conscious explanations of how we control bodily movements, and they rule out reflective theory in the normal case. That is, in the normal situation, we do not require a second-order representation of the bodily movement; we do not have to be reflectively conscious of the onset of the action or the course of the movement as we execute it. Rather, in moving, input from our perceptual experience of the objects that we target and perceptual-ecological feedback about our bodily performance contribute to motor control. In this context, some of the information required for motor control is consciously generated, as when I decide to reach and grasp this particular object rather than another, or when I have a general idea which way the beach is located. In addition, however, much of the information (for example, the precise visual information that guides the shape of my grasp) is generated non-consciously (Jeannerod 1997, 2003). In regard to these latter aspects, where conscious awareness adds nothing to motor control and may even interfere with the timing or smoothness of action, the epiphenomenalist view is correct.

We should expect that answers to questions about how I control my body or how I make my body move will be of this sort. That most of this control happens non-consciously is for the best. If, as in the case of deafferentation (which involves loss of proprioceptive feedback), we had to control our movement consciously or reflectively (Gallagher and Cole 1995), or if we were normally required to consciously represent our movements in a Cartesian mental space before we effected them in worldly space, we would have to exert great cognitive effort and slow things down to a significant degree.[7] Libet's results, then, are of no surprise unless we think that we control our bodily movements in a conscious and primarily reflective way. The Libetarian experiments are precisely about the control of bodily movement, and even in this regard they are limited insofar as they effect an atypical involution of the question of motor control. In the experimental situation, we are asked to pay attention to all the processes that we normally do *not* attend to, and to move our body in a way that we do not usually move it (in a rough sense, we are asked to act in a way that is similar to the way a deafferented subject is required to act).

These experiments, however, and more generally the broader discussions of motor control, have nothing to tell us about free will per se. If they contribute to a justification of perceptual or epiphenomenal theories of how we control our movement, these are not theories that address the question of free will. The question of free will is a different question.

4   The Question of Free Will

As in the experiments, something similar happens in standard philosophical contexts when philosophers try to find examples of free action. There is a long tradition of appealing to examples of bodily movements in discussions of free will, e.g., "Look how I can freely raise my arm" (Chisholm 1964; Searle 1984; Mohrhoff 1999).[8] Lowe (1999, pp. 235–236) makes the following claim:

> In the case of normal voluntary action, movements of the agent's body have amongst their causes intentional states of that agent which are 'about' just such movements. For instance, when I try to raise my arm and succeed in doing so, my arm goes up—and amongst the causes of its going up are such items as a desire of mine *that my arm should go up*. The intentional causes of physical events are always 'directed' upon the occurrence of just such events, at least where normal voluntary action is concerned.

Zhu, who characterizes free will as "a mediating executive mental process, which somehow puts the bodily parts into action," thinks of motor control as the "prototype" of free action (2003, p. 64). Such philosophical reflections, often cast in terms of interactionism (mind-body or mind-brain) and specifically framed by the mind-body problem, may be what send the neuroscientists looking for free will in the wrong place—namely, in the realm of motor control processes, which generally turn out to be subpersonal processes.[9]

The attempt to frame the question of free will in terms of these subpersonal, motor control processes—either to dismiss it or to save it—is misguided for at least two reasons. First, free will cannot be squeezed into time frames of 150–350 ms; free will is a longer-term phenomenon, is too slow for normal motor control, and, I will argue, depends on consciousness. Second, the notion of free will does not apply primarily to abstract motor processes or even to bodily movements that make up intentional actions; rather, it applies to intentional actions themselves, described at the highest pragmatic level of description. I have offered a clarification of these points in other places (Gallagher 2005; Gazzaniga and Gallagher 1998). Here I will provide a summary with the help of an example.

First, in regard to time frame, the kinds of processes associated with free actions are not made at the spur of the moment—they are not momentary, and they cannot fit within the thin phenomenology of the milliseconds between RP and movement. The following example reflects the distinction between fast movement under automatic control and slower voluntary action. Let me note, however, that automatic movement is not the opposite of voluntary movement. Fast automatic movement may be purely reflex, or it may be voluntary in the sense that it may fit into and serve an intentional action.

At time T something moves in the grass next to my feet. At $T + 150$ ms the amygdala in my brain is activated, and before I know why, at $T + 200$ ms, I jump and move several yards away. Here, the entire set of movements can be explained purely in terms of non-conscious perceptual processes, neurons firing and muscles contracting, together with an evolutionary account of why our system is designed in this way. My behavior, of course, motivates my awareness of what is happening, and by $T + 1,000$ ms I see that what moved in the grass was a small harmless lizard. My next move is not of the same sort. At $T + 5,000$ ms, after observing the kind of lizard it is, I decide to catch it for my lizard collection. At $T + 5,150$ ms I take a step back and *voluntarily* make a quick reach for the lizard.

My choice to catch the lizard is quite different from the reflex behavior. What goes into this decision involves awareness of what has just happened (I would not have decided to catch the lizard if I had not become conscious that there was a lizard there) and recognition of the lizard as something I could appreciate. At $T + 5,150$ ms I take a step back and reach for it. One could focus on this movement and say that at $T + 4,650$ ms, without my awareness, processes in my brain were already underway to prepare for my reaching action, before I had even decided to catch the lizard—therefore, what seemed to be my free decision was actually predetermined by my brain. But this ignores the context defined by the larger time frame, which involves previous movement and a conscious recognition of the lizard. Furthermore, it could easily happen that things don't go as fast as I have portrayed, and perhaps, waiting for the strategic moment, I don't actually reach for the lizard until 10 seconds after I made the decision that it would be a good addition to my collection. Now Libet and some philosophers might insist that an extra decision would have to be made to initiate my bodily movement precisely at that time. But it is clear that any such decision about moving is already under the influence of the initial conscious decision to catch the lizard. Although I do not deny that the bodily movement is intimately connected with my action, my action is not well described in terms of making bodily movements, but rather in terms of attempting to catch the lizard for my collection, and this is spread out over a larger time frame than the experimental framework of milliseconds.

This leads to the second point, which concerns the proper level of description relevant to free will. As I have been suggesting, and in contrast to the common understanding, the question of free will is not about bodily movements but about intentional actions. The kinds of actions that we freely decide are not the kinds of involuted bodily movements described by Libet's experiments. If I am reaching to catch the lizard and you stop and ask what I am doing, I am very unlikely to say any of the following: "I am activating my neurons." "I am flexing my muscles." "I am moving my arm." "I am reaching and grasping." These are descriptions appropriate for a discussion of motor control and bodily movement, but not for the action in which I am engaged. Rather, I would probably say "I am trying to catch this lizard for my collection." And this is a good description of what I freely decided to do.

I suggest that the temporal framework for the exercise of free will is, at a minimum, the temporal framework that allows for the process to be informed by a conscious reflection of a certain type. This conscious reflection is not of the sort described by the reflective theory. According to that theory, my reflective regard would be focused on my beliefs and desires and on how to move my body in order to achieve a goal. But when I am reaching for the lizard I am not at all thinking about either my mental states or how to move my body—if I'm thinking about anything, I'm thinking about catching the lizard. My decision to catch the lizard is the result of a conscious reflection that is *embedded* or *situated* in the particular context that is defined by the present circumstance of encountering the lizard and by the fact that I have a lizard collection. This embedded or situated reflection is neither introspective nor focused on my body. As described by Gallagher and Marcel (1999, p. 25), it is "a first-person reflective consciousness that is embedded in a pragmatically or socially contextualized situation" that "involves the type of activity that I engage in when someone asks me what I am doing or what I plan to do." In such reflection I do not make consciousness the direct introspective object of my reflection; I do not reflect on my beliefs and desires as states within a mental space; nor do I reflectively consider how I ought to move my arm or shape my grasp. Rather, I start to think matters through in terms of the object to which I am attending (the lizard), the collection I have, and the actions I can take (leave it or catch it). When I decide to catch the lizard, I make what, in contrast to a reflex action, must be described as a conscious free choice, and this choice shapes my actions.[10]

In conscious deliberation of the sort found in situated reflection, certain things in the environment begin to matter to the agent. Meaning and interpretation come into the picture. The conscious deliberation of the agent, which involves memory and knowledge about lizards and such things, is not epiphenomenal; it has a real effect on behavior. Why I reach to catch the lizard would be inexplicable without recourse to this kind of situated reflection. Some epiphenomenalists might object that this relegates the explanation to a "space of reasons" rather than a "space of causes," and at best explains the motivation, but not the cause of the action (cf. McDowell 1996). My reflective decision to catch the lizard does not *cause* me to try to do so. But this narrow definition of causality begs the question and limits the notion of causality to the determined mechanics of motor control. That is, as I am suggesting, it frames the question of free will in precisely the wrong way. If the notion of causality at stake in this debate is narrowly construed on the traditional billiard hall model of determined mechanisms, then the question of free will is not about causality at all. Yet it seems to me undeniable that the embedded reflection described here does have an effect on my action, and must play a role in the explanation of how (and not just why) that action is generated.

To the extent that consciousness enters into the ongoing production of action, and contributes to the production of further action, even if significant aspects of this action rely on automatic non-conscious motor control, our actions are voluntary. Voluntary actions are not about neurons, muscles, body parts, or even movement— each of which plays some part in what is happening, and for the most part non-consciously. Rather, all such processes are carried along by (and are intentional because of) my conscious decision to catch the lizard—that is, by what is best described on a personal level as my intentional action. The exercise of free will cannot be captured in a description of neural activity or of muscle activation or of bodily movement.

In contrast to the position I have just outlined, Daniel Dennett (2003) suggests that the processes that constitute free will need not be conscious and need not depend on conscious decision. Indeed, he considers it Cartesian to suggest that consciousness is necessary for free will (Dennett 2003, p. 242, n. 3). The notion of a situated reflection, however, is not at all Cartesian, nor is it opposed to a properly conceived epiphenomenalism. The truth of epiphenomenalism is narrowly circumscribed. It pertains to some of the specifics of motor control. When epiphenomenalist claims are made in regard to the question of free will, however, it's a different matter, as I have tried to show in this chapter.

I am not arguing here for a disembodied notion of free will, as something that occurs in a Cartesian mind, nor do I mean to imply that the non-conscious brain events that make up the elements of motor control are simply irrelevant to free will. Indeed, for two closely related reasons, such non-conscious embodied processes, including the kind of neurological events described by Libet, are essential to a free will that is specifically human. First, as I have suggested elsewhere (Gallagher 2005), non-conscious body-schematic mechanisms of motor control support intentional action and are structured and regulated by relevant intentional goals. Following Anscombe (1957), I would argue that these levels of operation are intentional, even if they are not intentional actions. All such relevant processes are structured and regulated by my intentional goals; they also limit and enable my action. When I decide to reach for the lizard, all the appropriate physical movements fall into place without my willing them to do so. These embodied mechanisms thus enable the exercise of free will. Second, precisely to the extent that we are not required to consciously deliberate about bodily movement or such things as autonomic processes, our deliberation can be directed at the more meaningful level of intentional action. Our possibilities for action are diminished to the extent that these supporting mechanisms fail. Nonetheless, proposals to answer the question of free will in terms of mind-body or mind-brain interaction are looking in the wrong place. The relevant interaction to consider is the interaction between a situated mind-body system and its physical-social environment, a level of interaction found in the collecting of lizards, the helping of friends, and in the variety of deliberate actions that we engage in everyday.

Thus, the exercise of free will should not be conceived as equivalent to those processes that contribute to motor control, or to something that is generated at a *purely* subpersonal level, or to something instantaneous, an event that takes place in a knife-edge moment located between being undecided and being decided. Free will involves temporally extended deliberative consciousness that is best described as a situated reflection. This doesn't mean that freely willed action is something that occurs in the head—whether that is conceived, following a long philosophical tradition, as in a mental space, or following a more recent neuroscientific conception, as in the brain. Nor is it accomplished in a mindless way. Freely willed action is something accomplished in the world, in situations that motivate embedded reflection, and among the things that I reach for and the people that I affect.

Notes

1. The idea that even if the animal were conscious nothing would be added to the production of behavior, even in animals of the human type, was first voiced by La Mettrie (1745), and then by Cabanis (1802), and was further explicated by Hodgson (1870) and Huxley (1874).

2. I will outline what I call the "common understanding" of this question below. By this I mean an understanding (or misunderstanding) that is found among many philosophers and scientists.

3. The roots of this modern idea go back at least as far as the Stoics. They helped to relocate certain important aspects of action. For Aristotle and other Ancient Greek thinkers, morally significant action was something that happened publicly, in the world, as a display of moral character (Arendt 1958). In Stoic philosophy, the better parts of action are moved into the interior of the person. It no longer matters whether the external expression of action is even possible—and it can be made impossible by the constraints of the situation (for example, being chained up in prison). What matters is the integrity and intentions of one's interior life; what one does, one does primarily within the space of one's own mental realm. As we find this thought developed in Augustine (395), one will be judged not simply by external behavior, but by one's internal intentions, which define the significance of one's actions. As is well known, Descartes' concept of the mind as an interior mental space in which the exercise of will means affirming or denying ideas, derives from this tradition. For Descartes it is difficult to speak of the freedom of mixed or composite actions, i.e., those involving mental states (volitions) followed by bodily movement (Gaukroger 1997; Chappell 1994).

4. "Now the action of the soul consists entirely in this, that simply by willing it makes the small [pineal] gland to which it is closely united move in the way requisite for producing the effect aimed at in the volition. . . . When we will to walk or to move the body in any manner, this volition causes the gland to impel the spirits toward the muscles which bring about this effect." (Descartes 1649, §§ xli, xliii) Concerning the will, Descartes also writes: "Our volitions, in turn, are also of two kinds. Some actions of the soul terminate in the soul itself, as when we will to love God, or in general apply our thought to some nonmaterial object. Our other actions terminate in our body, as when from our merely willing to walk, it follows that our legs are moved and that we walk." (1649, § xviii)

5. A recent example of this view can be found in Metzinger (2003: 422), explicated in Metzinger's own specialized terminology: "Conscious volition is generated by integrating abstract goal representations or concrete self-simulations into the current model of the phenomenal intentionality relations as object components, in a process of decision or selection." The self-simulation, which forms the object component of this process, is in fact a conscious "opaque simulation" of "a possible motor pattern" (ibid., p. 423), i.e., a possible movement of my own body. An opaque simulation is one of which we are explicitly conscious. "A *volitional first-person* perspective—the phenomenal experience of practical

intentionality—emerges if two conditions are satisfied. First, the object component must be constituted by a particular self-simulatum, by a mental simulation of a concrete behavioral pattern, for example, like getting up and walking toward the refrigerator. Second, the relationship depicted on the level of conscious experience is one of *currently selecting* this particular behavioral pattern, as simulated."

6. Haggard and Libet (2001, p. 47) frame the question in the same way, referring to it as the traditional concept of free will: "How can a mental state (my conscious intention) initiate the neural events in the motor areas of the brain that lead to my body movement?"

7. Jeannerod (2003: 159) notes: "The shift from automatic to [consciously monitored] controlled execution involves a change in the kinematics of the whole [grasping] movement; movement time increases, maximum grip aperture is larger, and the general accuracy degrades." See also Gallagher 2005.

8. Even Aristotle offers this example: "An agent acts voluntarily because the initiative in moving the parts of the body which act as instruments rests with the agent himself." (*Nicomachean Ethics* 1110a15)

9. I am reminded here of the airplane crash that occurred because the entire cockpit crew had focused their attention on a malfunctioning signal light in an attempt to fix it, but had lost track of the fact that the plane was losing altitude. They were clearly looking in the wrong place and at the wrong problem.

10. I think this view is consistent with the general sense of Josef Perner's (2003) "dual control" theory of action, setting aside his requirement for a higher-order-thought (HOT) account of consciousness. Embedded reflection need not be at a higher level, and the problem that Perner attempts to solve with the HOT theory can be addressed by the phenomenological notion of pre-reflective self-consciousness (Gallagher and Zahavi 2005). Perner's theory is helped along by Searle's widely cited distinction between prior intention and intention-in-action. The notion of embedded reflection does not have to be a matter of prior intention, but neither is it reducible to intention-in-action (if that is understood in terms of motor control, as in perceptual theory). Situated reflection contributes to the formation of what Pacherie (this volume) calls "present-directed intention," which initiates and sustains the action and which is distinct from motor intentions and from future-directed intentions.

References

Anscombe, G. E. M. 1957. *Intention*. Blackwell.

Arendt, H. 1958. *The Human Condition*. University of Chicago Press.

Augustine. 395. *De libero arbitrio voluntatis*. English translation: *On the Free Choice of the Will* (Hackett, 1993).

Bach, K. 1978. A representational theory of action. *Philosophical Studies* 34: 361–379.

Cabanis, P. 1802. *Rapports du physique et du moral de l'homme*. Crapart, Caille et Ravier.

Carpenter, W. B. 1874. *Principles of Mental Physiology, with their Applications to the Training and Discipline of the Mind, and the Study of its Morbid Conditions*. Henry S. King.

Chappell, V. 1994. Descartes's compatibilism. In *Reason, Will, and Sensation: Studies in Descartes's Metaphysics*, ed. J. Cottingham. Oxford University Press.

Chisholm, R. 1964. Human Freedom and the Self. Reprinted in *Reason and Responsibility: Readings in Some Basic Problems of Philosophy*, eleventh edition, ed. J. Feinberg and R. Shafer-Landau (Wadsworth, 2002).

Davidson, D. 1980. *Essays on Actions and Events*. Clarendon.

Dennett, D. 2003. *Freedom Evolves*. Viking.

Descartes, R. 1649. *The Passions of the Soul* (Hackett, 1989).

Eilan, N. 2003. The explanatory role of consciousness in action. In *Voluntary Action: Brains, Minds, and Society*, ed. S. Maasen et al. Oxford University Press.

Gallagher, S. 2005. *How the Body Shapes the Mind*. Oxford University Press.

Gallagher, S. 1995. Body schema and intentionality. In *The Body and the Self*, ed. J. Bermúdez et al. MIT Press.

Gallagher, S., and Cole, J. 1995. Body schema and body image in a deafferented subject. *Journal of Mind and Behavior* 16: 369–390.

Gallagher, S., and Marcel, A. J. 1999. The self in contextualized action. *Journal of Consciousness Studies* 6, no. 4: 4–30.

Gallagher, S., and Zahavi, D. 2005. Phenomenological approaches to self-consciousness. In *Stanford Encyclopedia of Philosophy*.

Gaukroger, S. 1997. *Descartes: An Intellectual Biography*. Clarendon.

Gazzaniga, M., and Gallagher, S. 1998. A neuronal Platonist: An interview with Michael Gazzaniga. *Journal of Consciousness Studies* 5: 706–717.

Goldman, A. 1970. *A Theory of Human Action*. Prentice-Hall.

Haggard, P. 2003. Conscious awareness of intention and of action. In *Agency and Self-Awareness*, ed. N. Eilan and J. Roessler. Clarendon.

Haggard, P., and Libet, B. 2000. Conscious intention and brain activity. *Journal of Consciousness Studies* 8, no. 11: 47–63.

Hodgson, S. 1870. *The Theory of Practice*. Longmans, Green, Reader, and Dyer.

Huxley, T. H. 1874. On the hypothesis that animals are automata, and its history. *Fortnightly Review*, n.s. 16: 555–580.

James, W. 1890. *Principles of Psychology*. Dover.

Jeannerod, M. 1997. *The Cognitive Neuroscience of Action*. Blackwell.

Jeannerod, M. 2003. Self-generated actions. In *Voluntary Action: Brains, Minds, and Sociality*, ed. S. Maasen et al. Oxford University Press.

La Mettrie, J. O. de. 1745. *Histoire naturelle de l'ame*. Jean Neaulme.

Libet, B. 1985. Unconscious cerebral initiative and the role of conscious will in voluntary action. *Behavioral and Brain Sciences* 8: 529–566.

Libet, B. 1992. The neural time-factor in perception, volition, and free will. *Revue de Métaphysique et de Morale* 2: 255–272.

Libet, B. 1996. Neural time factors in conscious and unconscious mental functions. In *Toward a Science of Consciousness: The First Tucson Discussions and Debates*, ed. S. Hameroff et al. MIT Press.

Libet, B. 1999. Do we have free will? *Journal of Consciousness Studies* 6, no. 8–9: 47–57.

Libet, B. 2003. Can conscious experience affect brain activity? *Journal of Consciousness Studies* 10, no. 12: 24–28.

Libet, B., Gleason, C. A., Wright, E. W., and Perl, D. K. 1983. Time of conscious intention to act in relation to cerebral activities (readiness potential): The unconscious initiation of a freely voluntary act. *Brain* 106: 623–642.

Lowe, E. J. 1999. Self, agency and mental causation. *Journal of Consciousness Studies* 6, no. 8–9: 225–239.

McDowell, J. 1996. *Mind and World*. Harvard University Press.

Mele, A. R. 1992. *Springs of Action*. Oxford University Press.

Metzinger, T. 2003. *Being No One: The Self-Model Theory of Subjectivity*. MIT Press.

Mohrhoff, U. 1999. The physics of interactionism. *Journal of Consciousness Studies* 6, no. 8–9: 165–184.

Perner, J. 2003. Dual control and the causal theory of action: The case of non-intentional action. In *Agency and Self-Awareness*, ed. N. Eilan and J. Roessler. Clarendon.

Proust, J. 2003. How voluntary are minimal actions? In *Voluntary Action: Brains, Minds, and Sociality*, ed. S. Maasen et al. Oxford University Press.

Searle, J. 1983. *Intentionality: An Essay in the Philosophy of Mind*. Cambridge University Press.

Searle, J. 1984. *Minds, Brains, and Science*. Harvard University Press.

Velmans, M. 2002. How could conscious experiences affect brains? *Journal of Consciousness Studies* 9, no. 11: 3–29.

Velmans, M. 2003. Preconscious free will. *Journal of Consciousness Studies* 10 no. 12: 42–61.

Wegner, D. 2002. *The Illusion of Conscious Will*. MIT Press.

Wegner, D., and Wheatley, T. 1999. Apparent mental causation—sources of experience of will. *American Psychology* 54: 480–492.

Williams, B. 1995. *Making Sense of Humanity*. Cambridge University Press.

Zhu, J. 2003. Reclaiming volition: An alternative interpretation of Libet's experiments. *Journal of Consciousness Studies* 10, no. 11: 61–77.

7 Empirical Constraints on the Problem of Free Will

Peter W. Ross

With the success of cognitive science's interdisciplinary approach to studying the mind, many theorists have taken up the strategy of appealing to science to address long-standing disputes about metaphysics and the mind. For example, in the 1980s C. L. Hardin's *Color for Philosophers* introduced perceptual psychology into the discussion of the metaphysics of color. Psychological research, Hardin showed, can provide constraints for the philosophical debate, ruling out certain positions on the nature of color. To provide an example of such a constraint, psychophysics shows that for any determinate color, physical objects in the same viewing condition may differ in indefinitely many ways with respect to their spectrally relevant physical properties, and nevertheless look precisely that color. Neurophysiology explains how such physically distinct objects, called metamers, can occur. These scientific findings now provide constraints on philosophical accounts of color—anyone writing on the philosophy of color must acknowledge these scientific findings, which rule out, for instance, the proposal that colors are properties of physical objects which are physical natural kinds.[1]

Recently, philosophers and psychologists have also begun to explore how science can be brought to bear on the debate about the problem of free will. Prominent examples have been Robert Kane's (1996, 1999) attempt to shore up libertarianism through an appeal to physics and neuroscience, Daniel Dennett's (2003) account of compatibilist freedom in evolutionary terms, and Daniel Wegner's (2002) psychological model of our experience of mental causation.

I take the problem of free will to be the problem of whether we control our actions.[2] (The problem of free will is best stated in terms of the first-person point of view. But in stating the problem this way I don't mean to endorse a necessary connection between consciousness and control, or to prejudge any theoretical positions at all.) Science has traditionally been central to the problem, for one standard way of viewing it is through considering whether we can fit ourselves as free agents into the natural world characterized by science. If our actions are brought about by a combination of genetic and environmental factors, we can fit ourselves into the natural world. But in that case, since we ultimately control neither our genes nor our environments,[3] it seems that we don't control our actions. The standard responses are that our actions are in fact brought about by genetic and environmental factors and this rules out control (hard determinism); that our actions are so brought about but nevertheless this doesn't rule out control (compatibilism); and that the bringing about of our actions involves a third factor, namely causal indeterminacy, which is necessary and in certain contexts sufficient for control (libertarianism).

Despite the centrality of science to the problem of free will, even Kane, Dennett, and Wegner do not consider the general question of how scientific research can provide constraints that serve to rule out certain positions on the problem; their use of empirical findings is tailored to support specific philosophical or psychological proposals. I will attempt to clarify the debate by taking up the general question of empirical constraints.

The debate can be viewed according to two basic dimensions: a dimension opposing compatibilism and incompatibilism, where the disagreement is about whether the bringing about of our actions by genetics and environment is compatible with control, and a dimension opposing indeterminism and determinism, where the dispute is about whether causal indeterminacy can ever be sufficient for control. I will argue that empirical findings don't apply at all to the dispute between compatibilism and incompatibilism. However, I will show that empirical research can provide constraints in connection with the other fundamental dimension, namely the dispute between libertarianism, which claims that causal indeterminacy is in certain contexts sufficient for controlling our actions, and the other positions, which deny this sufficiency claim. I will argue that psychological research into the accuracy of introspection has the potential to decide the truth of naturalized libertarianism, and thus that this research provides the source of the most powerful constraint, that is, the constraint that rules out the broadest category of positions.

1   Compatibilism versus Incompatibilism: A Semantic Debate

One of the fundamental issues associated with the problem of free will is whether the bringing about of our actions by genetic and environmental factors rules out control. A strong intuition supports the incompatibilist claim, embraced by hard determinists and libertarians, that it does. The intuition is that, despite our ordinary thought that we control least some of our actions, if our actions in fact are produced by genetics and environment—factors ultimately outside of our control—then this ordinary thought is mistaken.

But of course a strong intuition also supports the ordinary thought that we control at least some of our actions. The compatibilist accepts that our actions are brought about by genetics and environment and nevertheless attempts to hold on to the intuition of control. Consequently, the compatibilist seeks to counter the incompatibilist intuition by having us consider what we really mean by "control." If we mean *self-formation*, where some of our goal-directed states become causally efficacious in producing action in a way that is not the result of genetics and environment alone but is also the result of a third necessary factor (indeterminacy), then we don't have control in that sense.[4] But, compatibilists argue, why think that by "control" we mean self-formation?

As an alternative, compatibilists give a variety of sophisticated accounts of the psychological complexity that allows us to take a standpoint from which—they contend—it makes sense to say that we control our actions despite their being brought about by genetics and environment. So, for example, Harry Frankfurt (1971) claims that free will is a matter of taking a standpoint from which we reflectively want certain desires to be effective in producing action and acting on those desires (rather than on desires which we reflectively don't want to be effective). Thus we control our actions in the sense that we take a reflective standpoint from which we choose our effective desires. Dennett's recent account also characterizes a reflective standpoint from which we choose our effective desires, a standpoint from which our choice is "rational, self-controlled, and not wildly misinformed" (2003, p. 284). In addition, Dennett attempts to explain the development of the standpoint so characterized in evolutionary terms.

Yet no matter how sophisticated and persuasive an account of a reflective standpoint may be, the incompatibilist contends that its perspective on desire and action produces mere illusion. We have the psychological complexity enabling us to take a standpoint from which it *seems* to make sense to say that we control our actions. But, the incompatibilist insists, if our actions are brought about genetics and environment—a point to which the compatibilist is committed—then they are out of our control.[5]

The debate between these positions amounts to whether we should accept that "control" means self-formation—which takes indeterminacy as a necessary factor—or that it has a meaning consistent with the bringing about of our actions by genetics and environment alone. But nothing is at stake here except what we mean by "control."

Although the debate between compatibilism and incompatibilism is semantic, it is not trivial. Both the compatibilist meaning of "control" and the incompatibilist meaning have intuitive pull. Yet the question of which of these meanings is fundamental is not one that we can address through the empirical sciences. (It is interesting to consider whether this debate could be settled at all, and if so, how. In view of my limited purposes here, I will set these questions aside.)

To illustrate the point that the empirical sciences can't address which meaning of "control" is fundamental, consider that the issue dividing compatibilists and hard determinists is merely incompatibilism (the issue of whether the bringing about of our actions by genetics and environment is compatible with control) and not any aspect of a scientific description of the world. Rather than disagree about a scientific description of the world, they disagree about how a scientific description of the world relates to our normative terms.

While the hard determinist understands an interrelated set of normative terms on the basis of self-formation, the compatibilist understands a homophonic set on the basis of a meaning of control without self-formation. As a result, they often talk past each other. However, because a hard determinist can accept that there is an ersatz control (that is, control without self-formation) from which we can derive similarly ersatz but nevertheless useful justification for punishment, this theorist is in a position to accept both sets of terms.[6] As far as a hard determinist is concerned, compatibilism is correct in its account of ersatz control. Thus, a hard determinist can accept a compatibilist sense of "control" as practically indispensable, but retain a distinct sense of "control" which requires self-formation (and thus, by the hard determinist's lights is non-ersatz or genuine control); and, likewise, accept a compatibilist sense of "punishment" as justified in terms of its practical indispensability, but retain a distinct sense of "punishment" the justification of which requires self-formation (and thus, by the hard determinist's lights is genuine punishment); and so on.

Because these views do not differ on any aspect of a scientific description of the world with regard to ersatz control, and because they agree that we can't achieve self-formation, they don't differ on any aspect of a scientific description of the world at all. But then there is no way to address their dispute through the empirical sciences. Given any amount of empirical research, the compatibilist and the hard determinist will remain divided, flaunting different meanings of "control."[7]

Moreover, suggestions that compatibilists can refute hard determinism on non-semantic grounds are misguided, building more into hard determinism than an adherent of this view needs to accept. For instance, although Skinner's influential version of hard determinism was combined with a crude behaviorism, and the success of cognitive science has shown the empirical inadequacy of this behaviorism, hard determinism doesn't rely on Skinnerian behaviorism. Hard determinism merely claims that our actions are brought about by genetics and environment, and that this rules out control.

However, setting aside the dispute between hard determinism and compatibilism, whether libertarianism provides a tenable alternative is not a semantic issue. Libertarians are incompatibilists. But libertarians claim more than that what is meant by "control" is self-formation. They also contend that at least sometimes we *achieve* self-formation, and thus that the conditions sufficient for self-formation exist. It is at this point that empirical research becomes relevant, at least if the metaphysics of self-formation is *naturalistic*, that is, scientifically tractable.

Thus, empirical findings apply only to the dimension of the debate pitting libertarianism, which claims that indeterminacy is in certain contexts sufficient for control, against the other positions, which deny this. In what follows, I will consider how scientific research can provide constraints for the debate between naturalized libertarianism and the so-called determinist views.

2 Quantum Indeterminacy: At Best a Weak Constraint

The general area of the problem of free will is, of course, standardly characterized as a problem having to do with determinism. And determinism, which claims that at any point in time there is only one physically possible future and thus rules out causal indeterminacy, is an empirical claim. However, framing the debate in terms of determinism is a vestige of outmoded Newtonian science. By now the standard interpretation of quantum mechanics holds that determinism is false. But current versions of the so-called determinist views, hard determinism and compatibilism, don't reject quantum indeterminacy. Instead, "determinism" has in effect become a label for the idea that there is no context in which any indeterminacy that does exist is sufficient for control.[8] Thus the discovery of quantum indeterminacy has not had the impact of refuting the so-called determinist views.

Ironically, it is the naturalized libertarians, more so than the so-called determinists, who are vulnerable to the question of the existence of quantum indeterminacy. For while most who write on free will—including most so-called determinists—accept the standard interpretation of quantum mechanics, this interpretation might be false and the behavior of subatomic particles might be deterministic. If this were so, it would seem to be grounds for rejecting naturalized libertarianism since it would eliminate what seems to be the only indeterminacy purported to be scientifically acceptable.

Nevertheless, this appearance is deceiving. If the standard interpretation of quantum mechanics is false, this would be grounds to reject certain versions of naturalized libertarianism. But it would not affect all versions. For example, it would not affect Timothy O'Connor's version of naturalized libertarianism (discussed below), which doesn't appeal to quantum indeterminacy. Thus, the falsity of the standard interpretation of quantum mechanics would provide only a weak constraint, ruling out only a narrow range of views.

Yet, if the standard interpretation is correct, perhaps empirical considerations can establish a naturalized libertarianism which appeals to quantum indeterminacy.

Kane offers this strategy, attempting to turn the question of libertarian freedom into one for physics and neuroscience.

I will argue, however, that Kane's strategy fails. In fact, resolving the question of the standard interpretation does little to further the free will debate. If the standard interpretation is correct, the question remains whether it makes sense to think that quantum indeterminacy is sometimes sufficient for controlling our actions. If it is false, its falsity provides only a weak constraint.

Kane's Naturalized Libertarianism: Trying to Make Quantum Indeterminacy Matter

Traditionally, libertarianism has rejected the attempt to fit ourselves as free agents into the natural world characterized by science.[9] Over the past three decades, however, Robert Kane has developed libertarianism in new ways, striving to naturalize it (1996, pp. 17, 115–117; 1999, p. 163). Kane's hope is to lead us out of the mystery of older libertarian views, and he uses the strategy of rendering libertarianism scientifically innocuous as a measure of having done this. However, as Kane recognizes, a naturalized libertarianism continues to face the serious challenge of addressing how libertarian freedom, in holding that indeterminacy is sometimes sufficient for control, makes sense at all. Kane calls the issue of making sense of libertarian freedom the Intelligibility Question (1996, p. 13).

It is crucial to libertarianism that it doesn't hold that just any indeterminacy is sufficient for control. This claim would render libertarian freedom rather blatantly unintelligible. Instead, the libertarian claims that indeterminacy *in a certain context* is sufficient for control. The traditional libertarianism filled out the context (to the extent that this was possible) in terms of a scientifically intractable agent. Naturalizing libertarianism amounts to offering a naturalistic context. And the fundamental problem for naturalized libertarianism is whether it makes sense to think that there is a naturalistic context in which indeterminacy is sufficient for control.

Kane spells out the naturalistic context in terms of locating quantum indeterminacy at a particular point in deliberation involving a conflict of values (such as egoistic and altruistic values). When distinct values support different courses of action in a situation, and a conflict ensues where each course of action is supported by a set of reasons, Kane claims that there is "a kind of stirring up of chaos in the brain that makes it sensitive to the micro-indeterminacies at the neuronal level" (1999, p. 164). His idea is that being torn due to such conflicts creates chaotic conditions which amplify quantum indeterminacy so that its effects percolate up, that is, are manifested at the level of individual neurons, and then at the level of neural networks (1996, pp. 128–130). Kane claims that moral conflicts "create tensions that are

reflected in appropriate regions of the brain by movement further from thermody-
namic equilibrium, which increases the sensitivity to micro indeterminacies at the
neuronal level and magnifies the indeterminacies throughout the complex macro
process which, taken as a whole, is the agent's effort of will" (ibid., p. 130). Thus,
Kane's view isn't that moral conflicts create quantum indeterminacies, but rather
that they create the conditions in which quantum indeterminacies can be amplified
and manifested in our deliberative processes.[10]

In particular, this amplification of the effects of quantum indeterminacy makes
the outcome of our deliberation indeterminate, since it occurs in the physical basis
of the interaction among neurally realized goal-directed states which express our
values.[11] In addition, the feeling that in such cases branching paths are metaphysically open is a neural sensitivity to these amplified effects of quantum indeterminacy (1996, pp. 130, 132–133; 1999, p. 164). But even though the outcome of
deliberation in such cases is indeterminate, it is backed by reasons—since each of
the competing courses of action is. Kane's proposal is that the felt indeterminacy
and reasons backing of deliberative outcomes is necessary and sufficient for control
(1996, pp. 133–135, 141; 1999, pp. 174–176).

The proposal is sketchy and highly speculative. Yet, if Kane successfully addresses
the Intelligibility Question, he has converted the issue of libertarian freedom into
the empirical question of whether the effects of quantum indeterminacy are manifested in neural processes. If chaotic amplification of the effects of quantum indeterminacy were discovered, then, it seems, libertarianism would receive strong
empirical support.

Kane's strategy of naturalizing libertarianism has the effect of focusing our attention on empirical possibilities. Considering the naturalized libertarian's reconcilia-
tion of incompatibilism, freedom, and science, this position is attractive. And due to
the empirical possibilities and the position's attractiveness, one might be hopeful
that Kane's attempt to disarm the Intelligibility Question succeeds.

I will argue, however, that, despite Kane's ingenious strategy, his attempt to
disarm the Intelligibility Question and transform the question of libertarianism into
one for physics and neuroscience fails. Kane tries to reconcile the arbitrariness of
indeterminacy with libertarian freedom as follows:

An ultimate arbitrariness remains in all undetermined SFAs [self-forming actions] because
there cannot in principle be sufficient or overriding *prior* reasons for making one set of competing reasons prevail over the other. . . . The absence of an explanation of the difference in
choice in terms of prior reasons does not have the tight connection to issues of responsibility one might initially credit it with. . . . None of [the conditions necessary and sufficient for
responsibility] is precluded by the absence of an explanation of the difference in choice in
terms of prior reasons. (1999, pp. 176–177)

Having our attention distracted by the empirical possibilities, Kane's attempt may seem an adequate answer to the worry about the arbitrariness of indeterminacy which the Intelligibility Question poses. But, at best, Kane shows that indeterminacy is *consistent* with responsibility and, consequently, with the control necessary for responsibility. Thus, he claims, indeterminacy doesn't *preclude* control.[12]

Yet this approach is vulnerable to the following objection. (This objection was raised by Galen Strawson (1986, chapter 2).) Strawson, however, takes as his target libertarianism in general as opposed to just Kane's variety, and Strawson's overall aim is to show that libertarian freedom is incoherent whereas my aim is much more modest—it is merely to show that Kane's argument rests on a prior question with respect to introspective evidence.) The libertarian must render intelligible the idea that there is a context for indeterminacy where it is *sufficient* for control, not just one where it is consistent with control. Kane's approach involves enriching this context through the inclusion of the reasons backing of deliberative outcomes. But the question then becomes whether this inclusion allows us to understand Kane's claim of sufficiency by smuggling in the satisfaction of compatibilist sufficient conditions for control while pointing to an indeterminacy which, irrelevant to sufficiency for control, merely plays the role of satisfying the incompatibilist intuition that indeterminacy is necessary for control.

To make sense of libertarian freedom, and to free libertarianism of the charge that it is (in Galen Strawson's phrase) "a covert compatibilism with an idle incompatibilist premise danglingly subjoined" (1986, p. 32), Kane needs to demonstrate that the context for indeterminacy can be enriched in such a way that it is clear that indeterminacy has a role to play in sufficiency for control.

As a result, even if chaotic amplification of indeterminacy were found, the question would remain as to whether we can make sense of naturalized libertarian freedom. Alternatively, as I will discuss below, even if chaotic amplification of quantum indeterminacy were *not* found, the question would remain as to whether a naturalized libertarianism is true. Consequently, physical and neurophysiological research into chaotic amplification of quantum indeterminacy would provide only a weak constraint.

Resolving the question of quantum indeterminacy, either with regard to the correctness of the standard interpretation of quantum mechanics or with regard to chaotic amplification, does little to further the debate. If chaotic amplification of quantum indeterminacy exists, the question remains whether it makes sense to think that there is a context in which quantum indeterminacy is sufficient for control. If it doesn't exist, its absence provides only a weak constraint.

Kane's Appeal to Introspection

However, Kane suggests that enriching the context for indeterminacy must also include the first-person perspective:

... when described from a physical perspective alone, *free will looks like chance*. But the physical description is not the only one to be considered. ... the undetermined outcome of the process, [whether it is settled] one way or the other, is, experientially considered, the agent's choice. (1996, p. 147)

The claim is that when considered from the first-person perspective, it *is* clear that indeterminacy has a role to play in sufficiency for control. Thus, according to Kane, the contentions of Banks (this volume) and Prinz (this volume) that physical indeterminacy has no such role simply fail to consider this indeterminacy from the first-person perspective of introspection. But for this reasoning to be compelling, we have to decide as a prior issue how heavily we can rely on indetrospective evidence.

Furthermore, as I will show in the next section, Timothy O'Connor's defense of a version of naturalized libertarianism, which provides the major alternative to Kane's, also relies on an appeal to introspection. Thus a broad consideration of the tenability of naturalized libertarianism must take up the question of the accuracy of introspection.

3 O'Connor's Naturalized Libertarianism

O'Connor (2000, p. 67) claims to offer a characterization of libertarian freedom which is consistent with science, joining Kane in attempting to avoid the mystery of a scientifically intractable agent. Thus, he purports to offer a version of naturalized libertarianism. But O'Connor finds Kane's way of spelling out the naturalistic context for indeterminacy—in terms of the physical basis of the interaction among goal-directed states—unconvincing as an attempt to make sense of naturalized libertarian freedom (2000, pp. 36–42). Instead of attempting to explain libertarian freedom in terms of a certain context for quantum indeterminacy, O'Connor's strategy is to tailor his proposal to match our feeling of freedom as exactly as possible, and contend that agents *create* indeterminacy.

O'Connor's view is that free will is a macrodeterminative emergent property of agents, where a macrodeterminative emergent property is "a qualitatively new, macro-level feature" of the world (2000, p. 111). While he claims that such properties are "completely dependent on some set of properties or disjunctive range of properties in the [instantiating] object's microstructure" nevertheless, "[they] exert a causal influence on the micro-level pattern of events that is not reducible to the *immediate* causal potentialities of the subvening properties" (ibid., pp. 111–112). Thus, such properties are "radically new features of the world, in a sense 'transcending' the lower level properties from which [they] emerge" (2000, p. 112). In response to the concern that transcendence indicates that macrodeterminative emergent properties are not naturalistic, O'Connor counters that we need to expand our conception of scientifically acceptable causation to include causation at the macro-level which is not reducible to the causal properties of micro-level parts (top-down causation) as well causation at the macro-level which is reducible (bottom-up causation) (2000, pp. 115, 125).

But rather than address the Intelligibility Question, O'Connor's characterization of libertarian freedom as a macrodeterminative emergent property offers a promissory note. Furthermore, there is a serious worry as to whether payment can be made good. While he holds out the prospect that empirical research may discover other examples of macrodeterminative emergence, forcing us to enrich our conception of scientific causation (2000, pp. 110–115),[13] he provides no reason at all to think that we will be able to understand libertarian freedom as a macrodeterminative emergent property.

O'Connor claims that we are "not wholly moved movers" (2000, p. 67). This, of course, means that we are partly unmoved movers (ibid., p. 97); we are partly moved as well because our reasons influence our choices. Since O'Connor's case for macrodeterminative emergent properties appeals to the possibility of other examples of such properties than libertarian freedom, simply being a macrodeterminative emergent property isn't sufficient for libertarian freedom. Rather, libertarian freedom is a macrodeterminative emergent property of a distinctive sort: a macrodeterminative property that allows unmoved moving. Setting aside the question of whether macrodeterminative emergent properties are consistent with science, O'Connor gives no reason to think that unmoved moving is.

O'Connor's view is important, though, not only because it is a proposal of a purported naturalized libertarianism which doesn't appeal to quantum indeterminacy, but also because, as O'Connor points out, agent causation, in which agents create indeterminacy, is better tailored to the introspective evidence than Kane's view. As O'Connor states, we experience ourselves as creating gaps in causal necessitation by undeterminedly and directly forming a particular intention (2000, p. 124).

For O'Connor, as well as for Kane, the introspective evidence holds out the hope that libertarian freedom is intelligible. This reliance on introspection points to a powerful empirical constraint. I will argue that, because it directly addresses the Intelligibility Question, the question on which the tenability of naturalized libertarianism turns, psychological research into the accuracy of introspection is the source of the most powerful empirical constraint for the problem of free will.

4 Naturalized Libertarianism and Psychological Constraints

Introspection does seem to indicate that when we struggle with a conflict of values, branching paths are metaphysically open. Whatever the metaphysics turns out to be, we experience ourselves as undeterminedly and directly forming the particular intention which causes our action. Thus we feel that we could have done otherwise (in the same circumstances) if we had formed a different intention. This feeling of freedom is a type of introspective state—that is, it represents a mental state rather than the world—and this type of introspective state provides evidence in favor of libertarian freedom. Kane and O'Connor claim this introspective evidence strongly suggests that, despite our present inability to address the Intelligibility Question, libertarian freedom is nonetheless intelligible.[14]

Furthermore, aside from the fact that both Kane and O'Connor appeal to introspective evidence, all libertarians assign introspective evidence some role, for it is our feeling of metaphysically open branching paths that is the raison d'etre of libertarian freedom. It is the first-person perspective that at least seems to give self-formation meaning. Even if the naturalized libertarian has yet to achieve the goal of making sense of self-formation from the third-person perspective of science, we will not be in a position to confidently conclude that libertarian freedom is *unintelligible* until we address the accuracy of this introspective evidence.

Considering a case of a conflict of values, the libertarian's claim is that it is metaphysically indeterminate which intention is formed. According to the libertarian, some of our intentions are formed in a way that is not merely the result of mental causation, that is, causation by further mental states that are ultimately caused by genetics and environment, but is also the result of indeterminacy. Introspective evidence supports this claim by indicating an absence of sufficient mental causation. The question is whether this introspective evidence is accurate, or whether background beliefs and desires missed by introspection are causally sufficient with respect to which intention produces action. O'Connor suggests that introspection is accurate—that our experience of ourselves as undeterminedly and directly forming a particular intention is as accurate as our perception of ordinary physical objects:

> ... in the deliberate formation of an intention, the coming to be of my intention doesn't seem to me merely to occur at the conclusion of my deliberation; I seem to experience myself directly bringing it about. .... This apparent perception of [undetermined] causality could be mistaken, of course; our experience cannot furnish the basis of a 'demonstrative proof' of our having free will. By the same token, our apparent perception of ordinary physical objects also could (in this epistemic sense) be mistaken, yet few take that as a reason not to believe that we do perceive them. (2000, p. 124)

But any answer to the question of the accuracy of introspection is likely to be quite complex, taking into account such factors as the kind of mental state represented (for example, whether it is an intention or a background desire), and empirical research is needed to tease out the complexities. In this effort, psychological research could show that introspection provides a reliable indicator of (the existence or absence of) sufficient mental causation of intention, so that introspective evidence of an absence of sufficient mental causation should be taken seriously. This finding could at least spur us to continue to address the Intelligibility Question.

Or such research could show not only that introspection provides a poor indicator of mental causation of intention but also why it produces illusions of an absence of sufficient mental causation, so that introspective evidence of such an absence should be discarded. In this way, the strongest evidence in support of libertarian freedom would be undermined. As a result, the naturalists among us would have to take seriously the conclusion that libertarianism is refuted.

In addition, this research would provide a payoff with respect to a connection that some, for example Kane, draw between libertarian freedom and consciousness. According to Kane, in cases of libertarian freedom

indeterminism and the effort [of will] are 'fused': the indeterminacy is a property *of* the effort and the effort *is* indeterminate. To fully understand how this fusion could take place would be . . . to understand the nature of conscious experience and its unity . . . , as well as to understand how consciousness and mind are related, if at all, to the indeterminacy of natural processes. . . . (1998, p. 151)

While Kane rightly points out that understanding quantum indeterminacy and consciousness are problems for everyone, not just libertarians (1998, p. 151), his proposal of a fusion of indeterminacy and conscious effort of will is meant to make sense of libertarian freedom in particular. Given the heady level of speculation, however, the situation cries out for empirical constraints. Kane's proposal of this fusion presents the possibility that indeterminacy and consciousness combine to form something that on the face of it is unintelligible: control for which indeterminacy is necessary and sufficient. If introspection provides a reliable indicator of (the existence or absence of) sufficient mental causation of intention, then this possibility should be taken seriously. But if introspection provides a poor indicator of mental causation of intention, it may be that the introspective evidence in support of libertarian freedom is systematically illusory. If, in addition, research were to explain introspective illusions of an absence of sufficient mental causation, the idea that indeterminacy and consciousness combine to form libertarian freedom would be undermined. While consciousness may play a role in causing behavior (perhaps along the lines carefully and compellingly argued by Pacherie in this volume), it would not in the way that libertarians envision.

Wegner's *Illusion of Conscious Will* amasses psychological research which supports the idea that introspection is a poor indicator of mental causation, at least in the case of causation of action.[15] Wegner's main focus is not the problem of free will but the problem of whether the *feeling* of mental causation of action accurately tracks mental causation of action, a problem which intersects with the problem of free will only at certain points. He finds two broad categories of cases where this tracking goes wrong, which I will call type I and type II inaccuracies (Wegner 2002, pp. 8–11).

Type I inaccuracy (false alarm or false positive)   One has a feeling that one's mental states cause action where no such mental causation exists.

Type II inaccuracy (miss or false negative)   One does not have a feeling that one's mental states cause action where such mental causation does exist.

Wegner's elaborate "I Spy" experiment is an example of a type I inaccuracy. In the experiment, a subject and an experimental confederate sit at a computer, together controlling a mouse that moves a cursor around a screen which displays a variety of objects (for example, a swan). Both subject and confederate wear headphones; the subject hears 10 seconds of music at the end of each 40-second trial, and, at some point during each trial, also hears a word which in some cases would refer to an object on the screen (for example, "swan"). Subject and confederate are told to stop the cursor sometime during the music. However, the confederate, rather than hearing music or words, hears instructions including, for some trials, instructions on when to stop the cursor. After each stop, the subject rates it according to whether the subject had intended the stop or had allowed it to happen. The experiment found that for trials where the confederate forces the cursor to stop on an object, when the subject hears the word for the object 1 to 5 seconds before the stop (versus 30 seconds before or 1 second after the stop), the subject feels more strongly that he or she had intended the stop (Wegner 2002, pp. 74–78).

This experiment indicates that introspection sometimes misleads us into believing that we have an intention which causes our actions when they aren't caused by our mental states at all (in the experiment, actions are caused by an experimental confederate's forcing the subject to act in certain ways). (However, for reasons to be skeptical about the conclusiveness of this experiment, see Malle's chapter in this volume.) Since the experiment identifies an illusion of control, it might seem to tell against libertarian freedom. But its findings in fact don't help to constrain the problem of free will. For the illusion of control which results from a false alarm isn't relevant to the ordinary example of free will, that is, the case where one's intentions clearly do cause one's actions. Furthermore, the libertarian can accept that there are *some* types of illusions of control; rather, all the libertarian claims is that *not all* types of control are systematically illusory—that is, that there are also some types of control. The relevant question then is whether introspection systematically misses mental causation whenever we have a feeling of libertarian freedom.

Rather, it is the type II inaccuracies, the misses, that are relevant to the question of libertarian freedom, for it is in these sorts of cases that introspection misses mental causation. And, indeed, Wegner shows that these inaccuracies of introspection sometimes mislead us into believing that our mental states are not sufficient causes of our actions when in fact they are. Thus, in these cases, an absence of awareness of sufficient mental causation is erroneously taken to be an awareness of an absence of sufficient mental causation.

These examples include automatisms such as alien hand syndrome and automatic writing (Wegner 2002, pp. 4–6, 103–108). In cases of alien hand syndrome, one's hand can do things such as turn pages of a book or unzip a jacket while one isn't aware that one's intentions are sufficient to cause such actions, and one can even think that such intentions have no role in causing such actions. Automatic writing, documented in spiritualist writings in America and Europe in the middle of the nineteenth century, involves writing (including gibberish, reverse writing, or ordinary writing) which one isn't aware of intentionally producing, instead attributing its production to disembodied spirits. These cases vividly show that introspection can miss cases of sufficient mental causation.

Wegner's presentation of research skeptical of the accuracy of introspection is a descendant of Nisbett and Wilson's (1977) influential discussion.[16] Nisbett and Wilson gather research showing that introspection can misidentify or simply miss mental processes, as well as the external inputs and physiological and nonverbal behavioral outputs of mental processes. However, Nisbett and Wilson don't speak directly to the question of whether introspection sometimes misleads us into believing that our mental states don't cause actions when they in fact do. They consider cases where introspection misidentifies mental causes, and they also take up cases where there is an absence of awareness of mental causes (for example, in cases of problem solving), but they don't consider cases where an absence of awareness of sufficient mental causation is mistakenly taken to be an awareness of absence of sufficient mental causation. Wegner's discussion is interesting because it does speak directly to this question.

Yet on the face of it Wegner's examples of automatic writing and alien-hand syndrome have little to do with free will. After all, these are cases where one *lacks* a feeling of control. But the connection with free will is this: type II inaccuracies divide into two subgroups, one group of cases where one feels a lack of control and another where one feels a presence of control. In cases of the first subgroup (type IIa inaccuracies), introspection misses the *intention* producing action. Consequently, the action is not self-attributed and one feels a lack of control. Automatic writing and alien-hand syndrome are examples of type IIa inaccuracies.

However, in cases of the second subgroup (type IIb inaccuracies) introspection misses *mental states such as desires producing the intention* which produces action, rather than the intention itself. (Thus the distinction between subgroups appeals in part to the separation, stressed by both Mele and Malle in this volume, between desires and intentions.) In cases of type IIb inaccuracies, this ignorance of background mental states producing the intention creates the feeling that branching paths are metaphysically open—i.e., that it is metaphysically indeterminate which intention is formed. As a result, we feel that we initiate action in the strong sense of self-formation. Of course, even if introspection does systematically miss background mental states (an empirical question) and this account of the feeling of libertarian freedom is along the right lines, much more needs to be said, for the feeling withstands the appreciation of this point.

But now it is clear that Wegner's examples are of limited use with respect to the issue of libertarian freedom. Because Wegner's focus is introspective inaccuracies with respect to intentions that cause action, he gives examples of type IIa inaccuracies, but not type IIb inaccuracies, where introspection misses mental causes producing intentions.[17] And even setting this problem aside, Wegner's examples are of the wrong sort. His examples where introspection misses cases of sufficient mental causation involve neuropsychological disorders, as with alien hand syndrome, or specific unusual contexts, such as that set up by the spiritualist movement, which abetted introspective illusions. The libertarian could reasonably contend that the experience of metaphysical indeterminacy in a situation of a conflict of values is neither pathological nor particularly unusual. Wegner's examples might show that introspective evidence is fallible in some unusual cases, but they don't impugn its reliability in more ordinary cases such as the feeling of libertarian freedom.[18]

Moreover, the libertarian might claim that if the introspective evidence supporting libertarian freedom were mistaken, this would amount to a systematic illusion. But, the libertarian might assert, such a systematic illusion should be regarded as implausible. Nevertheless, as Wegner notes (2002, p. 137), illusions of the absence of sufficient mental causation can be explained by our background beliefs and desires, as the case of automatic writing in the context of the spiritualist movement suggests. And this explanation might be applied even to systematic illusions. Furthermore, libertarianism's provision of an absolute autonomy suggests a background motivation.[19]

Yet even if this point is along the right lines, again, much more needs to be said, for we can appreciate this point and yet the feeling of libertarian freedom remains. In any event, this isn't the place for armchair science.

My conclusion is that the only empirical research which provides constraints for the problem of free will is research relevant to the truth of libertarianism, and, that, because it directly addresses the Intelligibility Question, psychological research regarding the accuracy of introspection offers the most powerful empirical constraint. The libertarian claims that the best explanation of our feeling that there are metaphysically open branching paths is that we become aware of an absence of sufficient mental causes. A specific question for research is whether this is the best explanation. If psychologists were to provide an alternative explanation which not only indicates that there are sufficient mental causes even in ordinary cases where our introspection indicates otherwise, but also offers a model explaining the illusion of their absence, this would undermine any naturalized libertarianism.

Appendix

With respect to other research relevant to the accuracy of introspection, the physiologist Benjamin Libet's research (1985) can be interpreted as indicating that our control of our behavior is limited in a surprising way. Libet's studies (discussed by many of the authors in this volume) indicate the existence of two time gaps (measured in hundreds of milliseconds) in the mental process immediately preceding action: between unconscious brain activity called a readiness potential and the conscious intention to act, and between the conscious intention to act and the muscular motion involved in action. Also, these studies show that during the gap between conscious intention and muscular motion, one can veto the conscious intention and so block action. Furthermore, Libet argues that the veto is itself a "conscious control function" which need not be unconsciously initiated (1999, pp. 558–559).

Libet's finding of the first time gap can be interpreted to give the dizzying impression that our actions are initiated before we consciously intend to act, thus undercutting control at this stage; while the ability to veto conscious intentions during the second time gap provides us with control at a later stage. Thus our control is limited. Yet Dennett (2003, pp. 227–242) argues that this interpretation of the first time gap mistakenly assumes that conscious intentions immediately prior to action exhaust the mental processes involved in control, and thus that such processes don't also include unconscious processes or conscious deliberations long before action.

In any event, it is not clear that the possibility of a surprising limitation of control is a constraint on the problem of free will at all, in that it doesn't seem to rule out any positions on the problem. While Libet's findings show that some of the causes of our actions are not transparent to introspection, the libertarian needn't have claimed otherwise. Furthermore, the power to veto conscious intentions could be co-opted by libertarians as Campbellian resistance of temptation (a vivid image repeated by Kane (1996, pp. 126–128)); for this approach to Libet's data, see Kane 1996, p. 232, note 12. Libet's findings don't rule out any versions of compatibilism or hard determinism either, these views not being committed to the accuracy of introspection. (For extended discussions of reasons to be skeptical about the importance of Libet's findings to the issue of free will, see the chapters in this volume by Gallagher and Mele.)

In fact, Libet's conclusion about empirical constraints on the problem of free will is similar to mine, leaving the introspective evidence of libertarian freedom open to empirical study. After acknowledging that his findings don't rule out free will (1999, pp. 551 and 561), Libet states:

. . . we must recognize that the almost universal experience that we can act with a free, independent choice provides a kind of prima facie evidence that conscious mental processes can causatively control some brain processes. This creates, for an experimental scientist, more difficulty for a determinist than for a non-determinist option. The phenomenal fact is that most of us feel that we do have free will, at least for some of our actions and within certain limits that may be imposed by our brain's status and by our environment. The intuitive feelings about the phenomenon of free will form a fundamental basis for views of our human nature, and great care should be taken not to believe allegedly scientific conclusions about them that actually depend upon hidden ad hoc assumptions. A theory that simply interprets the phenomenon of free will as illusory and denies the validity of this phenomenal fact is less attractive than a theory that accepts or accommodates the phenomenal fact. (ibid., p. 563)

Wegner's claim is that the feeling of conscious control is illusory, and his goal is to accommodate—that is, explain in naturalistic terms—the phenomenal fact (2003, chapter 9, especially pp. 318 and 325–334), but, as I have argued, he doesn't provide adequate evidence to establish that conscious control in fact is illusory in a relatively ordinary case such as the feeling of libertarian freedom.

Acknowledgments

My greatest debt with respect to thinking through the issues of this chapter is to Dale Turner, with whom I taught a seminar on free will in the spring of 2003. I presented versions of this chapter at the 2004 APA Pacific Division Meeting in Pasadena and the 2004 Joint Meeting of the Society for Philosophy and Psychology and the European Society for Philosophy and Psychology in Barcelona. I am thankful to audience members at those events for comments, and in particular to Stephan F. Johnson for his comments at the Pasadena meeting. I also owe thanks to Dion Scott-Kakures, Michael Cholbi, and William P. Banks for extremely useful comments on earlier drafts.

Notes

1. See Hardin 1988. Also see Ross 2001 and peer commentary for further discussion.

2. The problem of free will is commonly stated in terms of whether we control our actions. Stated more fully, the problem is whether we control our actions through controlling the goal-directed states— intentions, desires, or other goal-directed states—which produce action. (Gallagher, in this volume, also emphasizes that the problem of free will should be characterized in terms of control of environmentally situated intentional actions rather than control of bodily movement.) If we call the mental capacity for producing goal-directed states "the will," then the problem is whether we control our goal-directed states, and consequently our actions, through controlling the will. (There are other uses of the word 'will'. For example, it is sometimes used to refer to the goal-directed states that are products of the mental capacity called the will—see Frankfurt 1971 for this usage.)

3. According to the claim that our actions are brought about by genetics and environment, even if we can in some ways manipulate our genes through gene therapy and in some ways manipulate our adult environments, ultimately we control neither our genes nor environments. For our manipulation of our genes and adult environments is brought about by goal-directed states, and such states are in turn ultimately brought about by aspects of our genetics and environments which we don't control.

4. For this idea of self-formation, see Kane 1996, pp. 74–77 and 124–125; Kane 1999, pp. 164–165. I have described self formation as a negative claim along with indeterminacy. Kane seems to suggest more of

a positive aspect: "Free will . . . is the power of agents to be the ultimate creators (or originators) and sustainers of their own ends or purposes." (1996, p. 4) But this description isn't helpful until we understand what it means to be an ultimate creator, and Kane's suggestion is largely negative: "Such a notion of *ultimate* creation of purposes is obscure. . . . Its meaning can be captured initially by an image: when we trace the causal or explanatory chains of action back to their sources in the purposes of free agents, these causal chains must come to an end or terminate in the willings (choices, decisions, or efforts) of the agents. . . . If these willings were in turn caused by something else, so that the explanatory chains could be traced back further to heredity or environment, to God, or fate, then the ultimacy would not lie with the agents but with something else." (1996, p. 4) However, Kane is clear that ultimate creation involves metaphysical indeterminacy. Thus, I take the involvement of indeterminacy in the production of actions to be the sole positive aspect of self formation. I will discuss the relation between indeterminacy and control below.

5. Derk Pereboom (2001, pp. 110–117) offers this argument. For a similar argument, see Taylor 1992, pp. 45–47.

6. For example, hard determinism can accept justification for punishment on the basis of social utility. For a discussion of a sophisticated hard determinist's account of ersatz normativity (that is, normativity without self formation), see chapters 5–7 of Pereboom 2001. Prinz (this volume) also comments on the social utility of ersatz ("invented") control.

7. Dennett admits that a sophisticated hard determinism's account of ersatz normativity is only "terminologically different" from compatibilism (2003, pp. 97–98).

8. Hard determinists and compatibilists divide as to whether indeterminacy is necessary for control, the hard determinists claiming that it is and the compatibilists claiming that it isn't. However, both sorts of determinism reject the libertarian's claim that indeterminacy is sometimes sufficient for control.

9. An example of a traditional non-naturalist libertarian view is Roderick Chisholm's proposal that "we have a prerogative which some would attribute only to God: each of us, when we act, is a prime mover unmoved" (1964, p. 34).

10. For a helpful discussion of quantum indeterminacy and chaotic amplification, see Bishop 2002, especially section 3.

11. As far as this discussion is concerned, the goal-directed states that express our values can be characterized as desires or, alternatively, as besires, which are hybrids of beliefs and desires. For discussions of besires, see van Roojen 1995 and Ross 2002.

12. Similarly, Kane states that "the core meaning of 'he got lucky,' which *is* implied by indeterminism, I suggest, is that 'he succeeded *despite the probability or chance of failure*'; and this core meaning does not imply lack of responsibility, if he succeeds" (1999, p. 171).

13. Pereboom (2001, pp. 74, 85–86) also considers the existence of top-down causation to be an empirical question, although he is pessimistic about its prospects.

14. Campbell (1957, pp. 176–178) states this point in classic fashion. Also see O'Connor 2000, p. 124. Kane puts the point in a way reminiscent of Campbell: ". . . when described from a physical perspective alone, *free will looks like chance*. But the physical description is not the only one to be considered. The indeterministic chaotic process is also, experientially considered, the agent's effort of will; and the undetermined outcome of the process, [whether it is settled] one way or the other, is, experientially considered, the agent's choice. From a free willist point of view, this experiential or phenomenological perspective is also important; it cannot simply be dispensed with." (1996, p. 147) At points Kane conflates epistemic and metaphysical indeterminacy. Kane states: "Every free choice (which is a [self formed willing]) is the initiation of a 'value experiment' whose justification lies in the future and is not fully explained by the past. It says, in effect 'Let's try this. It is not required by my past, but it is consistent with my past and is one branching pathway my life could now meaningfully take. I am willing to take responsibility for it one way or the other. . . .'" (1996, p. 145) Kane repeats this statement in a later work and continues as follows: "To initiate and take responsibility for such value experiments whose justification lies in the future, is to 'take chances' without prior guarantees of success. Genuine self-formation requires this sort of risk-taking and indeterminism is a part of it. If there are persons who need to be certain in advance just exactly what is the best or right thing to do in every circumstance (perhaps to be told so by some human or divine authority), then free will is not for them." (1999, p. 176) Claiming that my action is "not required by my past" suggests metaphysical indeterminacy. But a lack of certainty with

respect to the best future action is an epistemic matter. This point is important because while everyone has to accept that epistemic indeterminacy is involved in processes of deliberation leading to the production of action—uncertainty about what action is best is a fact of life—it is only the libertarian who claims that metaphysical indeterminacy involved in such processes is sufficient for controlling action. Thus, Kane's conflation tends to give libertarianism more credibility than it deserves. However, Kane's misleading description of the indeterminacy doesn't detract from the point that libertarians use introspective evidence to support metaphysical indeterminacy.

15. In addition to supporting the idea that introspection is fallible, Wegner puts forth the further claim that such introspective states are causally inefficacious (2002, pp. 317–318). For a careful elucidation of Wegner's claim and a convincing argument that it is false, see Nahmias 2002; also see, in the present volume, Bayne's trenchant criticism of this aspect of Wegner's work. Some of Wegner's claims seem to place him in the compatibilist camp (see, for example, pp. 318–319). But because he never makes clear what he means by "control" in the way that philosophers in the free literature do, it is not clear whether Wegner is a compatibilist or a hard determinist.

16. Wegner (2002, p. 67) notes this heritage.

17. In addition, while Wegner (2002, pp. 65–95) offers a psychological model for the experience of mental causation of action, unfortunately it has features that make it specific to causation of action and so doesn't straightforwardly apply to the existence or absence of mental causation of mental states.

18. Wegner (2002, p. 327) acknowledges that introspection is accurate much of the time. While Nisbett and Wilson (1977) offer a more sweeping skepticism about the accuracy of introspection (contending that the accuracy of first-person verbal reports of mental processes is no better than third-person guesses (pp. 248–251)), White's 1988 review of the psychological literature shows that their claims needed to be modified, and that introspection may be highly accurate in some cases (pp. 36–37).

19. Kane notes that his conception of self formation is closely connected to our " 'life-hopes'—including dispositions to view ourselves as ultimately responsible for our own characters and achievements rather than as pawns of nature, fate, or the whims of others, including God" (1996, p. 4).

References

Bishop, R. C. 2002. Chaos, indeterminism, and free will. In *The Oxford Handbook of Free Will*, ed. R. Kane. Oxford University Press.

Campbell, C. A. 1957. Has the self 'free will'? In Campbell, *On Selfhood and Godhood*. Allen and Unwin.

Chisholm, Roderick M. 1964. Human freedom and the self. The Lindley Lecture. Reprinted in Watson 2003. Page numbers refer to reprint.

Dennett, Daniel C. 2003. *Freedom Evolves*. Viking.

Ekstrom, Laura, ed. 2001. *Agency and Responsibility: Essays on the Metaphysics of Freedom*. Westview.

Frankfurt, Harry 1971. Freedom of the will and the concept of a person. *Journal of Philosophy* 68: 5–20.

Hardin, C. L. 1988. *Color for Philosophers: Unweaving the Rainbow*. Hackett.

Kane, R. 1996. *The Significance of Free Will*. Oxford University Press.

Kane, R. 1999. Responsibility, luck, and chance: Reflections on free will and indeterminism. *Journal of Philosophy* 96: 217–240. Reprinted in Ekstrom 2001. Page numbers refer to reprint.

Kane, R., ed. 2002. *The Oxford Handbook of Free Will*. Oxford University Press.

Libet, B. 1985. Unconscious cerebral initiative and the role of conscious will in voluntary action. *Behavioral and Brain Sciences* 8: 529–566.

Libet, B. 1999. Do we have free will? *Journal of Consciousness Studies* 6, no. 8–9: 47–57. Reprinted in Kane 2002. Page numbers refer to reprint.

Nahmias, E. 2002. When consciousness matters: A critical review of Daniel Wegner's *The Illusion of Conscious Will*. *Philosophical Psychology* 15: 527–541.

Nisbett, R. E., and Wilson, T. D. 1977. Telling more than we can know: Verbal reports on mental processes. *Psychological Review* 84: 231–259.

O'Connor, T. 2000. *Persons and Causes: The Metaphysics of Free Will.* Oxford University Press.

Pereboom, D. 2001. *Living without Free Will.* Cambridge University Press.

Ross, P. W. 2001. The location problem for color subjectivism. *Consciousness and Cognition* 10: 42–58.

Ross, P. W. 2002. Explaining motivated desires. *Topoi* 21, no. 1–2: 199–207.

Strawson, G. 1986. *Freedom and Belief.* Oxford University Press.

Taylor, R. 1992. *Metaphysics*, fourth edition. Prentice-Hall.

van Roojen, M. 1995. Humean motivation and Humean rationality. *Philosophical Studies* 79: 37–57.

Watson, G. ed. 2003. *Free Will*, second edition. Oxford University Press.

Wegner, D. M. 2002. *The Illusion of Conscious Will.* MIT Press.

White, P. A. 1988. Knowing more about what we can tell: "Introspective access" and causal report accuracy 10 years later. *British Journal of Psychology* 79: 13–45.

8 Toward a Dynamic Theory of Intentions

Elisabeth Pacherie

In this chapter, I shall offer a sketch of a dynamic theory of intentions. I shall argue that several categories or forms of intentions should be distinguished based on their different (and complementary) functional roles and on the different contents or types of contents they involve. I shall further argue that an adequate account of the distinctive nature of actions and of their various grades of intentionality depends on a large part on a proper understanding of the dynamic transitions among these different forms of intentions. I also hope to show that one further benefit of this approach is to open the way for a more perspicuous account of the phenomenology of action and of the role of conscious thought in the production of action.

I take as my point of departure the causal theory of action (CTA). CTA is the view that behavior qualifies as action just in case it has a certain sort of psychological cause or involves a certain sort of psychological causal process. In the last decades, CTA has gained wide currency. Yet it covers a variety of theories with importantly different conceptions of what constitutes the requisite type of cause or causal process qualifying a piece of behavior as an action. Broadly speaking, CTA takes actions to be associated with sequences of causally related events and attempts to characterize them in terms of certain causal characteristics they have. Versions of CTA can take different forms depending on what they take the elements of the action-relevant causal sequence to be and on what part of the sequence they identify as the action.

The earlier belief/desire versions of CTA, made popular most notably by Davidson (1980, essay 1) and Goldman (1970), held that what distinguishes an action from a mere happening is the nature of its causal antecedent, conceived as a complex of some of the agent's beliefs and desires. However, it soon appeared that simple belief/desire versions of the causal theory are both too narrow and too unconstrained. On the one hand, they do not deal with "minimal" actions, those that are performed routinely, automatically, impulsively, or unthinkingly. On the other hand, they are unable to exclude aberrant manners of causation when specifying the causal connection that must hold between the antecedent mental event and the resultant behavior for the latter to qualify as an (intentional) action.

Belief/desire versions of CTA are also largely incomplete. They account at best for how an action is initiated, but not for how it is guided, controlled, and monitored until completion. They provide no analysis of the role of the bodily movements that ultimately account for the success or failure of an intended action. They say next to nothing about the phenomenology of action, and what they say does not seem right. On their accounting, the phenomenology of passive and active bodily movements could be exactly the same, which implies that an agent would know that she is performing an action not in virtue of her immediate awareness that she is moving, but only because she knows what the antecedent conditions causing her behavior are.

In order to overcome some of these difficulties and shortcomings, many philosophers have found it necessary to introduce a conception of intentions as distinctive, sui generis mental states with their own complex and distinctive functional role that warrants considering them as an irreducible kind of psychological state on a par with beliefs and desires. Bratman (1987) stresses three functions of intentions. First, intentions are *terminators of practical reasoning* in the sense that once we have formed an intention to A we will not normally continue to deliberate whether to A or not; in the absence of relevant new information, the intention will resist reconsideration. Second, intentions are also *prompters of practical reasoning*, where practical reasoning is about means of A-ing. This function of intentions thus involves devising specific plans for A-ing. Third, intentions also have a *coordinative function* and serve to coordinate the activities of the agent over time and to coordinate them with the activities of other agents.

Brand (1984) and Mele (1992) point out further functions of intentions. They argue that intentions are motivators of actions and that their role as motivators is not just to trigger or initiate the intended action (*initiating function*) but also to sustain it until completion (*sustaining function*). Intentions have also been assigned a guiding function in the production of an action. The cognitive component of an intention to A incorporates a plan for A-ing, a representation or set of representations specifying the goal of the action and how it is to be arrived at. It is this component of the intention that is relevant to its *guiding function*. Finally, intentions have also been assigned a *monitoring function* involving a capacity to detect progress toward the goal and to detect, and correct for, deviations from the course of action as laid out in the guiding representation.

The first three functions of intentions—their roles as terminators of practical reasoning about ends, as prompters of practical reasoning about means and as coordinators—are typically played in the period between initial formation of the intention and initiation of the action. In contrast, the last four functions (initiating, sustaining, guiding, and monitoring) are played in the period between the initiation of the action and its completion. Let me call the first set of functions *practical-reasoning functions* for short and the second set *executive functions*.

Attention to these differences has led a number of philosophers to develop dual-intention theories of action—that is, theories that distinguish between two types of intentions. For instance, Searle (1983) distinguishes between prior intentions and intentions-in-action, Bratman (1987) between future-directed and present-directed intentions, Brand (1984) between prospective and immediate intentions, Bach (1978) between intentions and executive representations, and Mele (1992) between distal and proximal intentions.[1]

My own stance is that all seven functions are proper functions of intentions. I also think that at least two levels of guiding and monitoring of actions must be distinguished, and that taking into account this distinction of levels is important in order to make sense of certain intuitive differences between intentional actions of varying grades. Furthermore, although important, a characterization of intentions uniquely in terms of their different functions remains insufficient. One must also take into account the different types of content intentions may have, their dynamics, their temporal scales, and their explanatory roles.

This leads me to draw a more complex picture of the situation. I will try to motivate a threefold distinction among categories or levels of intentions: future-directed intentions (F-intentions), present-directed intentions (P-intentions), and motor intentions (M-intentions). I shall also distinguish between two levels of dynamics in the unfolding of intentions: the local dynamics specific to each level of intention and the global dynamics involved in the transition from one level to the next. It is also useful to distinguish for each type of intention two phases of its internal dynamics: the upstream dynamics (which culminate in the formation of the intention) and the downstream dynamics (manifested once the intention has been formed). I have tried to show elsewhere (Pacherie 2003) how certain shortcomings of the more traditional versions of the causal theory may be overcome in this dynamic framework. Here I will focus on the phenomenology of action and on the role of conscious thought in the generation and control of action.

1 Future-Directed Intentions (F-Intentions)

Bratman stressed three functions of F-intentions: as terminators of practical reasoning about ends, as prompters of practical reasoning about means and plans, and as intra- and interpersonal coordinators. The upstream dynamics of F-intentions—the dynamics of decision making that leads to the formation of an intention—are associated with the first of these three functions. Practical reasoning has been described by Davidson as a two-step process of evaluation of alternative courses of action. The first step consists in weighting possible alternative actions and reasons for and against each, and forming a judgment that, all things considered, some course of action is the best. The second step in the process consists in moving from this prima facie judgment to an unconditional or all-out judgment that this action is the best simpliciter. With this move we reach the end point of the upstream dynamics: to form an all-out judgment is to form an intention to act.

The downstream dynamics of F-intentions are linked to their functions as prompters of practical reasoning about means and as intra- and interpersonal coordinators. This reasoning must be internally, externally, and globally consistent. All the intentions that are the building blocks of an action plan must be mutually consistent (*internal consistency*). The plan as a whole should be consistent with the agent's beliefs about the world (*external consistency*). Finally the plan must take into account the wider framework of activities and projects in which the agent is also involved and be coordinated with them in a more global plan (*global consistency*).

The dynamics of F-intentions, although not completely context-free, are not strongly dependent on the particular situation in which the agent finds himself when he forms the F-intention or reasons from it. I can form an F-intention to act an hour from now, next week, two years from now, or once I retire from work. This temporal flexibility makes it possible for an agent to form an F-intention to perform an action of a certain type even though his present situation does not allow its immediate performance. An F-intention is therefore in principle detachable from the agent's current situation and is indeed commonly detached from it.

The rationality constraints that bear on F-intentions both at the stage of intention-formation and at the stage of planning and coordination require the presence of a network of inferential relations among intentions, beliefs, and desires. Concepts are the inferentially relevant constituents of intentional states. Their sharing a common conceptual representational format is what makes possible a form of global consistency, at the personal level, of our desires, beliefs, intentions and other prepositional attitudes. If we accept this common view, what follows is that for F-intentions to satisfy the rationality constraints to which they are subject they must have conceptual content.

In a nutshell, then, the content of F-intentions is both conceptual and descriptive; it specifies a type of action rather than a token of that type. Because many aspects of an intended action will depend on unpredictable features of the situation in which it is eventually carried out, the description of the type of action leaves indeterminate many aspects of the action. An F-intention therefore always presupposes some measure of faith on the part of the agent, in the sense that the agent must trust herself at least implicitly to be able, once the time to act comes, to adjust her action plan to the situation at hand.

2 Present-Directed Intentions (P-Intentions)

Philosophers who draw a distinction between future-directed intentions and present-directed intentions typically assign four functions to the latter: they trigger or initiate the intended action (the *initiating function*), sustain it until completion (the *sustaining function*), guide its unfolding (the *guiding function*), and monitor its effects (the *monitoring function*). We may call the first two functions motivational or volitional functions and the latter two control functions. Although there seems to be some consensus as to what the initiating and sustaining functions amount to, the situation is much less clear where the guiding and monitoring or control functions are concerned. My impression is that the disagreements among philosophers on these issues stem in a large part from the fact that they do not always distinguish clearly between two levels of guidance and monitoring. I will defend the view that higher-level guidance and monitoring are indeed functions of P-intentions and are therefore subject to strong rationality constraints, whereas lower-level guiding and monitoring functions should properly be assigned to M-intentions.

As we did with F-intentions, we can distinguish two stages in the dynamics of P-intentions. Their upstream dynamics are concerned with the transformation of an F-intention into an intention to start acting now. The downstream dynamics are concerned with the period between the initiation of the action and its completion.[2]

A P-intention often inherits an action plan from an F-intention. Its task is then to anchor this plan in the situation of action. The temporal anchoring, the decision to start acting now, is but one aspect of this process. Once the agent has established a perceptual information-link to the situation of action, she must ensure that the action plan is implemented in that situation. This means that she must effect a transformation of the purely descriptive contents of the action plan inherited from the F-intention into indexical contents anchored in the situation. When I decide to act now on my F-intention to go to the hairdresser, I must think about taking this bus, getting off at that stop, walking down that street to the salon, pushing this door to enter the salon, and so on. As I do this I am anchoring my plan in the situation, making it more specific. When I formed the F-intention to go to the hairdresser a few days ago, I did not necessarily know where I would be when the time to act would come and which bus line would be most convenient. Only now, in the situation of action, can the "getting there" element of the action plan be specified in detail.

Another essential function of P-intentions is to ensure the rational control of the ongoing action. It is important to emphasize that what is specifically at stake here is the *rational* control of the action, since, as we shall see, motor intentions also have a control function (although of a different kind).

What should we understand rational control to be? Here I will follow Buekens, Maesen, and Vanmechelen (2001),[3] who describe rational control as taking two forms, the second of which is often ignored in the literature. The first type of rational control Buekens et al. describe is what they call "tracking control." Tracking control enables an agent to keep track of her way of accomplishing an action and to adjust what she does to maximize her chances of success. The second type of rational control is "collateral control": control of the side effects of accomplishing an action. The agent may notice undesirable side effects of her ongoing action, and may correct her way of accomplishing it in order to minimize them, or may even abort the action. For instance, if I intended to surprise a friend by, for once, being on time for our appointment, but I find that the traffic is such that I could only do it by speeding madly in the crowded streets, I might renounce trying to arrive on time and leave that surprise for some other occasion. Both types of control are rational insofar as what the agent does in both cases is connect her indexical conception of her ongoing action to general principles of means-end reasoning, to her desires, values, general policies, and rules of conduct. The agent exercises rational control over her action insofar as (1) she is in a position to judge whether or not her way of accomplishing her action is likely to lead to success and adjusts it so as to maximize her chances of success (tracking control) and (2) she is also in a position to judge whether or not it brings about undesirable side effects and corrects it accordingly (collateral control). P-intentions are thus, like F-intentions, subject to strong rationality constraints. Unlike F-intentions, however, P-intentions don't have much temporal flexibility. Rather, insofar as a P-intention is tied to a corresponding ongoing action and gets deployed concurrently with it, it is subject to severe temporal constraints.

These temporal constraints are of two kinds: cognitive and action-related. First, P-intentions are responsible for high-level forms of guidance and monitoring—they are concerned with aspects of the situation of action and of the activity of the agent that are both consciously perceived and conceptualized. Therefore the time scale of P-intentions is the time scale of conscious perception and rational thought. Their temporal grain is a function of the minimal time required for conscious rational thought. Second, their temporality is also constrained by what we may call the tempo of the action. This is literally the case when, say, one is playing a piece of music on the piano and must respect the tempo and rhythm of the piece. It is also the case in many other kinds of actions. In a game of tennis, one is allowed very little time to decide on how to return a serve. A slow tempo offers better conditions for online rational guidance and control of the action, since the agent has more time to decide on adjustments or to consider and evaluate possible side effects. When the tempo is extremely fast, possibilities for online rational control may be very limited. In a nutshell, for a P-intention to play its role of guidance and control, it must be the case that the tempo of the action is not faster then the tempo of conscious rational thought; more accurately, it is only on those aspects of an action the tempo of which does not exceed the tempo of conscious rational thought that P-intentions can have rational control.

3   Motor Intentions (M-Intentions)

I claimed in the previous section that it was important to distinguish between two levels of action: guidance and control. P-intentions are responsible for high-level forms of guidance and monitoring, applying to aspects of the situation of action and of the activity of the agent that are both consciously perceived and conceptualized. However, work in the cognitive neuroscience of action shows that there also exist levels of guidance and control of an ongoing action that are much finer-grained, responsible for the precision of the action and the smoothness of its execution. P-intentions and M-intentions are both responsible for the online control of action, but whereas the time scale at which the former operate is the time scale of the consciously experienced present, the latter's time scale is that of a neurological micropresent, which only partially overlaps the conscious present.

We have seen that the move from F-intention to corresponding P-intention involves a transformation of a descriptive, conceptual content into a perceptual, indexical content. The role of an M-intention is to effect a further transformation of perceptual into sensory-motor information. M-intentions therefore involve what neuroscientists call motor representations.

I will not attempt here to review the already considerable and fast-growing empirical literature on motor representations.[4] A brief description of the main characteristics of these representations will suffice. It is now generally agreed that there exist two visual systems, dedicated respectively to vision for action and vision for semantical perception (i.e., the identification and recognition of objects and scenes).[5] The vision-for-action system extracts from visual stimuli information about the properties of objects and situations that is relevant to action, and uses this to build motor representations used in effecting rapid visuo-motor transformations. The motor representations produced by this system have three important characteristics. First, the attributes of objects and situations are represented in a format useful for the immediate selection of appropriate motor patterns. For instance, if one wants to grab an object, its spatial position will be represented in terms of the movements needed to reach for it and its shape and size will be represented in terms of the type of hand grip it affords. Second, these representations of the movements to be effected reflect an implicit knowledge of biomechanical constraints and the kinematic and dynamic rules governing the motor system. For instance, the movements of the effectors will be programmed so as to avoid awkward or uncomfortable hand positions and to minimize the time spent at extreme joint angles. Third, a motor representation normally codes for transitive movements, where the goal of the action determines the global organization of the motor sequence. For instance, the type of grip chosen for a given object is a function not just of its intrinsic characteristics (its shape and size) but also of the subsequent use one wants to make of it. The same cup will be seized in different ways depending on whether one wants to carry it to one's lips or to put it upside down. A given situation usually affords more than just one possibility for action and can therefore be pragmatically organized in many different ways. Recent work suggests that the affordances of an object or a situation are automatically detected even in the absence of any intention to act. These affordances automatically prepotentiate corresponding motor programs (Tucker and Ellis 1998; Grèzes and Decety 2002).

One can therefore also distinguish two moments in the dynamics of M-intentions. The upstream dynamics constitute the process that leads to the selection of one among (typically) several prepotentialized motor programs. When an M-intention is governed by a P-intention and inherits its goal from it, the presence of the goal tends to increase the salience of one of these possible pragmatic organizations of the situation and thus allow for the selection of the corresponding motor program. But it can also be the case that M-intentions are formed in the absence of a P-intention. In such cases, the upstream dynamics work in a different way. According to the model proposed by Shallice (1988), there is then a competition among motor programs, with the program showing the strongest activation being triggered as a result of a process Shallice calls "contention scheduling."

The guidance and monitoring functions of M-intentions are exercised as part of their downstream dynamics. According to the neuro-computational models of action control developed in the last two decades, the motor system makes use of internal models of action in order to simulate the agent's behavior and its sensory consequences.[6] The internal models that concern us here are of two kinds: inverse models and forward or predictive models. Inverse models capture the relationships between intended sensory consequences and the motor commands yielding those consequences. They are computational systems, taking as their inputs representations of (a) the current state of the organism, (b) the current state of its environment, and (c) the desired state and yielding as their outputs motor commands for achieving the desired state. In contrast, the task of predictive or forward models is to predict the sensory consequences of motor commands. Although strictly speaking it is an oversimplification,[7] one might say that inverse models have a guiding function (to specify the movements to be performed in order to achieve the intended goal) and that forward models have a monitoring function (to anticipate the sensory consequences of the movements and adjust them so that they yield the desired effect). In most sensory-motor loops there are large delays between the execution of a motor command and the perception of its sensory consequences, and these temporal delays can result in instability when trying to make rapid movements and a certain jerkiness and imprecision in the action. It is hypothesized that predictive models allow the system to compute the expected sensory consequences in advance of external feedback and thus make faster corrections of the movements, preventing instability.

P-intentions and F-intentions must maintain internal, external, and global consistency of an action plan and are therefore subject to strong rationality constraints. M-intentions are not subject to these constraints. This is a consequence of the fact that the motor system exhibits some of the features considered by Fodor (1983) as characteristic of modular systems. It is informationally encapsulated, with only limited access to information from other cognitive systems or subsystems. A well-known illustration is the following: When you move your eye using your eye muscles, the sensory consequences of this movement are anticipated, and the displacement of the image on the retina is not interpreted as a change in the world; but when you move your eye by gently pressing on the eyelid with the finger, the world seems to move. When we press on our eyeball with our finger, we are well aware that it is our eye that is moving and not the world, but the forward model in charge of predicting the sensory consequences of our motor performances has no access to that information. Similarly, the fact that the motor system does not seem to be sensitive to certain perceptual illusions suggests that the inverse models that operate online do not typically have access to conscious perceptual representations (non-veridical in the case of illusions) constructed by the vision for perception or semantical visual system.[8]

Obviously the motor system cannot be fully encapsulated. If it were, it would be impossible to explain how a P-intention can trigger motor behavior, or that the way we grasp an object depends not just on immediate sensory affordances but also on our prior knowledge of the function of the object. But it is likely that the motor system has only limited access to the belief/desire system and that this access is typically mediated by P-intentions. I can have mistaken beliefs about the pattern of muscular contractions involved in my raising my arm, but when I raise my arm the motor system does not exploit this belief to produce some weird gesticulation.

A second feature of the motor system is its limited cognitive penetrability. Conscious access to the contents of our motor representations is limited. The motor system does not seem to fall squarely on either side of the divide between the personal and the subpersonal. Some aspects of its operation are consciously accessible; others do not seem to be. Several studies (Jeannerod 1994; Decety and Michel 1989; Decety et al. 1993; Decety et al. 1994) have shown that we are aware of selecting and controlling our actions and that we are capable of imagining ourselves acting. Moreover, the awareness we have of the movements we intend to perform is not based solely on the exploitation of sensory reafferences, because paralyzed subjects can have the experience of acting. However, other studies indicate that we are not aware of the precise details of the motor commands that are used to generate our actions, or of the way immediate sensory information is used for the fine-tuning of those commands (Fourneret and Jeannerod 1998). For instance, several pointing experiments (Goodale et al. 1986; Castiello et al. 1991) have shown that subjects can point a finger at a target accurately even on trials where the target is suddenly displaced by several degrees and they have to adjust their trajectories. Moreover, they can do so while remaining completely unaware both of the displacement of the target and of their own corrections. One series of experiments (Pisella et al. 1998) is especially instructive. In one condition, a green target was initially presented and subjects were requested to point at it at instructed rates. On some trials the visual target was altered at the time of movement onset. It could jump to a new location, change color, or both. Subjects were instructed to point to the new location when the target simply jumped, but to interrupt their ongoing movement when the target changed color or when it both changed color and jumped. The results showed that when the target changed both color and position in a time window of about 200–290 milliseconds, the subjects would point at the displaced target instead of interrupting their ongoing movement. The very fast in-flight movement corrections made by the visuo-motor system seem to escape conscious voluntary control. According to the explanatory scheme proposed here, this experiment may be interpreted as showing that M-intentions have dynamics of their own, which are not entirely under the control of P-intentions.

These kinds of experiments also illustrate the fact that P-intentions and M-intentions operate at different time scales. The type of control exercised by P-intentions is, as we have seen, both rational and conscious. Temporal constraints on conscious processes set a minimal temporal threshold for information to become consciously accessible. The experiments of Pisella et al. illustrate that there is at least some incompatibility between the temporal constraints the motor system must satisfy to perform smooth online corrections and adjustments of an action and the temporal constraints on conscious awareness.

4   General Dynamics of Intentions

I distinguished earlier between two levels of dynamics: the local or micro-level dynamics specific to each type of intention and the global or macro-level dynamics of the transition from F-intentions to P-intentions and M-intentions. Some characteristics of the macro-level dynamics can easily be inferred from what was said of the local dynamics of each type of intention. In particular, the global dynamics of the transition from F-intentions to P-intentions and M-intentions involve transformation of the contents of these respective intentions. We move from contents involving descriptive concepts to contents involving demonstrative and indexical concepts, and from there to sensori-motor contents. This transformation also involves a greater specification of the intended action. Many aspects of the action that were initially left indeterminate are specified at the level of the P-intention and further specified at the level of the M-intention.

Yet one may want to know what it is that ensures the unity of the intentional cascade from F-intentions to P-intentions and to M-intentions if their respective contents differ. In a nutshell, the answer is that what ensures this unity is the fact that each intention inherits its goal from its predecessor in the cascade. However, such an answer may seem to raise a question: If the mode of presentation (MP) of the goal differs from one level of intention to the next, in what sense can we talk of an identity of goal? Suppose my F-intention is to get rid of the armchair I inherited from my uncle. A conversion of this F-intention into a corresponding P-intention requires (among other things) a transformation of the purely descriptive MP of this target object into a perceptual MP. But one problem is that being inherited from one's uncle is not an observational property. At the level of the P-intention, the target object of the action will have to be recaptured under a different MP—for instance, as the red armchair next to the fireplace. Similar problems will arise when moving from P-intentions to M-intentions where goals are encoded in sensory-motor terms.

To ensure the unity of the intentional cascade, the transformation of the MPs of the action goal must be rule-governed. By a rule-governed transformation, I mean a transformation of MPs that exploits certain identities. More precisely, if we consider the transition from an F-intention to a P-intention—a transition that is subject to strong rationality constraints—identities should not just be exploited, they should be recognized as such by the agent. For instance, it is because I judge that the armchair I inherited from my uncle is the same object as the red armchair next to the fireplace that the unity of my F-intention to get rid of the armchair I inherited from my uncle with my P-intention to get rid of the red armchair I visually perceive next to the fireplace is warranted. In contrast, when we consider the transition from P-intentions to M-intentions, it seems that certain identities are hardwired in the motor system and are, as a result, systematically exploited. For instance, in the experiment by Pisella et al. discussed earlier, the target to which the subject should point is identified both by its color and by its position. Information on color is processed by the system for semantical perception but is not directly accessible by the visuomotor system. Yet the visuomotor system can directly process information on position. When the subject is instructed to point to the green target, the transition from the P-intention to the M-intention exploits the following identity: the green target = the target located at p. In other words, the P-intention to point to the green target unless it changes color gets transformed into an M-intention to point to the target located at p. At the motor level, the movement will be controlled by the position of the target and not its color, and it will be automatically adjusted in response to a change of position.

What I have said so far about the dynamics of the three types of intentions in no way implies that all actions require the presence of the entire intentional cascade. Some decisions to act are made on the fly and do not warrant a distinction between an F-intention and a P-intention. If a colleague knocks at my office door around noon and asks me if I want to join him for lunch now, I may just say Yes and follow him to the cafeteria. I may deliberate for a minute: Am I really hungry? Is the thing I am doing now really so urgent that I should get over with it before going for lunch? But once I have made up my mind, I immediately start acting. In such cases, there is not really room for a distinction between an F-intention and a P-intention.

The existence of automatic, spontaneous, or routine actions suggests that it is not even always necessary that I form a P-intention in order to start acting. When, while trying to make sense of some convoluted sentence I am reading, I automatically reach for my pack of cigarettes, my action seems to be triggered by the affordances offered by the pack of cigarettes and need not be controlled by a P-intention. It is interesting to note that even when a certain action happens to be controlled by a P-intention, it is not necessarily this P-intention that triggered the action. If I am a heavy smoker and am completely absorbed by some philosophical argument I am trying to unravel, I can take a cigarette and light it without even noticing what I am doing. If, while this action unfolds, I become aware of what I am doing, I may decide whether or not I should go on with the action. If I decide to carry on, the action that had been initially triggered by an M-intention is now also controlled by a P-intention. Finally, it should be noted that P-intentions can have varying degrees of control on the unfolding of an action. Well-practiced actions require little online control by P-intentions. In contrast, novel or difficult actions are typically much more closely controlled by P-intentions.

5   Conscious Agency

I now turn to the problems of conscious agency and the bearing the dynamic theory of intentions presented here may have on them. Let me start by distinguishing three issues. The first issue is concerned with the phenomenology of action, understood as the experience of acting one may have at the time one is acting. The second issue concerns mental causation, i.e. whether or not mental states play a causal role in the production of actions. The third issue concerns the phenomenology of mental causation, or (to use Wegner's phrase) the experience of the conscious will, conceived as the experience we have that our actions are caused and controlled by our conscious states. The latter two issues are often confused, with the unfortunate consequence that evidence that experiences of mental causation are sometimes non-veridical is taken as evidence that the very notion of mental causation is mistaken. Similarly, the phenomenology of action in the sense outlined above should not be confused with the phenomenology of mental causation. One's awareness that one is acting is not the same thing as one's awareness that one's action is caused by one's conscious mental states. The experience of acting may well be an ingredient in the experience of mental causation, but it is not all there is to it. I will first try to provide an analysis of the experience of acting. I will then turn to the issue of mental causation and argue that Libet's experiments provide no conclusive reasons to think that mental causation is generally illusory. Finally, I will move on to the phenomenology of mental causation and argue that Wegner's experiments are similarly inconclusive in ruling out actual mental causation.

As was mentioned above, one objection to the earlier belief/desire versions of CTA was that they failed to account for the phenomenology of action. Their central claim is that what distinguishes actions from other events is the nature of their mental antecedents, namely complexes of beliefs and desires. An agent would know that she is performing an action not in virtue of her immediate awareness that she is moving, but because she knows what the antecedent conditions causing her behavior are. Such an inferential approach seems unable to account for the specificity and the immediacy of the phenomenology of bodily action. One reason the phenomenology of action may have been neglected is that it is much less rich and salient than the phenomenology of perception. Typically, when we are acting, our attentional focus is on the outside world we are acting on rather than on the acting self. Our awareness of our active bodily involvement is only marginal. Typically also, the representational content of the experience of acting is relatively unspecific and elusive.

In the model proposed here, three types of intentions are distinguished. F-intentions, insofar as they are temporally separated from the action, make no direct contribution to the experience of acting, although they may contribute indirectly to a sense of personal continuity and to a temporally extended sense of one's agency. In contrast, P-intentions and M-intentions are simultaneous with the action they guide and control and hence are immediately relevant to the phenomenology of agency. Here I follow Wakefield and Dreyfus (1991) and distinguish between knowing what we are doing and knowing that we are acting. As they point out, "although at certain times during an action we may not know what we are doing, we do always seem to know during an action that we are acting, at least in the sense that we experience ourselves as acting rather than as being passively moved about" (p. 268). One may further distinguish between knowing what we are doing in the sense of being aware of the goal of our action (and its general form) and knowing it in the sense of being aware of our specific manner of bringing about this desired result. In the framework proposed here, this distinction between three aspects of the experience of acting—which may be termed *that-experience*, *what-experience*, and *how-experience*—may be accounted for as follows: On the one hand, it is P-intentions, through their role of rational and perceptual guidance and monitoring of the ongoing action, that are mainly responsible for what-experience. What-experience, that is, is awareness of the content of P-intentions. On the other hand, M-intentions are responsible for the most basic aspect of action phenomenology (that-experience) and for the most specific form it can take (how-experience). These two forms of the experience of acting nevertheless depend on rather different mechanisms.

As we have seen, motor control involves mechanisms of action anticipation and correction. According to recent neurocomputational models of motor control, motor control exploits internal models of action used to predict the effects of motor commands as well as comparators that detect mismatches between predicted effects, desired effects, and actual effects in order to make appropriate corrections. Although these mechanisms operate largely at the subpersonal level, in the sense that the representations they process are typically unavailable to consciousness, they may nevertheless underlie the experience of acting in its most basic form. In other words, our awareness that we are acting—the sense of bodily implication we experience—may result from the detection by the comparison mechanisms used in motor control of a coherent sensory-motor flow. On this view, the basic experience that one is acting need not involve conscious access to the contents of the motor and sensory representations used for the control of the ongoing action. That is why, as Wakefield and Dreyfus remark, we may experience ourselves as acting without knowing what it is exactly we are doing. This is also why the representational content of the experience of acting may appear so thin. This is especially so when one is engaged in what I termed minimal actions—actions that are performed routinely, automatically, impulsively, or unthinkingly. These actions unfold with little or no conscious control by P-intentions. Their phenomenology may therefore involve nothing more than the faint phenomenal echo arising from coherent sensory-motor flow.

In contrast, our awareness of the specific form our bodily implication in action takes—say, the exact trajectory of my arm, or the precise way I am shaping my hand—requires conscious access to the content of at least some of our current sensory-motor representations. It therefore requires that these normally unconscious representations be transformed into conscious ones. As Jeannerod (1994) points out, these representations are usually too short-lived to become accessible to consciousness. During execution, they are normally canceled out as soon as the corresponding movements have been performed. Converting them into conscious representations therefore requires that they be kept in short-term memory long enough to become available to consciousness. This can happen when the action is blocked or when it is delayed. To a degree, it also can happen through top-down attentional amplification.

In a series of experiments, Jeannerod and co-workers (Fourneret and Jeannerod 1998; Slachewsky et al. 2001) investigated subjects' awareness of their movements. Subjects were instructed to move a stylus with their unseen hand to a visual target. Only the trajectory of the stylus was visible as a line on a computer screen, super-imposed on the hand movement. A directional bias (to the right or to the left) was introduced electronically, such that the visible trajectory no longer corresponded to that of the hand, and the bias was increased from trial to trial. In order to reach the target, the hand-held stylus had to be moved in a direction opposite to the bias. In other words, although the line on the computer screen appeared to be directed to the target location, the hand movement was directed in a different direction. At the end of each trial, subjects were asked in which direction they thought their hand had moved by indicating the line corresponding to their estimated direction on a chart presenting lines oriented in different directions.

These experiments revealed several important things. Subjects accurately corrected for the bias in tracing a line that appeared visually to be directed to the target. When the bias was small, this resulted from an automatic adjustment of their hand movements in a direction opposite to the bias. Subjects tended to ignore the veridical trajectory of their hand in making a conscious judgment about the direction of their hand. Instead, they adhered to the direction seen on the screen and based their report on visual cues, thus ignoring non-visual (e.g., motor and proprioceptive) cues. However, when the bias exceeded a mean value of about 14°, subjects changed strategy and began to use conscious monitoring of their hand movement to correct for the bias and to reach the target. The general idea suggested by this result is that it is only when the discrepancy between the seen trajectory and the felt trajectory becomes too large to be automatically corrected that subjects become aware of it and use conscious compensation strategies. Thus, the experience of acting may become vivid and be endowed with detailed representational content only when action errors occur that are large enough that they can't be automatically corrected.[9]

With respect to the issues of mental causation and its phenomenology, the main conclusion to be drawn from this discussion of the experience of doing is that such an experience need not and indeed should not be thought of as the experience of one's conscious mental states causing one's actions. In its most basic form, exemplified in minimal actions, the experience of doing may reduce to the faint background buzz of that-experience. During the action, I am peripherally aware that I am acting rather than being acted upon. Minimal actions may be experienced as doings without being experienced as purposive, intended, or done for reasons. Something more than mere that-experience is required for an experience of mental causation. What-experience and how-experience may be further ingredients of the experience of mental causation by contributing a sense of purposiveness. But other factors may still be required as the experience of purposiveness may yet fail to qualify as an experience of mental causation.

Before I dwell further on this topic, let me be clear about what I think conscious mental causation is. First, the notion of a conscious state can be understood in at least two ways. We may want to say that a mental state is conscious if, in virtue of being in that state, the creature whose state it is is conscious of the object, property, or state of affairs the state represents or is about (first-order consciousness). Or we may want to say that a state is conscious if the creature whose state it is is conscious of being in that state, that is, has a representation of that state as a specific attitude of hers toward a certain content (second-order consciousness). Thus, an intention of mine will be conscious in the first of these two senses if I am conscious of the goal or means-goal relation the intention encodes (say, I raise my hand to catch a ball). For my intention to be conscious in the second sense, I must be aware of my intention as an intention of mine, where the state of awareness is distinct from the intention itself. I take it that the issue of mental causation is first and foremost concerned with whether or not conscious states understood in the first of these two senses are causally efficacious in the production of actions. Second, there is more to causation than the mere triggering of effects. Many other factors can contribute to shaping the effect triggered, and there are no good reasons to deny them the status of causal factors. Similarly, an effect is often not the result of a single causal event but the result of a chain of such events, and there is usually no good reason to single out the first element of the chain as the cause. To claim that something can only qualify as a cause if it is some sort of prime mover unmoved is to cling to a doubtful tenet of Aristotelian metaphysics. Third, in a naturalistic, non-dualistic framework, personal-level mental states are constituted or realized by complex physical states, and a personal-level account of behavior must be backed up by a subpersonal explanation of how mental causation works. Subpersonal and personal-level explanations are pitched at different levels of generality and should therefore be seen as complementary rather than mutually exclusive.

For the notion of conscious mental causation to be vindicated, two conditions must be satisfied. First, it must be the case that conscious mental states and conscious intentions (in the first-order sense) can be elements in the causal chain of information processing that translates beliefs, desires, and goals into motor behavior and effects in the world. Second, it must be the case that the causal chains that include such conscious states as elements have distinctive functional properties. The first condition may be taken as a necessary condition for conscious mental causation. If conscious intentions were always post hoc reconstructions, they would be effects of actions rather than causes thereof. Note, though, that for a conscious intention to qualify as a causal contributor to an action it is not necessary that it be the very first element in the causal chain leading to the performance of the action. The second condition may be taken as a sufficient condition for the causal efficacy of conscious mental states. If it makes a difference whether or not a causal chain contains conscious mental states as elements, in particular if there are differences in the kinds of actions that can be the outcome of such chains or in the conditions in which such actions can be successfully performed, then it is fair to say that conscious mental states make a difference and are causally efficacious.

With respect to the first condition, although there may be cases where conscious intentions are retrospective illusions, no one has ever offered convincing evidence for the claim that this is always the case. With respect to the second condition, there is plenty of evidence that automatic and non-automatic actions are not produced by the same mechanisms, that the performance of novel, difficult, complex or dangerous actions requires conscious guidance and monitoring,[10] and that recovery from error in certain circumstances is not possible unless one switches from automatic to consciously guided correction procedures.[11] In particular, the fact that the same action may sometimes be performed automatically and sometimes consciously does not show that conscious states are causally idle. When the circumstances are favorable, the performance goes smoothly, and no breakdown occurs, one may indeed be under the impression that appealing to conscious mental states adds nothing of value to an explanation of why the action unfolds as it does and is successfully completed. To better see the causal import of conscious mental states, one should reason counterfactually and ask what would have happened had something gone wrong, had unexpected events occurred, or had the world or our body not behaved as predicted. The distinction I introduced earlier between the rational guidance and monitoring exerted at the level of conscious P-intentions and the automatic guidance and monitoring exerted at the level of unconscious M-intentions was meant to capture the important difference in how automatic and non-automatic actions are produced. As I tried to make clear, each mode of guidance and monitoring has its specific strengths and limitations, linked to their respective representational formats, to their temporal dynamics, and to their modular or nonmodular character. Conscious guidance and monitoring in no way displaces the need for automatic motor guidance and monitoring. Indeed, because there are limits to how much of an action one can consciously monitor without interfering with its performance, conscious monitoring can be only partial, and we must tacitly rely in large part on automatic control processes. Thus, conscious and unconscious processes necessarily coexist and play complementary roles in the control of non-automatic actions. They are not separate parallel streams; rather, they interact in complex ways, with control being passed up (for instance, when action errors are too large to be automatically corrected and control is passed to conscious processes) and down (as when we consciously focus on one aspect of an action and delegate control over other aspects to automatic motor processes).

Many people have seen in Libet's famous studies on the "readiness potential" evidence that favors a skeptical attitude toward conscious mental causation. Libet et al. (1983) asked subjects to move a hand at will and to note when they felt the urge to move by observing the position of a dot on a special clock. While the participants were doing this, the experimenters recorded their readiness potential (the brain activity linked to the preparation of movement). What they found was that the onset of the readiness potential (RP) predated the conscious awareness of the urge to move (W) by about 350 ms, whereas the actual onset of movement measured in the muscles of the forearm occurred about 150 ms after conscious awareness. Libet (1985) and others have claimed that these results suggest that, since the conscious awareness of the urge to move occurs much later than the onset of the brain activity linked to the preparation of movement occur, the conscious urge to move plays no causal role in the production of the intentional arm movement.

There are serious reasons to doubt that these results warrant such a conclusion. First, the conscious urge to move may lag behind the onset of brain activity but it still precedes the actual onset of movement. As I mentioned earlier, there is no good reason to think that only the initial element in a causal chain may genuinely qualify as a cause. A conscious mental state may play a causal role in the production of an action even though it doesn't trigger the whole causal process. Besides, the unconscious processes that precede conscious awareness are not themselves uncaused, and by parity of reasoning Libet should also deny that they initiate the action. Second, as Mele (2003) points out, it is not clear whether the readiness potential constitutes the neural substrate of intentions or decisions rather than that of desires or urges. If the latter, it should indeed be expected to precede conscious intentions. Indeed, in a more recent experiment involving a task similar to Libet's, Haggard and Eimer (1999) showed that the readiness potential can be divided into two distinct phases: an early phase in which the readiness potential is equally distributed over both hemispheres (RP) and a latter phase in which it lateralizes, becoming larger contralateral to the hand that the subject will move. This second phase is known as the lateralized readiness potential (LRP). The first stage corresponds to a general preparation phase preceding movement selection, and a second with a specific preparation phase that generates the selected action. The data of Haggard and Eimer suggest that, whereas RP onset precedes the onset of conscious awareness, LRP onset coincides with conscious awareness and may constitute the neural correlate of the conscious decision to act. Third, Libet's analysis focuses on what I termed P-intentions and their relation to neural activity and neglects F-intentions. Yet his experiments involve F-intentions. The participants must at the very least have formed the F-intention to comply with the experimenter's instructions and to produce hand movements when they felt the urge. This F-intention has two uncommon features: it concerns a very simple hand action, of a kind one does not ordinarily need to plan for in advance, and, more strikingly, the initiation condition for the action takes a rather unusual form. Participants are asked to act at will or when they feel the urge, rather than when some external condition obtains. This could be achieved in at least two ways. The F-intention may cause it to be the case that the initiation condition is satisfied by generating an urge to move. Or, if such urges occur spontaneously on a more or less regular basis, the F-intention may direct attention toward them and initiate a process of attentional amplification. In either case, F-intentions are not causally inert. Haggard and Eimer's claim that the conscious intention to move one's hand coincides with the onset of LRP, the specific preparation phase that generates the selected action, is consistent with my claim that the content of a P-intention must be more specific than the content of a corresponding F-intention—it represents a specific act-token, e.g. that this hand move in such and such a way, rather than an action type. Finally, because the action the participants were requested to perform was such a simple and well-rehearsed element of their motor repertoire, it required little or no conscious planning and control. It is therefore not surprising that conscious awareness arises, on average, only 200 ms before onset of movement. My bet is that for more complex or less familiar actions more time should elapse between onset of awareness and onset of movement.

Let me now turn to the third and last issue: the phenomenology of conscious mental causation, or, as Wegner calls it, the experience of conscious will. Some of Wegner's experiments suggest that the experience of conscious will can be non-veridical. For instance, in his I-spy experiment (Wegner and Wheatley 1999), a participant and a confederate have joint control of a computer mouse that can be moved over any one of a number of pictures on a screen. When participants had been primed with the name of an item on which the mouse landed, they showed a slightly increased tendency to self-attribute the action of stopping on that object (when in fact the stop had been forced by the confederate). In other words, they experienced conscious will for an action they had not actually controlled. Some authors, including Wegner himself on occasion,[12] seem to think that the fact that the experience of conscious will can be non-veridical is evidence for the claim that conscious mental causation is an illusion. This inference appears less than compelling. To show that the experience of willing is not always errorless is certainly not to show that it is always in error.

It has long been recognized that, although we can be aware of the contents of our thoughts, we have little or no direct conscious access to the mental processes these thoughts are involved in.[13] Mental processes, in other words, are not phenomenally transparent. Wegner may well be right that the experience of conscious will is typically not a direct phenomenal readout of our mental processes and must be theoretically mediated. In his view, the experience of consciously willing our actions seems to arise primarily when we believe that our thoughts have caused our actions. For this to happen, "the thought should be consistent with the action, occur just before the action, and not be accompanied by other potential causes" (Wegner 2003, p. 3). Bayne (this volume) raises doubts as to whether, as Wegner's model suggests, a mere match between thought and action suffices to generate the experience of conscious will. Bayne suggests that it may further be required that one be aware of the prior state as one's own. It may also be required that one identifies this state as a state of intention. As I mentioned earlier, a state may be conscious in the sense that one is conscious of its content without being conscious in the sense that one is conscious of being in that state. While acting, one should normally be expected to attend to the world in which one is acting, rather than to one's state of intending. Intentions may therefore be conscious in the first sense but not being conscious in the second. One's conscious intentions (in the first sense) may therefore cause an action without one having an experience of conscious will. One may simply have an experience of doing while performing the action caused by the conscious intention. Thus, conscious F-intentions or P-intentions may well play a role in the production of an action without this action giving rise to an experience of conscious will if the agent is focusing on the situation of action rather than on his or her mental states and thus is not conscious of these F-intentions and P-intentions as states of intention she is in.

Moreover, our second-order awareness of our first-order conscious states, understood as the awareness of one's attitude toward a certain content, may well be inferentially mediated and fallible. We may be mistaken in identifying a first-order conscious state as a state of intention rather than, say, as a mere thought. For instance, as Bayne suggests, we may identify a prior thought as an intention because its content is consistent with an action performed in its wake. We can therefore have a non-veridical experience of conscious will, when a conscious thought that is not a conscious intention is mistaken for one. This seems to be what is happening in Wegner's I-spy experiment.

Yet it is not certain that the participants in this experiment would have had an experience of conscious will, veridical or non-veridical, simply in virtue of a correspondence between their consciously experienced prior thought and the target action and of a misidentification of this prior thought as an intention. One further element that may be necessary is an experience of doing. As I argued earlier, this experience can be very unspecific and reduce to a that-experience. Of course, the veridicality of an experience of doing does not guarantee the veridicality of the experience of conscious will of which it may be a component. The participants in the I-spy experiment who were tricked into thinking that they were responsible for stopping the cursor on a certain item were wrong about that but were at least right that they had been acting. Had they not been acting at all, it is not clear whether they would have had an experience of conscious will. There are therefore several reasons why experiences of conscious will and actual mental causation may fail to coincide. Conscious intentions may be causally efficacious without giving rise to an experience of conscious will and an experience of conscious will may be present where conscious intentions are not causally involved. The dynamic theory of intentions I have sketched certainly leaves both possibilities open. Yet, as we have independent reasons to think that conscious intentions (in the first-order sense) are causally efficacious in the production of actions and no good reasons to think that our second-order awareness of intentions is always or most of the time the result of a misidentification of mere thoughts with actual intentions, we can, I think, remain confident that the experience of conscious will is a reliable indicator of actual mental causation.

Notes

1. For more detailed analyses of the difficulties and shortcomings of the belief/desire versions of CTA and for an evaluation of some of the proposals made by dual-intention theorists, see Pacherie 2000 and Pacherie 2003.

2. Note that here by completion I simply mean the end of the action process, whether the action is successful or not.

3. Buekens, Maesen, and Vanmechelen (2001) are to my knowledge the only authors who distinguish three categories of intentions. They call them future-directed intentions, action-initiating intentions and action-sustaining intentions, respectively. However, their typology differs from the typology presented here. Their action-initiating intention corresponds to the upstream phase of the dynamics of P-intention and their action-sustaining intention to its downstream phase. Another difference between their scheme and mine is that they make no room for motor intentions. They are also perfectly explicit that they are concerned with personal-level phenomena and that both action-initiating intentions and action-sustaining intentions present the action to the agent via observation and not experience. These authors defend two very interesting claims to which I fully subscribe. The first is that the content of 'action-sustaining intentions' is essentially indexical and action-dependent; the second is that the control these intentions have over the action is concerned not just with the way in which the intended goal is accomplished but also with the side effects generated by this way of accomplishing this goal.

4. For a review and synthesis of recent work in the cognitive neuroscience of action, see Jeannerod 1997.

5. This of course does not mean that the two systems do not interact in some ways. For discussions of these interactions, see Milner and Goodale 1995; Rossetti and Revonsuo 2000; Jacob and Jeannerod 2003.

6. On neurocomputational approaches to motor control, see Wolpert 1997; Jordan and Wolpert 1999; Wolpert and Ghahramani 2000.

7. This is an oversimplification insofar as there exist complex internal loops between inverse models and predictive models. In practice, it is therefore difficult, if not impossible, to draw the line between guidance and control.

8. Regarding this latter case, caution is required however, first because the interpretation of the various experiments reporting such data is still a matter of debate (Aglioti et al. 1995; Gentilucci et al. 1996; Haffenden and Goodale 1998; Jacob and Jeannerod 2003) and second because the experiments that have been conducted also suggest that illusory perceptions can influence action when a delay is introduced between the sensory stimulation and the action.

9. For further discussion of these issues, see Jeannerod and Pacherie 2004.

10. Here it may be useful to introduce Block's conceptual distinction between phenomenal consciousness and access-consciousness, where the former refers to the experiential properties of consciousness, for instance what differs between experiences of green and red, and the latter to its functional properties, access-conscious content being content made available to the global workspace and thus for use in reasoning, planning, and verbal report (Block 1995). When one speaks of conscious guidance or monitoring, it is the notion of access-consciousness that is, at least primarily, at stake. Block himself think that phenomenal consciousness and access-consciousness are dissociable, hence independent, thus leaving open the possibility that phenomenal consciousness is causally idle. Others, however, have argued that phenomenal consciousness provides a basis for wide availability to the cognitive system and is thus a precondition of access-consciousness (Kriegel, forthcoming).

11. See, for instance, Shallice 1988; Jeannerod 1997.

12. See, for instance, Wegner 2002, p. 342; Wegner 2003, p. 261. See also Libet 2004; Pockett 2004.

13. See, e.g., Nisbett and Wilson 1977.

References

Aglioti, S., DeSouza, J. F. X., and Goodale, M. A. 1995. Size-contrast illusions deceive the eye, but not the hand. *Current Biology* 5: 679–685.

Bach, K. 1978. A representational theory of action. *Philosophical Studies* 34: 361–379.

Block, N. 1995. On a confusion about a function of consciousness. *Behavioral and Brain Sciences* 18: 227–247.

Brand, M. 1984. *Intending and Acting*. MIT Press.

Bratman, M. E. 1987. *Intention, Plans, and Practical Reason*. Cambridge University Press.

Buekens, F., Maesen, K., and Vanmechelen, X. 2001. Indexicaliteit en dynamische intenties. *Algemeen Nederlands Tijdschrift voor Wijsbegeert* 93: 165–180.

Castiello, U., Paulignan, Y., and Jeannerod, M. 1991. Temporal dissociation of motor responses and subjective awareness: A study in normal subjects. *Brain* 114: 2639–2655.

Davidson, D. 1980. *Essays on Actions and Events*. Oxford University Press.

Decety, J., and Michel, F. 1989. Comparative analysis of actual and mental movement times in two graphic tasks. *Brain and Cognition* 11: 87–97.

Decety, J., Jeannerod, M., Durozard, D., and Baverel, G. 1993. Central activation of autonomic effectors during mental simulation of motor actions. *Journal of Physiology* 461: 549–563.

Decety, J., Perani, D., Jeannerod, M., Bettinardi, V., Tadary, B., Woods, R., Mazziotta, J. C., and Fazio, F. 1994. Mapping motor representations with PET. *Nature* 371: 600–602.

Fodor, J. A. 1983. *The Modularity of Mind*. MIT Press.

Fourneret, P., and Jeannerod, M. 1998. Limited conscious monitoring of motor performance in normal subjects. *Neurospychologia* 36: 1133–1140.

Gentilucci, M., Chiefffi, S., Daprati, E., Saetti, M. C., and Toni, I. 1996. Visual illusion and action. *Neuropsychologia* 34: 369–376.

Goldman, A. 1970. *A Theory of Human Action*. Prentice-Hall.

Goodale, M. A., Pélisson, D., and Prablanc, C. 1986. Large adjustments in visually guided reaching do not depend on vision of the hand or perception of target displacement. *Nature* 320: 748–750.

Grèzes, J., and Decety, J. 2002. Does visual perception afford action? Evidence from a neuroimaging study. *Neuropsychologia* 40: 1597–1607.

Haffenden, A. M., and Goodale, M. A. 1998. The effect of pictorial illusion on perception and prehension. *Journal of Cognitive Neuroscience* 10: 122–136.

Haggard, P., and Eimer, M. 1999. On the relation between brain potentials and the awareness of voluntary movements. *Experimental Brain Research* 126: 128–133.

Jacob, P., and Jeannerod, M. 2003. *Ways of Seeing: The Scope and Limits of Visual Cognition*. Oxford University Press.

Jeannerod, M., and Pacherie, E. 2004. Agency, simulation and self-identification. *Mind and Language* 19, no. 2: 113–146.

Jeannerod, M. 1994. The representing brain: Neural correlates of motor intention and imagery. *Behavioral and Brain Sciences* 17: 187–246.

Jeannerod, M. 1997. *The Cognitive Neuroscience of Action*. Blackwell.

Jordan, M. I., and Wolpert, D. M. 1999. Computational motor control. In *The Cognitive Neurosciences*, ed. M. Gazzaniga. MIT Press.

Kriegel, U. Forthcoming. The concept of consciousness in the cognitive sciences. In *Handbook of Philosophy of Psychology and Cognitive Science*, ed. P. Thagard. Elsevier.

Libet, B. 1985. Unconscious cerebral initiative and the role of conscious will in voluntary action. *Behavioral and Brain Sciences* 8: 529–566.

Libet, B. 2004. *Mind Time*. Harvard University Press.

Libet, B., Gleason, C. A., Wright, E. W., and Pearl, D. K. 1983. Time of conscious intention to act in relation to onset of cerebral activities (readiness potential): The unconscious initiation of a freely voluntary act. *Brain* 106: 623–642.

Mele, A. R. 1992. *Springs of Action*. Oxford University Press.

Mele, A. R. 2003. *Motivation and Agency*. Oxford University Press.

Milner, A. D., and Goodale, M. A. 1995. *The Visual Brain in Action*. Oxford University Press.

Nisbett, R. E., and Wilson, T. D. 1977. Telling more than we can know: Verbal reports on mental processes. *Psychological Review* 84: 231–259.

Pacherie, E. 2000. The content of intentions. *Mind and Language* 15, no. 4: 400–432.

Pacherie, E. 2003. La dynamique des intentions. *Dialogue* 42: 447–480.

Pisella, L., Arzi, M., and Rossetti, Y. 1998. The timing of color and location processing in the motor context. *Experimental Brain Research* 121: 270–276.

Pockett, S. 2004. Does consciousness cause behaviour? *Journal of Consciousness Studies* 11, no. 2: 23–40.

Rossetti, Y., and Revonsuo, A., eds. 2000. *Beyond Dissociation: Interaction between Dissociated Implicit and Explicit Processing*. John Benjamins.

Searle, J. 1983. *Intentionality*. Cambridge University Press.

Shallice, T. 1988. *From Neuropsychology to Mental Structure*. Cambridge University Press.

Slachewsky, A., Pillon, B., Fourneret, P. Pradat-Diehl, Jeannerod, M., and Dubois, B. 2001. Preserved adjustment but impaired awareness in a sensory-motor conflict following prefrontal lesions. *Journal of Cognitive Neuroscience* 13: 332–340.

Tucker, M., and Ellis, R. 1998. On the relations between seen objects and components of potential actions. *Journal of Experimental Psychology: Human Perception and Performance* 24: 830–846.

Wakefield, J., and Dreyfus, H. 1991. Intentionality and the phenomenology of action. In *John Searle and His Critics*, ed. E. Lepore and R. Van Gulick. Blackwell.

Wegner, D. M. 2002. *The Illusion of Conscious Will*. MIT Press.

Wegner, D. M. 2003. The mind's self-portrait. *Annals of the New-York Academy of Sciences* 1001: 1–14.

Wegner, D. M., and Wheatley, T. 1999. Apparent mental causation: Sources of the experience of will. *American Psychologist* 54: 480–492.

Wolpert, D. M., and Ghahramani, Z. 2000. Computational principles of movement neuroscience. *Nature Neuroscience Supplement* 3: 1212–1217.

Wolpert, D. M. 1997. Computational approaches to motor control. *Trends in Cognitive Sciences* 1, no. 6: 209–216.

9 Phenomenology and the Feeling of Doing: Wegner on the Conscious Will

Timothy Bayne

Given its ubiquitous presence in everyday experience, it is surprising that the phenomenology of doing—the experience of being an agent—has received such scant attention in the consciousness literature. But things are starting to change, and a small but growing literature on the content and causes of the phenomenology of first-person agency is beginning to emerge.[1] One of the most influential and stimulating figures in this literature is Daniel Wegner. In a series of papers and in his book *The Illusion of Conscious Will* (henceforth cited as *ICW*), Wegner has developed an account of what he calls "the experience of conscious will." In this chapter I assess Wegner's model of the conscious will and the claims that he makes on the basis of it. Although my focus is on Wegner's work, many of the issues I raise are relevant to the study of the phenomenology of agency more generally.

I regard Wegner's work on the phenomenology of agency as comprising two components. First, Wegner provides a model of how the experience of conscious will is generated. Roughly speaking, Wegner's view is that we experience conscious will with respect to an action when we have an introspective preview of it:

The experience of consciously willing our actions seems to arise primarily when we believe our thoughts have caused our actions. This happens when we have thoughts that occur just before the actions, when these thoughts are consistent with the actions, and when other potential causes of the actions are not present. (2005, p. 23)

I will call this the *matching model* of the experience of conscious will. The second component of Wegner's account is his claim that the conscious will is an illusion. Exactly what Wegner might mean by describing the conscious will as an illusion is open to some debate (see section 3 below), but I take his central claim to be this: The experience of conscious will misrepresents the causal path by means of which one's own actions are generated.

How are the two components of Wegner's work related? The most straightforward way to read Wegner is to take him to be offering the matching model as *evidence* for the claim that the conscious will is an illusion. I will argue that if this is indeed Wegner's view then it is mistaken. The matching model might explain why people experience a sense of agency, but it does not show that this sense of agency is an illusion. I proceed as follows: In section 1, I explore the notion of the conscious will. In section 2, I examine Wegner's matching model of the conscious will. In sections 3 and 4, I turn my attention to his claim that the conscious will is an illusion.

1   What Is the Conscious Will?

The notion of the experience of conscious will is anything but straightforward, and there is ample room for terminological confusion in these waters. One issue concerns the relationship between the experience of conscious will and the will itself. It is natural to suppose that acts of the will are the intentional objects of experiences of conscious will. On this view, the logical relationship between experiencing oneself as willing something and actually willing it is akin to the relationship between, say, experiencing something as being blue and it actually being blue. The experience is one thing, the property or object experienced is another. Although much of what Wegner says can be read in these terms, there are passages in his work that suggest a very different conception of the relationship between experience of the will and the will itself. For example, Wegner states that "will is a feeling, not unlike happiness or sadness or anger or anxiety or disgust" (*ICW*, p. 326; see also pp. 3 and 29). Referring to the will as a feeling threatens to collapse the distinction between the will itself and experiences of the will.

A second issue concerns the representational content of the experience of conscious will. For the most part Wegner leaves the notion of the experience of conscious will at an intuitive level, often describing it simply as "the experience of doing." He does, however, link the experience of conscious will with various other aspects of the phenomenology of agency, such as the experience of *authorship* (Wegner 2005, p. 27), the experience of *intentionality* (Wegner and Erskine 2003, p. 688), the experience of *effort* (*ICW*, p. 39), the experience of experience of *free will* (*ICW*, p. 318), and the experience of *mental causation* (Wegner 2005, p. 23).

This terminological proliferation presents us with something of a challenge. Are these terms meant to be (rough) synonyms for a single type of experience, or are they meant to refer to distinct experiential types? Wegner does not tell us. One could of course stipulate that these terms are being used synonymously, but Wegner does not appear to have made this stipulation, and so we are left to rely on our pretheoretical grasp of these notions. Although recent writers on the phenomenology of agency often seem to assume that these terms are synonyms, it is far from obvious that this is the case.[2] Prima facie, at least some of these terms appear to refer to different experiential contents. To take just one contrast, the experience of authorship appears to differ from the experience of effort (Bayne and Levy 2006). But if these various terms refer to distinct types of experiences then it is entirely possible that the matching model might apply to some of them but not others. Furthermore, it might turn out that some of these experiential types are illusory but others are not.

Wegner appears to regard the experience of conscious will as most intimately associated with two kinds of experience: the experience of "mental causation" and the experience of authorship. Let me take these two notions in turn.

Wegner often refers to his account of the conscious will as "the theory of apparent mental causation." He writes: "Intentions that occur just prior to action . . . do seem to compel the action. This is the basic phenomenon of the experience of will." (*ICW*, p. 20) The view, I take it, is that an experience (as) of conscious will *just is* an experience (as) of one's intentions causing the action in question.[3] Frith has a similar view: "Our sense of being in control derives from the experience that our actions are caused by our intentions." (2002, p. 483)

But is there really such a thing as the experience of mental causation? To put the question slightly differently, does the *normal* phenomenology of agency include an experience of mental causation? The experience of being an agent is certainly imbued with a sense of intentionality and purposiveness—we experience ourselves as acting in light of our beliefs and desires and as realizing our intentions—but is this experience really *causal*? A number of authors have suggested that it is not (Horgan, Tienson, and Graham 2003; Searle 2001; Wakefield and Dreyfus 1991). We do not typically experience ourselves as being *caused* to move by our intentions. Arguably, if there is a causal component to the phenomenology of agency (and it is not clear to me that there is), it involves an experience of oneself, rather than one's mental states, as the cause of one's movements.[4] At any rate, the experience of will does not seem to involve an experience of one's intentions *compelling* one's actions. Leaving aside questions about whether the experience of "mental causation" is really causal, it is certainly true that it occupies a central place in the phenomenology of agency.

Consider now the experience of authorship. I am not sure whether Wegner thinks of the experience of authorship as identical to (or included within) the experience of conscious will, but he does suggest that the matching model of the experience of conscious will (also) functions as a model of the experience of authorship: "When the right timing, content, and context link our thought and our action, this construction yields a feeling of authorship of the action. It seems that we did it." (2005, p. 27)

What exactly *is* the feeling of authorship? The feeling of authorship, I take it, is the experience that you yourself are the agent or author of an event—the doer of the deed. The contrary of the feeling of authorship is the feeling that the event was done by someone else or had no agent as its source. But although it is helpful as an intuitive starting point, this gloss on the notion of authorship gets us only so far; we also need to know what the satisfaction conditions of experience of authorship are. What is it to author an action?

The quandaries that confront us here can be illustrated by considering Penfield actions (Penfield 1975). When Wilder Penfield directly stimulated the exposed brains of conscious patients, he triggered a variety of actions. But Penfield's patients reported that they did not "do" the action in question, and instead felt that Penfield had pulled it out of them. According to Wegner, Penfield actions show that it is possible to author an action without experiencing oneself as authoring it (*ICW*, p. 47). But should we accept that Penfield actions were authored by Penfield's patients? Perhaps they were authored by Penfield. Or perhaps they were not authored at all. More generally, there is a range of pathologies—utilization behavior, the anarchic hand syndrome, and hypnotically induced movement—where there is some obscurity about whether the subject in question stands in the authoring relation to the movement. But if we are in the dark as to when an action is authored then we are also in the dark as to when experiences of authorship are veridical, and, to the extent that the experience of conscious will includes the experience of authorship, we are also in the dark as to when the experience of conscious will is veridical.

The question of what Wegner might mean by "the experience of conscious will" is further complicated by the distinction between willed and unwilled actions (Jahanshahi and Frith 1998). Wegner himself invokes this distinction, often describing willed actions as "controlled" (or "voluntary") and unwilled actions as "automatic." The distinction between willed and unwilled actions is roughly the distinction between those actions that derive from the agent's plans and goals and those actions that are stimulus-driven. (I say "roughly" because at times the distinction between controlled and automatic actions seems to involve the rather different distinction between those actions that are accompanied by a sense of doing and those that are not.) Given the distinction between willed and automatic action, one might wonder whether Wegner is using "the experience of conscious will" to refer to an experience of the target action as willed rather than automatic. But this cannot be what Wegner has in mind. On this reading, the claim that the experience of conscious will is an illusion would amount to the claim that there are no willed (plan-driven) actions—all actions are automatic. Not only is this an implausible reading on its own terms, it also runs counter to Wegner's own work on the phenomenon of mental control. Just how the experience of conscious will might be related to the distinction between controlled and automatic actions is, I think, something of an open question.

We have seen that Wegner draws a close connection between the experience of conscious will and the experiences of mental causation and authorship. This gives us an intuitive grip on what the experience of conscious will might be, but it also raises unresolved questions. Not only are there questions about exactly how the experiences of mental and mental causation are related to the experience of conscious will (and to each other), there are also questions about how the experiences of mental causation and authorship should themselves be understood. Much more could be said here, but I turn now to Wegner's account of how the experience of conscious will might be produced.

2 The Matching Model

According to Wegner's matching model, "the experience of consciously willing our actions seems to arise primarily when we believe our thoughts have caused our actions. This happens when we have thoughts that occur just before the actions, when these thoughts are consistent with the actions, and when other potential causes of the actions are not present." (Wegner 2005, p. 23) Three questions can be raised here: What kind of thoughts are involved in generating the experience of will? What kind of consistency is needed between the target thoughts and the target actions? How is the presence of "other potential causes of the action" incorporated into the model? Let me take these questions in turn.

Matching models can be pitched at a number of explanatory levels. Some are *sub-personal*; that is, the target thoughts are not full-fledged mental states, such as beliefs or intentions, but sub-personal states, such as motor commands (Blakemore and Frith 2003; Haggard and Johnson 2003). Other matching models are pitched at a *personal* level, where it is a match between the agent's beliefs about what they are doing (or their intentions to do such-and-such) and their awareness of what they are doing that generates the experience of agency. Wegner's model operates at a personal level of explanation. He says that the experience of conscious will is generated when the prior thought appears in consciousness, which suggests that the conscious will is generated by full-blown mental states of the person—intentions, presumably—rather than sub-personal states of the motor system (2003b, p. 67).

But what exactly is the relationship between the awareness of a match between one's intentions and one's actions (on the one hand) and the experience of doing? Consider the following thought experiment, inspired by Davidson (1973): Chloe wants to rid herself of the weight and danger of holding another climber on a rope, and she knows that by loosening her hold on the rope she could satisfy this desire. This belief and this want lead her to form the intention to loosen her hold on the rope, but before she has the chance to act on this intention the contemplation of it so unnerves her that she loses her grip on the rope and the climber she is holding falls to his death. Chloe might experience the loosening of her hold as caused by her intention to loosen her hold, but she does not experience the loosening of her hold as an action—she does not experience this event as something that she does.

The case of Chloe the climber appears to show that one can experience one's movements as caused by (and realizing) one's intentions without experiencing a sense of agency toward them. It seems that the experience of doing cannot be generated simply by an awareness of a match between one's intentions and one's movements. Something more is needed. What might that be?

There are a number of ways in which one might respond to the case of Chloe. I have space here to examine just one line of response. Perhaps Chloe fails to experience a sense of agency with respect to her movements because she is not aware of them as implementing *fine-grained* intentions. Chloe experiences herself as having an intention to let go of the rope, but she is not aware of herself as having an intention to let go of the rope *in any particular way*. But note that this response incurs a certain cost. It suggests a model of the feeling of doing on which this feeling depends on awareness of *movement*-directed intentions, rather than an awareness of *goal*-directed intentions. And it is doubtful that we are normally conscious of having movement-direct intentions. We are normally aware of the goals of our actions, but we are not normally aware of how we intend to move our body in order to realize those goals.[5] So the proponent of Wegner's matching model might want to explore other responses to the case of Chloe the climber.

What light do Wegner's experiments shed on the nature of target thoughts?[6] Consider the I-Spy experiment of Wegner and Wheatley (1999), in which participants and an experimental confederate had joint control of a computer mouse that could be moved over any one of a number of pictures on a board (e.g., a swan). When participants had been primed with the name of the picture on which the mouse landed they showed a slightly increased tendency to self-attribute the action even when the landing was guided by the confederate and not by the participant. Did the subjects in this experiment experience themselves as having the intention to land on the primed object, as some of Wegner's commentators have suggested (Blakemore and Frith 2003, p. 220)? I see no reason to think that this was the case.[7] Rather than assume that participants formed an intention to land on the swan, it seems to me, one need suppose only that their representation of swans was activated.

Wegner's automatic typing priming experiment (2003a) also points toward an account of the experience of conscious will that need not involve intentions. Participants in this experiment were primed with various words (e.g. 'deer'), then required to type letters randomly without seeing the computer screen. They were then asked to rate a series of words, none of which they had actually written, according to the degree to which they felt they had authored them. Wegner and colleagues found that participants were more likely to judge that they had authored the presented word when it had been a prime than when it had not been a prime. Again, this experiment suggests that one can experience a sense of agency (at least retrospectively) without experiencing oneself as having (had) an intention to perform the action. Presumably the subjects experienced a sense of agency because they had had thoughts with content that had some semantic connection with the action.[8]

But there is, I suspect, a good reason why Wegner presents his model in terms of matches between intentions and actions. We know what it is for an intention to match an action: An intention matches an action when and only when the action realizes (satisfies) the intention. It is less clear what it is for "thoughts" that consist merely of heightened activation of certain concepts to match an action. Perhaps the natural thing to say here is that a semantic activation matches an action when they have common content. But this, of course, won't do as an account of the phenomenology of agency. Consider someone who experiences himself as intending not to have a hamburger for lunch, only to find his hands reaching for a juicy hamburger. Despite common semantic content between the intention and the target action, the person's actions are unlikely to be accompanied by the feeling of doing. In short, by moving away from a conception of target thoughts as intentions we problematize the matching component of the matching model.

Finally, let me turn to the "exclusivity condition"—the claim that the experience of conscious will is heightened when other potential causes of the actions are not present. Wegner includes the exclusivity condition in order to account of the finding that experiences of authorship can be modulated by the awareness of rival causes of agency (Wegner 2003a, p. 5f.). But there is also something puzzling about including the exclusivity condition in the basic model of how the experience of consciousness will is generated, for in order to apply the exclusion condition an agent must already know whether or not someone (or something) else is a potential cause of the action in question. Consider a schizophrenic suffering from delusions of control who reports that God (or the government, or the Devil) is causing him to raise his hand. Why does this person regard these (unobservable) agents as potential causes of his movements, and why does he regard them as exercising this potentiality on this particular occasion? This, it seems to me, is the really difficult question for accounts of the phenomenology of agency. Normally, of course, we do not regard God, the government, or the Devil as a potential cause of our movements. (And if, like Malebranche, we do regard these agents as potential causes of our movements, this does not undermine our experience of authorship.) All the heavy lifting appears to be done by an account of those systems responsible for identifying an entity as a potential cause of one's movements and by the principles by means of which we regard one agent as a more plausible cause of our actions than another. Of course, it is no criticism of Wegner that he fails to provide such an account, but insofar as these questions go unanswered any model of authorship-processing will be incomplete.

3 What Is Illusory about the Experience of Conscious Will?

Wegner's work suggests more than one reading of the claim that the conscious will is an illusion.[9] Consider the following passage:

We often consciously will our own actions. This experience is so profound that it tempts us to believe that our actions are caused by consciousness. It could also be a trick, however—the mind's way of estimating its own apparent authorship by drawing causal inferences about relationships between thoughts and actions. Cognitive, social and neuropsychological studies of apparent mental causation suggest that experiences of conscious will frequently depart from actual causal processes and so might not reflect direct perceptions of conscious thought causing action. (2003b, p. 65)

This passage seems to contain three ideas: (1) We experience our actions as caused by consciousness, but this experience is non-veridical (misleading). (2) We have a mistaken model of how experiences of conscious will are generated: We think that they are based on direct perception of their objects, but they are in fact theoretically mediated. (3) Experiences of conscious will are often non-veridical. The first two of these ideas can be dealt with fairly quickly; the third will prove more troublesome.

Do We Experience Our Actions as Caused by Consciousness?

Do we believe that our own actions are caused by consciousness? The first thing to ask here is "Consciousness *of what*?" Wegner appears to have consciousness of agency in mind. For example, he says that although we believe that our experiences of conscious will cause our actions, they do not (*ICW*, p. 318). Do we believe that experiences of conscious will cause our actions? More precisely, do we believe that the experience of consciously willing an action causes the movement (or action) that is the target of that experience? Some people appear to believe this. Searle says that it is part of the intentional content of an experience of acting that the experience itself causes the bodily movement in question (1983, p. 124; see also pp. 88, 95). I do not share Searle's view. It does not seem to me that my experience of raising my hand causes my hand to go up (or causes me to raise my hand). I might experience my hand as rising in virtue of my intention to raise it, but I do not experience my hand as rising in virtue of my *experience* of my intention to raise it. (Nor do I experience it as rising in virtue of my having an experience of agency directed toward its motion.)

Note that nothing in what I have just said involves a commitment to the view that consciousness is epiphenomenal. (Nor, of course, does it involve a rejection of epiphenomenalism!) To deny that experiences of agency bring about their target actions is not to deny that experiences of agency are causally efficacious—indeed, it is not even to deny that we experience experiences of agency as causally efficacious. It is perfectly possible that experiences of agency play various causal roles—such as generating beliefs about what we are doing. The point is that they do not cause those movements that are their intentional objects; or at least, if they do, we do not experience them as doing so.

The Experience of the Will as Theoretically Mediated

A second reason Wegner gives for regarding experiences of conscious will as illusory is that they are theoretically mediated: "[Conscious will is an illusion] in the sense that the experience of consciously willing an action is not the direct indication that the conscious thought has caused the action." (*ICW*, p. 2) It is not clear to me what "direct indication" might mean in this context. One possibility is that a direct-indication view of the phenomenology of agency involves thinking that one's experiences of (and beliefs about) one's own agency involve no sub-personal processing or inferential mechanisms of any kind. I suppose that some folk might hold such a view of the phenomenology of (first-person) agency, but I do not know of anyone who does, and I do not know of any reason for thinking that this view is plausible. More to the point, I do not know of any reason for thinking that experiences of agency could be reliable only if the direct-indication theory were true. The rejection of direct-indication views of visual perception has not led theorists to reject visual experiences as illusory, nor should it have. I don't see why the rejection of direct-indication accounts of the phenomenology of agency should lead us to reject the phenomenology of agency as an illusion.

4 The Conscious Will as Non-Veridical

I turn now to the third and, I think, central sense in which Wegner thinks of the conscious will as an illusion. On this view, the conscious will is an illusion in the sense that experiences of doing are systematically, or at least often, *non-veridical*: Experiences of doing misrepresent our agency and the structure of our actions. I detect two lines of argument in Wegner's work for this thesis. The main argument involves dissociations between the phenomenology of agency and the exercise of agency. A subsidiary argument involves an appeal to eliminativism.

The Dissociation Argument

The Illusion of Conscious Will contains extensive discussion of dissociations between the exercise of agency and the phenomenology of agency. Some of these cases appear to demonstrate that we can experience ourselves as doing something that someone else is doing (and that we are not doing). Wegner calls such cases *illusions of control*. The I-Spy experiment is an example of an illusion of control. Other dissociations involve experiencing someone (or something) else as the agent of what one is doing. Wegner calls such phenomena *illusions of action projection*. Among the most fascinating of the various illusions of action projection that he discusses is facilitated communication, a practice that was introduced as a technique for helping individuals with severe speech disorders. Facilitators would rest their hands on the hands of their clients as the clients typed messages. Although the facilitators experienced no sense of authorship of the typed messages, there is ample evidence that the contents of "facilitated" messages derived from the facilitators rather than the clients (Felce 1994; Jacobson, Mulick, and Schwartz 1995; Wegner, Fuller, and Sparrow 2003).

Although these dissociations clearly play an important role in Wegner's argument for the illusory nature of the conscious will, it is possible to provide different interpretations of that role. On one reading Wegner is mounting an inductive generalization: Since some experiences of conscious will are non-veridical it is reasonable to infer that most such experiences—perhaps even all of them—are non-veridical.[10] The problem with this argument is obvious: The fact that experiences of agency *can* be non-veridical shows that the mechanisms responsible for generating such experiences are fallible, but it does not show that they are unreliable.

Another way to read the argument from dissociations is as an inference to the best explanation.[11] The argument proceeds as follows: Since the phenomenology of agency plays no direct role in the genesis of action where such experiences are absent, we have good reason to think that it plays no direct role in the genesis of action when such experiences are present. This idea, I take it, lies behind the following claim: "If conscious will is illusory, automatisms are somehow the 'real thing,' fundamental mechanisms of mind that are left over once the illusion has been stripped away. Rather than conscious will being the rule and automatism the exception, the opposite may be true." (*ICW*, p. 143; see also p. 97).

I share Wegner's suspicion that automatisms may, in some sense, be "the real thing"—the "fundamental mechanisms of mind." But I don't share Wegner's view that this result would be inconsistent with the phenomenology of agency. Of course, much depends on what precisely it means to say that automatisms are the "fundamental mechanisms of mind." There may be a tension between automaticity and the experience of conscious will to the extent that automatisms are action-generation procedures that do not involve intentional states of any kind, but Wegner provides little evidence for the view that our actions are usually automatistic in *this* sense of the term. If, on the other hand, automatisms are action-generating procedures that are merely non-consciously initiated then there is ample reason to describe much of what we do as automatic in nature. But on this conception of an automatism there is, I claim, no conflict between automaticity and the feeling of doing. So there is no argument from automaticity (thus conceived) to the claim that the experience of conscious will is an illusion.

I do not deny that the phenomenology of agency *can* be illusory. Consider, for example, the experience of intentionality. An experience of intentionality will be non-veridical if the action in question is not guided by an intention, or if it is guided by an intention other than the one by which it seems to be guided. The phenomenon of confabulation suggests that at least one (if not both) of these conditions can occur. But I think there is little reason to assume that either kind of mistake is at all common in everyday life. Confabulation is striking precisely because it is unusual. In fact, Wegner's own account of the genesis of the experience of doing suggests that such experiences are normally veridical. According to the matching model, we experience ourselves as doing X when we are aware of our intention to X as being immediately prior to our X-ing, and when we are not aware of any rival causes of our X-ing. Now, if we experience ourselves as having an intention to X then it probably is the case that we do have the intention to X. (After all, it seems reasonable to suppose that introspection is generally reliable. At any rate, Wegner is in no position to challenge the reliability of introspection, for he himself assumes the reliability of introspection insofar as he takes subjects to be reliable in reporting their experiences of conscious will.) But if one has an intention to X, and if one has in fact X-ed, and if one's intention to X is immediately prior to one's X-ing, then it is highly likely that one's intention to X is involved in bringing about one's X-ing. It would be remarkable if one had an intention to raise one's hand just prior to raising one's hand but the intention played no causal role in the raising of one's hand. Far from showing that experiences of agency are illusory, Wegner's own model of how such experiences are generated predicts that they will normally be veridical.

The Argument from Eliminativism

A further and quite different line of argument for thinking that experiences of the conscious will are non-veridical can be found in Wegner's work. I call it *the argument from eliminativism*. Consider the following passages:

> . . . it seems to each of us that we have conscious will. It seems we have selves. It seems we have minds. It seems we are agents. It seems we cause what we do. *Although it is sobering and ultimately accurate to call all this an illusion*, it is a mistake to conclude that the illusion is trivial. On the contrary, the *illusions piled atop apparent mental causation* are the building blocks of human psychology and social life. (*ICW*, p. 342; emphasis added)

> The agent self cannot be a real entity that causes actions, but only a *virtual* entity, an *apparent* mental causer. (Wegner 2005, p. 23; emphasis added)

> The theory of apparent mental causation turns the everyday notion of intention on its head. . . . The theory says that people perceive that they are intending and that they understand behavior as intended or unintended—but they do not really intend. (Wegner 2003a, p. 10)

There are two closely related thoughts here. The first is that the experience of conscious will must be an illusion because there are no selves. The second is that the experience of conscious will must be an illusion because there is no intentional (mental) causation. How committed Wegner is to either of these claims is something of an open question, for he also says that the conscious will is a "fairly good sign" of our own causation (*ICW*, p. 333; see also pp. 334 and 327). How, one wonders, could the experience of conscious will be a "fairly good sign" of our own causation if we are merely virtual entities? There seems to be a deep tension between Wegner's eliminativism and his willingness to allow that experiences of conscious will are often veridical. This tension can be resolved by regarding Wegner as ambivalent about how much to build into the conception of the self as it is represented in the experience of authorship. In some passages Wegner seems to be working with a fairly weak conception of authorship—one according to which the experience of authorship merely tracks those actions that are mine and those that are produced by other people. Those passages in which Wegner claims that the experience of conscious will is generally reliable might be understood along these lines. After all, we are pretty good at working out whether we are raising our arms or someone else is raising them for us, and it would be hard to take an argument for the denial of this claim seriously. In other passages, however, Wegner appears to be working with a much stronger conception of authorship—one according to which an experience of authorship represents one's actions as caused by a homunculus of some kind: a substantival entity inside one's brain that is the ultimate (uncaused) cause of one's actions. And here, of course, there is ample room for eliminativist worries. There are no homunculi, and we are not ultimate causes.

But in acting do we experience ourselves as homunculi—as uncaused causes? I think the answer to this question is quite unclear. There is certainly a tradition of thought within philosophy that would reconstruct the phenomenology of authorship in terms of agent causation—that is, in terms of the experience of oneself as a sui generis cause. Timothy O'Connor writes: "[Agent causation] is appealing because it captures the way we experience our own activity. It does not seem to me (at least ordinarily) that I am caused to act by the reasons which favour doing so; it seems to be the case, rather, that I produce my own decisions in view of those reasons. . . ." (1995, p. 196) And, although he himself does not endorse agent causation, Carl Ginet also gives an agent causal gloss on the phenomenology of agency: "My impression at each moment is that *I* at that moment, and nothing prior to that moment, determine which of several open alternatives is the next sort of bodily exertion I voluntarily make." (1990, p. 90)

One might attempt to characterize the sense in which we experience ourselves as causes in a manner that does not involve any commitment to agent causation—or, at least, in such a way that does not involve any commitment to the idea that the agent cause must be an homunculus. Perhaps we experience our actions as caused by, well, ourselves, where this experience makes no commitment to any particular view of what kinds of things we are. Rather than conceive of the agent causal relation as holding between a Cartesian self and its actions, perhaps the agent-causation theorist should think of it as holding between an organism and its actions (Bishop 1983). If such a view can be defended, perhaps it is also possible that agent-causation accounts of the experience of authorship can resist the threat of eliminativism.

Of course, we still need an account of when agents stand in the authoring relation to their movements. Consider again the phenomenology of the anarchic hand, in which the patient fails to experience any sense of authorship with respect to the movements of her anarchic hand. Is this patient the author of these movements? Do these movements constitute *actions*, and if so, are the actions *her* actions? (See Peacocke 2003.) Her movements are clearly caused by events within her, but are they caused in such a way as to constitute an action that she performs? These are very difficult questions. Not only are their answers unclear, it is also unclear how we ought to go about answering them. But unless we have some handle on them we don't really have an adequate grip on the phenomenology of authorship.

Much more could be said about eliminativism and the experience of authorship, but I turn now to eliminativism about mental causation. Consider the following passage:

> When we apply mental explanations to our own behavior-causation mechanisms, we fall prey to the impression that our conscious will causes our actions. The fact is, we find it enormously seductive to think of ourselves as having minds, and so we are drawn into an intuitive appreciation of our own conscious will. . . . The real causal sequence underlying human behavior involves a massively complicated set of mechanisms. (*ICW*, p. 26)

To contrast intentional causation with "real causal sequences" is to suggest that intentional causation is not real—that it is merely ersatz or virtual. Wegner's argument for this view seems to be a version of the argument from explanatory exclusion: Lower levels of explanation exclude (eliminate) higher levels of explanation.

There is a lively debate in the philosophy of mind about what, if anything, is wrong with the exclusion argument. (See e.g. Block 2003; Kim 1998.) The debate is a complex one, and here is not the place to enter into it. Suffice it to say that it proceeds against the backdrop of a general—although far from universal—commitment to the causal efficacy of mental content.[12] Mental causation is no more undermined by the presence of underlying neuropsychological processes than neuropsychological causation is undermined by the presence of underlying neurochemical processes. To put the point slightly differently, it remains to be shown why neurochemical (or quantum, for that matter) explanations don't threaten the causal efficacy of neuropsychological states if, as proponents of the exclusion argument claim, neuropsychological explanations threaten the causal efficacy of mental states. If each explanatory level undermines the levels above it, then the only real causal explanations are those of fundamental physics, and we're *all* out of a job.

It seems to me that there something particularly puzzling about *Wegner* suggesting that mental causation is merely virtual, for his own work on thought suppression and mental control highlights just how potent (and surprising) mental causation can be (1989). Indeed, Wegner's model of the conscious will is itself committed to the causal efficacy of mental content, for according to the model it is a match between the content of one's intentions and one's actions that generates—that is, *causes*—the experience of doing.

Conclusion

In order to know whether the experience of conscious will is an illusion we need both an account of the content of the phenomenology of agency and an account of the structure of agency itself. We are still some way short of achieving either of these goals. This is perhaps most obvious with respect to the phenomenology of agency. As I suggested at the outset of this chapter, the content of the "experience of conscious will"—if we are to take this expression in its widest sense to refer to the phenomenology of first-person agency in general—is vastly more complex than is usually assumed within the cognitive sciences. It may well turn out that some components of the phenomenology of agency are systematically misleading and other components are highly reliable. It may even turn out that some components—such as the experience of libertarian free will, if there is such an experience—are logically incapable of being satisfied. The recent literature on the phenomenology of agency has brought into focus some of the issues that must be addressed here, but it also demonstrates just how much work remains to be done before we know, in the relevant sense, what it is like to be an agent.

We are also some way short of an adequate account of agency itself. Even so basic a distinction as the distinction between controlled and automatic actions is obscure and contested, with various theorists drawing the distinction in importantly different ways. And, of course, the roles of the self and of intentional states in the genesis of agency are even less clear. We will not know how much of the phenomenology of agency might be illusory until we know what role intentional states play in the explanation of human behavior. Despite these lacunae in our understanding it seems to me highly unlikely that the phenomenology of agency is systematically misleading. We experience ourselves as agents who do things for reasons, and there is little serious reason to suppose that we are mistaken on either count.

Acknowledgments

An earlier version of this chapter was presented at a workshop on the phenomenology of agency organized by Terry Horgan at the University of Arizona and at a workshop at Johannes Gutenberg-Universität organized by Thomas Metzinger. I am grateful to the audiences on both occasions for their comments. I am also grateful to David Chalmers, Tim Crane, Frédérique de Vignemont, Patrick Haggard, Neil Levy, Al Mele, Thomas Metzinger, Eddy Nahmias, Elisabeth Pacherie, and Sue Pockett for very helpful comments. This work was supported by Australian Research Council Discovery Grant DP0452631.

Notes

1. Recent examples of this work include Haggard et al. 2004; Haggard 2006; Haggard and Johnson 2003; Hohwy, in press; Metzinger 2006; Nichols 2004; Horgan, Tienson, and Graham 2003; Nahmias, Morris, Nadelhoffer, and Turner 2004; Pockett 2004.

2. Consider the following: "Most of us navigate through our daily lives with the belief that we have free will: that is, we have conscious intentions to perform specific acts, and those intentions can drive our bodily actions, thus producing a desired change in the external world." (Haggard and Libet 2001, p. 47) I think this equation of the free will with mental causation is implausible. It leads to the counter-intuitive conclusion that those who deny the reality of free will are thereby forced to deny the reality of mental causation.

3. This is the view suggested by *most* of Wegner's work. However, Preston and Wegner (2005) suggest that intention confabulation can occur when we ascribe intentions to ourselves in order to account for our experience of willing an action. This suggests that Wegner may now think that we can have an experience of conscious will in the *absence* of an experience of mental causation.

4. For useful discussions of these issues, see Horgan et al. 2003; Nahmias et al. 2004.

5. Note that by focusing on movement-direct intentions rather than object-direct intentions Wegner might be able to respond to an objection to his model raised by Zhu (2004). Zhu points out that one can experience a sense of agency with respect to failed actions. There is something it is like to try (but fail) to push over a heavy boulder. But if one can have a sense of agency with respect to failed intentions, then the sense of agency cannot rest on an awareness of a match between one's intentions and one's actions. In response to this objection one might point out that even in failed attempts at action one is usually aware that one has successfully implemented an intention to move one's muscles, even if one has failed to achieve the goal state (moving the boulder). Of course, this is only a first step in answering Zhu's objection. Perhaps it is possible to experience a sense of agency without having any sense of successfully implementing an intention. I suspect that some episodes of mental agency might have this form.

6. For more on the I-Spy experiment, see Hohwy (in press) and the chapters by Malle and Pacherie in the present volume.

7. Furthermore, even if participants had an intention to land the mouse on the swan, there is no reason to think that this intention was *conscious*.

8. This experiment also raises questions about what the other relatum of Wegner's matching relation is, for participants in this experiment did not have a perceptual experience of the action in question, they were only presented with an image of the results of the action.

9. For further discussion of what Wegner might mean by calling the conscious will an illusion, see Nahmias 2002; Holton 2004.

10. Bayne (2001) presents Wegner's argument in these terms. Nahmias (2002) also suggests that one can read Wegner as advancing an inductive generalization of this kind.

11. I thank Sue Pockett for drawing this reading of Wegner's work to my attention.

12. On the problem(s) of mental causation, see Heil and Mele 1995; Walter and Heckmann 2003.

References

Bayne, T. J. 2002. Review of D. M. Wegner, *The Illusion of Conscious Will. Journal of Consciousness Studies* 9, no. 7: 94–96.

Bayne, T. J., and Levy, N. 2006. The feeling of doing: Deconstructing the phenomenology of agency. In *Disorders of Volition*, ed. N. Sebanz and W. Prinz. MIT Press.

Bishop, J. 1983. Agent causation. *Mind* 92: 61–79.

Blakemore, S. J., and Frith, C. D. 2003. Freedom to act. In *Essays on Actions and Events*, ed. D. Davidson. Clarendon.

Block, N. 2003. Do causal powers drain away? *Philosophy and Phenomenological Research* 67, no. 1: 110–127.

Felce, D. 1994. Facilitated communication: Results from a number of recently published evaluations. *Mental Handicap* 22: 122–126.

Frith, C. 2002. Attention to action and awareness of other minds. *Consciousness and Cognition* 11: 481–487.

Ginet, C. 1990. *On Action*. Cambridge University Press.

Haggard, P. 2006. Conscious intention and the sense of agency. In *Disorders of Volition*, ed. N. Sebanz and W. Prinz. MIT Press.

Haggard, P., and Johnson, H. 2003. Experiences of voluntary action. *Journal of Consciousness Studies* 10, no. 9–10: 72–84.

Haggard, P., and Libet, B. 2001. Conscious intention and brain activity. *Journal of Consciousness Studies* 8, no. 11: 47–63.

Haggard, P., Cartledge, P., Dafydd, M., and Oakley, D. A. 2004. Anomalous control: When "free-will" is not conscious. *Consciousness and Cognition* 13: 646–654.

Heil, J., and Mele, A., eds. 1995. *Mental Causation*. Oxford University Press.

Hohwy, J. In press. The experience of mental causation. *Behavior and Philosophy*.

Holton, R. 2004. Review of *The Illusion of Conscious Will. Mind* 113, no. 449: 218–221.

Horgan, T., Tienson, J., and Graham, G. 2003. The phenomenology of first-person agency. In *Physicalism and Mental Causation: The Metaphysics of Mind and Action*, ed. S. Walter and H.-D. Heckmann. Imprint Academic.

Jacobson, J. W., Mulick, J. A., and Schwartz, A. A. 1995. A history of facilitated communication: Science, pseudoscience, and antiscience. *American Psychologist* 50: 750–765.

Jahanshahi, M., and Frith, C. D. 1998. Willed action and its impairments, *Cognitive Neuropsychology* 15, no. 6/7/8: 483–533.

Kim, J. 1998. *Mind in a Physical World: An Essay on the Mind-Body Problem and Mental Causation*. MIT Press.

Metzinger, T. 2006. Conscious volition and mental representation: Towards a more fine-grained analysis. In *Disorders of Volition*, ed. N. Sebanz and W. Prinz. MIT Press.

Nahmias, E. 2002. When consciousness matters: A critical review of Daniel Wegner's *The Illusion of Conscious Will. Philosophical Psychology* 15, no. 4: 527–541.

Nahmias, E., Morris, S. Nadelhoffer, T., and Turner, J. 2004. The phenomenology of free will. *Journal of Consciousness Studies* 11, no. 7–8: 162–179.

Nichols, S. 2004. The folk psychology of free will: Fits and starts. *Mind and Language* 19: 473–502.

O'Connor, T. 1995. Agent causation. In *Agents, Causes, Events*, ed. T. O'Connor. Oxford University Press.

Peacocke, C. 2003. Action: awareness, ownership, and knowledge. In *Agency and Self-Awareness*, ed. J. Roessler and N. Eilan. Oxford University Press.

Penfield, W. 1975. *The Mystery of Mind*. Princeton University Press.

Pockett, S. 2004. Does consciousness cause behaviour? *Journal of Consciousness Studies* 11: 23–40.

Preston, J., and Wegner, D. M. 2005. Ideal agency: On perceiving the self as an origin of action. In *On Building, Defending, and Regulating the Self*, ed. A. Tesser et al. Psychology Press.

Wakefield, J., and Dreyfus, H. 1991. Intentionality and the phenomenology of action. In *John Searle and His Critics*, ed. E. Lepore and R. van Gulick. Blackwell.

Wegner, D. M. 1989. *White Bears and Other Unwanted Thoughts: Suppression, Obsession, and the Psychology of Mental Control*. Viking/Penguin.

Wegner, D. M. 2002. *The Illusion of Conscious Will*. MIT Press.

Wegner, D. M. 2003a. The mind's self-portrait. *Annals of the New York Academy of Sciences* 1001: 1–14.

Wegner, D. M. 2003b. The mind's best trick: How we experience conscious will. *Trends in Cognitive Science* 7, no. 2: 65–69.

Wegner, D. M. 2005. Who is the controller of controlled processes? In *The New Unconscious*, ed. R. Hassin et al. Oxford University Press.

Wegner, D. M., Fuller, V. A., and Sparrow, B. 2003. Clever hands: Uncontrolled intelligence in facilitated communication. *Journal of Personality and Social Psychology* 85: 5–19.

Wegner, D. M., Sparrow, B., and Winerman, L. 2004. Vicarious agency: Experiencing control over the movements of others. *Journal of Personality and Social Psychology* 86, no. 6: 838–848.

Wegner, D. M., and Wheatley, T. 1999. Apparent mental causation: Sources of the experience of will. *American Psychologist* 54: 480–491.

Searle, J. 1983. *Intentionality*. Cambridge University Press.

Searle, J. 2001. *Rationality in Action*. MIT Press.

Zhu, J. 2004. Is conscious will an illusion? *Disputatio* 16: 59–70.

10 Free Will: Theories, Analysis, and Data

Alfred R. Mele

It is a truism that whether or not anyone has free will depends on what free will is. In section 1, I describe two competing theories about the nature of free will. In section 2, I sketch some conceptual background relevant to some striking claims Benjamin Libet has made about decisions and free will. The experiments on which Libet bases these claims are the topic of sections 3 and 4. I argue there that Libet's data do not justify his claim that "the brain 'decides' to initiate or, at least, to prepare to initiate the act before there is any reportable subjective awareness that such a decision has taken place" (Libet 1985, p. 536) and do not justify associated worries about free will. I conclude with some remarks about the relevance of another experiment.

1 Free Will: Conceptual and Theoretical Background

Free will may be defined as the power to act freely. But what is it to act freely? Familiar philosophical answers fall into two groups: compatibilist and incompatibilist. Compatibilism and incompatibilism are theses about the relationship between free action and determinism. Determinism is the thesis that a complete statement of the laws of nature together with a complete description of the condition of the entire universe at any point in time logically entails a complete description of the condition of the entire universe at any other point in time. Compatibilism is the thesis that free action is compatible with the truth of determinism. Because they attend to what contemporary physics tells us, the overwhelming majority of contemporary compatibilists do not believe that determinism is true, but they do believe that even if it were true people would be able to act freely. Incompatibilism is the thesis that free action is incompatible with the truth of determinism. In the incompatibilist group, most answers to the question what it is to act freely come from libertarians. Libertarianism is the conjunction of incompatibilism and the thesis that some people sometimes act freely. Some incompatibilists argue that no one acts freely (Pereboom 2001) and that even the falsity of determinism creates no place for free action.

The compatibilist thesis usually sounds strange to nonspecialists. When people first encounter the pair of expressions "free will" and "determinism" they tend to get the impression that the two ideas are defined in opposition to each other, that they are mutually exclusive by definition. This is one reason that it is useful to think of free will as the power to act freely and to regard acting freely as the more basic notion—that is, as a notion in terms of which free will is to be defined. Consider the following conversation between two Detroit police officers who have a notoriously stingy friend named Stan. Ann: "Stan gave $20 to a homeless man today." Bill: "Why? Did he hold a gun to Stan's head?" Ann: "No, Stan gave him the money freely." Surely it is not necessary for Ann and Bill to have an opinion about whether determinism (as defined above) is true in order for them to have this conversation. If what Ann says is true (that is, if Stan freely gave away $20) and free will is the power to act freely, then Stan has free will (or had it at that time). Even if "free will" is typically opposed to "determinism" in ordinary speech, "he did it freely" seems not to be. And even if "he did it freely" were typically opposed to determinism in ordinary speech, that would settle nothing. After all, in ordinary speech deductive reasoning seems to be defined as reasoning from the general to the particular, and that certainly would only jokingly be said to constitute an objection to a logician's definition of deduction (according to which "Ann is a police officer; Bill is a police officer; therefore Ann and Bill are police officers" is a valid deductive argument).

Compatibilist theories of free action emphasize a distinction between deterministic causation and compulsion (Frankfurt 1988; Smith 2003). If determinism is true, then my eating toast for breakfast today and my working on this chapter today were deterministically caused; and so were a certain compulsive hand-washer's washing his hands dozens of times today, a certain delusional person's spending the day trying to contact God with his microwave oven, a certain addict's using his favorite drug while in the grip of an irresistible urge to do so, and a certain person's handing over money to gunmen who convincingly threatened to kill him if he refused. But there is an apparent difference. I am sane and free from addiction, and I received no death threats today. The basic compatibilist idea is (roughly) that when mentally healthy people act intentionally in the absence of compulsion and coercion they act freely, and an action's being deterministically caused does not suffice for its being compelled or coerced.

Many compatibilists have been concerned to accommodate the idea that, for example, if I freely spent the day working, I could have done something else instead. They grant that, if determinism is true, then there is a sense in which people could never have done otherwise than they did: they could not have done otherwise in the sense that their doing otherwise is inconsistent with the combination of the past and the laws of nature. But, these compatibilists say, the fact that a person never could have done otherwise in that sense is irrelevant to free action. What is relevant is that people who act freely are exercising a rational capacity of such a kind that, had their situation been different in any one of a variety of important ways, they would have responded to the difference with a different suitable action (Smith 2003). For example, although I spent the day working, I would have spent the day relaxing if someone had bet me $500 that I would not relax all day. This truth is consistent with determinism.[1] (Notice that if someone had made this bet with me the past would have been different from what it actually was.) And it reinforces the distinction between deterministic causation and compulsion. Offer a compulsive handwasher $500 not to wash his hands all day and see what happens.

Like compatibilists, libertarians tend to maintain that when mentally healthy people act intentionally in the absence of compulsion and coercion they act freely, but they insist that the deterministic causation of an action is incompatible with the action's being freely performed. Some libertarian theories of free action assert that agents never act freely unless some of their actions are indeterministically caused by immediate antecedents (Kane 1996). Whereas the laws of nature that apply to deterministic causation are exceptionless, those that apply most directly to indeterministic causation are instead probabilistic.[2] Typically, events like deciding to help a stranded motorist—as distinct from the physical actions involved in actually helping—are counted as mental actions. Suppose that Ann's decision to help a stranded motorist is indeterministically caused by, among other things, her thinking that she should help. Because the causation is indeterministic, she might not have decided to help given exactly the same internal and external conditions. In this way, some libertarians seek to secure the possibility of doing otherwise that they require for free action.

There are a variety of kinds of libertarian and compatibilist theories about free will. Each kind has been challenged, of course. Reviewing the major details is a project for a separate essay. My brief remarks in this section provide enough theoretical background on free will to set the stage for what follows.

2 Some Conceptual Distinctions

A 1983 article by Benjamin Libet and colleagues (Libet, Gleason et al. 1983) has been described as "one of the most philosophically challenging papers in modern scientific psychology" (Haggard et al. 1999, p. 291).[3] A striking thesis of that 1983 article is that "the brain . . . 'decides' to initiate or, at the least, prepare to initiate [certain actions] at a time before there is any reportable subjective awareness that such a decision has taken place" (p. 640; also see Libet 1985, p. 536).[4] In a recent

article, Libet pointedly asserts that "if the 'act now' process is initiated unconsciously, then conscious free will is not doing it" (2001, p. 62; also see 2004, p. 136).

Because Libet uses 'decision', 'intention', 'wanting', 'wish', and 'urge' interchangeably, some conceptual preliminaries are in order.[5] Most people recognize that
deciding to do something differs from having an urge or wanting to do something.
For example, you might have an urge to scream at an irritating colleague but decide
not to. And you might want to have a second helping of dessert but decide to stop
at one. If, as I believe, to decide to *A* is to perform a momentary mental action of
forming an intention to *A* (Mele 2003, chapter 9), then in deciding to stop at one
dessert you form an intention to stop at one. Your having that intention also differs
from your merely wanting to stop at one dessert. You might want to have another
dessert (it is very tempting) while also wanting to refrain from having it (you are
concerned about your weight); but intending to have a second helping of dessert
while intending to refrain from doing that, if it is possible at all, would be a sign of
a serious disorder. Similarly, you might want to meet one friend at a 7 o'clock movie
tonight, want to meet another at a 7 o'clock play, and be unsettled about what to
do. At this point, you want to do each of these things and lack an intention about
which of them to do.[6]

In saying that deciding is momentary, I mean to distinguish it from, for example,
a combination of deliberating and deciding. Someone who is speaking loosely may
say "I was up all night deciding to sell my house" when what he means is that he
was up all night deliberating or fretting about whether to sell his house and eventually decided to sell it. Deciding to *A*, on my view, is not a process but a momentary mental action of forming an intention to *A*, 'form' being understood as an action
verb.

Not all intentions are formed in acts of deciding. Example: "When I intentionally
unlocked my office door this morning, I intended to unlock it. But since I am in the
habit of unlocking my door in the morning and conditions . . . were normal, nothing
called for a *decision* to unlock it." (Mele 1992, p. 231) If I had heard a fight in my
office, I might have paused to consider whether to unlock the door or walk away,
and I might have decided to unlock it. But given the routine nature of my conduct,
there is no need to posit an act of intention formation in this case. My intention to
unlock the door may have been acquired without having been actively formed. If,
as I believe, all decisions are prompted partly by uncertainty about what to do (Mele
2003, chapter 9), no decisions will be made in situations in which there is no such
uncertainty.

Some of our decisions and intentions are for the non-immediate future and others
are not. I might decide on Monday to attend a lecture on Friday, and I might decide
now to phone my sister now. The intention formed in the former decision is aimed
at action four days in the future. The intention I form when I decide to phone my

sister now is about what to do now. I call intentions and decisions of these kinds, respectively, *distal* and *proximal* intentions and decisions (Mele 1992, pp. 143–44, 158). Proximal decisions and intentions also include decisions and intentions to continue doing something that one is doing and decisions and intentions to start *A*-ing (e.g., start climbing a hill) straightaway.

A distinction between *relatively specific* and *relatively unspecific* intentions also is in order. Ann now intends to buy a particular Ford Escort that she saw yesterday. That is a more specific intention than the intention she had 3 months ago, in January, to buy a new car this year. In another illustration, Bob has agreed to be a subject in an experiment in which subjects are instructed to salute whenever they feel like it on at least 40 occasions in 2 hours. When Bob begins his participation in the experiment he has a relatively unspecific intention to salute many times during the next two hours. At various times during the experiment he has specific proximal intentions to salute.

3   Libet's Work

This section develops an interpretation of Libet's work that is sensitive to the conceptual points just made.[7] In some of his studies, subjects are instructed to flex their right wrists or the fingers of their right hands whenever they wish. Electrical readings from the scalp—averaged over at least 40 flexings for each subject—show a "negative shift" in "readiness potentials" (RPs) beginning at about 550 milliseconds before the time at which an electromyogram shows relevant muscular motion to begin (1985, pp. 529–530). Subjects are also instructed to "recall . . . the spatial clock position of a revolving spot at the time of [their] initial awareness" (ibid., p. 529) of something, *x*, that Libet variously describes as an "intention," an "urge," a "wanting," a "decision," a "will," or a "wish" to move. On average, "RP onset" preceded what subjects reported to be the time of their initial awareness of *x* (time *W*) by 350 ms. Time *W*, then, preceded the beginning of muscle motion by about 200 ms. These data may be represented as follows:

−550 ms: RP onset

−200 ms: time *W*

0 ms: muscle begins to move

Libet (ibid., pp. 531, 534) finds independent evidence of a slight error in subjects' recall of the times at which they first become aware of sensations. Correcting for that error, time *W* is −150 ms.

At what point, if any, does a specific intention to flex arise in Libet's subjects? According to Libet, "the brain 'decides' to initiate or, at least, to prepare to initiate the act before there is any reportable subjective awareness that such a decision has taken place" (1985, p. 536). If we ignore the second disjunct, this quotation (given its context) appears to offer the answer that a specific intention to flex appears on the scene with "RP onset," about 550 ms before relevant muscular motion and about 350–400 ms before the agent becomes aware of the intention (ibid., p. 539), for to decide to initiate an act is to form an intention to initiate it.[8] But are decision and intention the most suitable mental items to associate with RP onset? Again, Libet describes the relevant occurrence of which the agent later becomes aware not only as a "decision" and the onset of an "intention" to move but also as the onset of an "urge," a "wanting," and a "wish" to move. This leaves it open that at −550 ms, rather than acquire an intention or make a decision of which he is not conscious, the person instead acquires an urge or a desire of which he is not conscious—and perhaps an urge or a desire that is stronger than any competing urge or desire at the time—a *preponderant* urge or desire. It is also left open that what emerges around −550 ms is a pretty reliable causal contributor to an urge.

I believe that if Libet himself were to distinguish between intending and wanting (including having an urge) along the lines I sketched, he might find it more credible to associate the readiness potentials with the latter than with the former. To explain why, I turn to another experiment reported in Libet 1985 (and elsewhere).

Libet proposes that "conscious volitional control may operate not to initiate the volitional process but to select and control it, either by permitting or triggering the final motor outcome of the unconsciously initiated process or by vetoing the progression to actual motor activation" (1985, p. 529; also see 1999, p. 54, 2004, pp. 139, 142–143, 149). "In a veto," Libet writes, "the later phase of cerebral motor processing would be blocked, so that actual activation of the motoneurons to the muscles would not occur" (1985, p. 537). Libet offers two kinds of evidence to support the suggestion about vetoing. One kind is generated by an experiment in which subjects are instructed both to prepare to flex their fingers at a prearranged time (as indicated by a revolving spot on a clock face) and to "veto the developing intention/preparation to act . . . about 100 to 200 ms before the prearranged clock time" (ibid., p. 538). Subjects receive both instructions at the same time. Libet writes:

. . . a ramplike pre-event potential was still recorded . . . resembl[ing] the RP of self-initiated acts when preplanning is present. . . . The form of the 'veto' RP differed (in most but not all cases) from those 'preset' RPs that were followed by actual movements [in another experiment]; the main negative potential tended to alter in direction (flattening or reversing) at about 150–250 ms before the preset time. . . . This difference suggests that the conscious veto interfered with the final development of RP processes leading to action. . . . The preparatory cerebral processes associated with an RP can and do develop even when intended motor action is vetoed at approximately the time that conscious intention would normally appear before a voluntary act. (1985, p. 538)[9]

Keep in mind that the subjects were instructed in advance *not* to flex their fingers, but to prepare to flex them at the prearranged time and to "veto" this. The subjects intentionally complied with the request. They intended from the beginning not to flex their fingers at the appointed time. So what is indicated by the RP? Presumably, not the acquisition or presence of an *intention* to flex; for then, at some point in time, the subjects would have both an intention to flex at the prearranged time and an intention not to flex at that time. And how can a normal agent simultaneously be settled on *A*-ing at *t* and settled on not *A*-ing at *t*?[10] That is, it is very plausible that Libet is mistaken in describing what is vetoed as "*intended* motor action" (p. 538, emphasis added).

If the RP in the veto scenario is not associated with an intention to flex at the appointed time, with what might it be associated? In the passage I quoted from Libet 1985, p. 538, Libet compares "the 'veto' RP" with (a) "'preset' RPs that were followed by actual movements" and (b) "the RP of self-initiated acts when preplanning is present." The RP referred to in (a) is produced in experiments in which subjects are instructed to watch the clock and to flex when the revolving spot reaches "a pre-set 'clock time'" (Libet et al. 1982, p. 325): "The subject was encouraged to try to make his movement coincide as closely as possible with the arrival of the spot at the pre-set time." The RP referred to in (b) is produced in two kinds of studies: studies in which subjects are neither instructed to flex at a prearranged time nor explicitly told to flex spontaneously (ibid., p. 326), and studies in which subjects instructed to flex spontaneously reported that they experienced "some 'preplanning'," even if only in "a minority of the 40 self-initiated acts that occurred in the series for that averaged RP" (ibid., p. 328). "Even when some pre-plannings were recalled and reported, subjects insisted that the more specific urge or intention to actually move did not arise in that pre-planning stage" (p. 329). Reports of "preplanning" seem to include reports of thoughts about when to flex and reports of anticipations of flexing (pp. 328–329). Libet and his co-authors remark that "subject S.B. described his advance feelings [of pre-planning] as 'pre-tensions' rather than pre-plannings to act" (p. 329). This subject may have meant that he experienced tension that he expected to result in flexing.

The RPs referred to in (a) and (b) have a very similar form (Libet et al. 1982, pp. 330, 333–34; Libet 1985, p. 532). RPs with that form are called "type I RPs" (Libet et al. 1982, p. 326). They have significantly earlier onsets than the RPs produced in studies in which subjects instructed to flex spontaneously report that they experienced no "pre-planning"—"type II RPs." "The form of the 'veto' RP" is the form of type I RPs until "about 150–250 ms before the preset time" (Libet 1985, p. 538). What does the veto group (group V) have in common until that time with the three kinds of subjects who produce type I RPs: those with a pre-set time for flexing (group PS), those who are neither told to flex at a pre-set time nor instructed to flex spontaneously (group N), and those who are instructed to flex spontaneously but who report some "pre-planning" (group PP)?

Presumably, subjects in group PS are watching the clock with the intention of flexing at the pre-set time. But it certainly does not follow from that and the similar RPs in groups N and PP—and V for a time—that members of each of these groups are watching the clock with a similar intention to flex. For one thing, as I have explained, it is very likely that group V—subjects instructed in advance to prepare to flex and then veto the preparation—are watching the clock *without* an intention to flex at the targeted time. Given that the members of group V lack this intention, we should look for something that groups V and PS actually have in common that might be signified by the similarity in the RPs until "about 150–250 ms before the preset time." One possibility is that members of both groups have *urges* to flex (or to prepare to flex)—or undergo brain events that are pretty reliable relatively proximal causal contributors to such urges—that are associated with an RP and regularly play a role in generating subsequent flexings in the absence of "vetoing."[11] In the case of group V, perhaps a subject's wanting to comply with the instructions—including the instruction to prepare to flex at the appointed time—together with his recognition that the time is approaching produces a growing urge to (prepare to) flex, or a pretty reliable causal contributor to such an urge, or a simulation of such an urge, or the motor preparedness typically associated with such an urge. And the "flattening or reversing" of the RP "at about 150–250 ms before the preset time" might indicate a consequence of the subject's "vetoing" his preparation.

What about groups N and PP? It is possible that they, along with the subjects in groups PS and V, begin acquiring urges to flex at a greater temporal distance from 0 ms than do subjects instructed to flex spontaneously who report no pre-planning. That difference may be indicated by type I RPs' having significantly earlier onsets than type II RPs. Another possibility is consistent with this (see note 1). Earlier I distinguished proximal from distal intentions, and Libet himself recognizes the distinction (Libet et al. 1982, pp. 329, 334; Libet 1989, pp. 183–184). Presumably, subjects in group PS respond to the instruction to flex at a pre-set time with an intention to flex at that time. This is a distal intention. As the pre-set time for flexing draws very near, that intention may become, may help produce, or may be replaced by a proximal intention to flex—an intention to *flex now*, as one naturally says (Libet 1989, p. 183; 1999, p. 54; 2004, p. 148). That may happen around the time subjects in group V veto their urge to flex or closer to 0 ms. And it may happen at or around the time subjects in groups N and PP acquire a proximal intention to flex. They may acquire such an intention without having had a distal intention to flex soon: recall that members of group V probably had no distal intention to flex soon and that their RPs are very similar to those of groups N, PP, and PS until "about 150–250 ms before the preset time." All this is consistent (see note 1) with the similarities in RPs in the various groups of subjects, on the assumption that no segment of the RPs before about −150 to −250 ms for subjects in group PS specifically represents subjects' distal intentions to flex at the pre-set time—as opposed, for example, to something that such intentions have in common with distal urges to flex (or to prepare to flex) at the pre-set time—even though those intentions are present.

The main difference between type I and type II RPs, in Patrick Haggard's words, is that the former have "earlier onsets than" the latter (Haggard and Libet 2001, p. 49). The earlier onsets may be correlated with earlier acquisitions of urges to flex soon—urges that may be brought on, variously, by the instruction to flex at a pre-set time (group PS), the instruction to prepare to flex at a pre-set time and to veto that later (group V), unsolicited conscious thoughts about when to flex (groups N and PP), or unsolicited conscious anticipations of flexing (groups N and PP). (Of course, it is possible that some such thoughts and anticipations are instead products, in part, of urges to flex soon.) These urge inciters (or perhaps urge products, in the case of some experiences in groups N and PP) are absent in subjects instructed to flex spontaneously who report no "pre-planning"—at least, if their reports are accurate. If type I RPs indicate urges, or urges together with proximal intentions that emerge later than the urges do, the same may be true of type II RPs. The difference in the two kinds of RP may mainly be a matter of when the urge emerges—that is, how long before 0 ms. Once again, Libet describes in a variety of ways the mental item that is indicated by RPs. Even if "intention" and "decision" (to flex) are not apt choices, "urge" and "wanting" are still in the running.

If "RP onset" in cases of "spontaneous" flexing indicates the emergence of an urge to flex soon, proximal intentions to flex may emerge at some point between RP onset and time W, *at* time W, or *after* time W: at time W the agent may be aware only of an urge that has not yet issued in a proximal intention. Again, Libet asserts that "in a veto, the later phase of cerebral motor processing would be blocked, so that actual activation of the motoneurons to the muscles would not occur" (1985, p. 537). Perhaps, in non-veto cases, activation of these motoneurons is the direct result of the acquisition of a proximal intention (Gomes 1999, pp. 68, 72; Mele 1997, pp. 322–324). Libet suggests that this activation event occurs between 10 and 90 ms before the muscle begins moving and appears to favor an answer in the 10–50 ms range (p. 537). Elsewhere, he asserts that the activation event can occur no later than 50 ms before the onset of muscle motion (2004, pp. 137–138).

Although I will not make much of the following point, it should be observed that urges that may be correlated with RP onset at −550 ms might not be *proximal* urges, strictly speaking. Possibly, they are urges to flex *very soon*, as opposed to urges to flex straightaway. And perhaps they evolve into, or produce, proximal urges. Another possibility is that urges to flex very soon give rise to proximal intentions to flex without first evolving into or producing proximal urges to flex. Some disambiguation is in order. A smoker who is rushing toward a smoking section in an airport with the intention of lighting up as soon as he enters it wants to smoke soon. That want or desire has a specific temporal target: the time at which he enters the smoking section. A smoker walking outside the airport may want to smoke soon without having a specific time in mind. Libet's subjects, like the latter smoker, might at times have urges or desires to flex that lack a specific temporal target. Desires to A very soon, or to A, beginning very soon, in this sense of "very soon," are *roughly proximal* action-desires.

Libet's experimental design promotes consciousness of urges and intentions to flex, since his subjects are instructed in advance to be prepared to report on them—or something like them—later, using the clock to pinpoint the time they are first noticed. For my purposes, what is of special interest are the relative times of the emergence of a (roughly) proximal urge or desire to flex, the emergence of a proximal *intention* to flex, and initial consciousness of the intention.[12] If RP onset indicates the emergence of proximal, or roughly proximal, urges to flex, and if acquisitions of corresponding proximal intentions directly activate the motoneurons to the relevant muscles, we have the following picture of subjects instructed to flex "spontaneously" who report no "pre-planning"—subjects who produce type II RPs:

−550 ms: proximal or roughly proximal urge to flex emerges

−90 to −50 ms: acquisition of corresponding proximal intention[13]

0 ms: muscle begins to move.

Possibly, the intention is *consciously* acquired. My point here is simply that this picture is *consistent* (see note 1) with Libet's data on type II RPs and on time *W*.

In an alternative picture, the acquisition of a proximal intention to flex sends a signal that may be regarded as a command to flex one's wrist (or finger), and that signal helps produce finer-grained command signals that directly activate the motoneurons to the relevant muscles. This picture moves the time of the acquisition of a proximal intention further from 0 ms than −90 to −50 ms, but it does not move it anywhere near −550 ms. On this, see section 5 below.[14]

I mentioned that Libet offered a second kind of evidence for "veto control." Subjects instructed to flex "spontaneously" (in non-veto experiments) "reported that during some of the trials a recallable conscious urge to act appeared but was 'aborted' or somehow suppressed before any actual movement occurred; in such cases the subject simply waited for another urge to appear, which, when consummated, constituted the actual event whose RP was recorded" (1985, p. 538). RPs were not recorded for suppressed urges. But if these urges fit the pattern of the unsuppressed ones in cases of "spontaneous" flexing, they appeared on the scene about 550 ms before the relevant muscles would have moved if the subjects had not "suppressed" the urges, and subjects did not become conscious of them for about another 350–400 ms. Notice that it is *urges* that these subjects are said to report and abort or suppress. This coheres with my "urge" hypothesis about groups V, PS, N, and PP. In group V (the veto group), as I have explained, there is excellent reason to believe that no proximal *intention* to flex is present, and the RPs for this group resembled the type I RPs for these other three groups until "about 150–250 ms before the preset time." If it is assumed that these RPs represent the same thing for these four groups until the RPs for group V diverge from the others, these RPs do *not* represent a *proximal intention* to flex before the point of divergence, but they might represent a growing urge to (prepare to) flex, or a pretty reliable relatively proximal causal contributor to such an urge, or the motor preparedness typically associated with such an urge. And if at least until about the time of divergence there is no proximal intention to flex in any of these groups, we would need a special reason to believe that the type II RPs of the spontaneous flexers indicate that proximal intentions to flex emerge in them around −550 ms. In section 5, I show that there is independent evidence that their proximal intentions emerge much later.

Does the brain decide to initiate actions "at a time before there is any reportable subjective awareness that such a decision has taken place" (Libet, Gleason et al. 1983, p. 640)? Libet and his colleagues certainly have not shown that it does, for their data do not show that any such decision has been made before time *W* or before the time at which their subjects first are aware of a *decision* or *intention* to flex. Nothing justifies the claim that what a subject becomes aware of at time *W* is a *decision* to flex that has already been made or an *intention* to flex that has already been acquired (as opposed, for example, to an *urge* to flex that has already arisen). Indeed, the data about vetoing, as I have explained, can reasonably be used to argue that the "urge" hypothesis about what the RPs indicate is less implausible than the "decision" or "intention" hypothesis. Now, there certainly seems to be a connection between what happens at −550 ms and subsequent muscle motion in cases of "spontaneous" flexing. But it obviously is not a temporally direct connection. Between the former and latter times, subjects apparently form or acquire proximal intentions to flex, in those cases in which they do intentionally flex. And, for all Libet's data show, those intentions may be consciously formed or acquired.

4 Free Will

When Libet's work is applied to the theoretically subtle and complicated issue of free will, things can quickly get out of hand. The abstract of Haggard and Libet 2001 opens as follows: "The problem of free will lies at the heart of modern scientific studies of consciousness. An influential series of experiments by Libet has suggested that conscious intentions arise as a result of brain activity. This contrasts with traditional concepts of free will, in which the mind controls the body." Now, only a certain kind of mind-body dualist would hold that conscious intentions do *not* "arise as a result of brain activity." And such dualist views are rarely advocated in contemporary philosophical publications on free will. Moreover, contemporary philosophers who argue for the existence of free will typically shun substance dualism. If Libet's work is of general interest to philosophers working on free will, the source of the interest must lie elsewhere than the theoretical location specified in this passage.

In a recent article, Libet writes: "It is only the final 'act now' process that produces the voluntary *act*. That 'act now' process begins in the brain about 550 ms before the act, and it begins unconsciously." (2001, p. 61)[15] "There is," he says, "an unconscious gap of about 400 ms between the onset of the cerebral process and when the person becomes consciously aware of his/her decision or wish or intention to act." (A page later, he identifies what the agent becomes aware of as "the intention/wish/urge to act.") Libet adds: "If the 'act now' process is initiated unconsciously, then conscious free will is not doing it."

I have already explained that Libet has not shown that a decision to flex is made or that an intention to flex is acquired at −550 ms. But even if the intention emerges much later, that is compatible with an "act now" process having begun at −550 ms. One might say that "the 'act now' process" in Libet's spontaneous subjects begins with the formation or acquisition of a proximal intention to flex, much closer to the onset of muscle motion than −550 ms, or that it begins earlier, with the beginning of a process that issues in the intention. We can be flexible about that (just as we can be flexible about whether the process of my baking my frozen pizza began when I turned my oven on to pre-heat it, when I opened the oven door five minutes later to put the pizza in, when I placed the pizza on the center rack, or at some other time). Suppose we stipulate that "the 'act now' process" begins with the unconscious emergence of an urge to flex—or with a pretty reliable relatively proximal causal contributor to urges to flex—at about −550 ms and that the urge plays a significant role in producing a proximal intention to flex many milliseconds later. We can then agree with Libet that, given that the "process is initiated unconsciously, . . . conscious free will is not doing it"—that is, is not initiating "the 'act now' process." But who would have thought that conscious free will has the job of producing urges? In the philosophical literature, free will's primary locus of operation is typically identified as deciding (or choosing); and for all Libet has shown, if his subjects decide (or choose) to flex "now," they do so consciously.

"How," Libet asks (2001, p. 62), "would the 'conscious self' initiate a voluntary act if, factually, the process to 'act now' is initiated unconsciously?" In this paragraph, I offer an answer. As background, recall that, according to Libet, an "'act now' process" that is initiated unconsciously may be aborted by the agent; that apparently is what happens in instances of spontaneous vetoing, if "'act now' processes" start when Libet says they do.[16] Now, processes have parts, and the various parts of a process may have more and less proximal initiators. A process that is initiated by the welling up of an unconscious urge may have a subsequent part that is directly initiated by the conscious formation or acquisition of an intention. "The 'conscious self'"—which need not be understood as something mysterious—might more proximally initiate a voluntary act that is less proximally initiated by an unconscious urge. (Readers who, like me, prefer to use 'self' only as an affix may prefer to say that the acquisition or formation of a relevant proximal intention, which intention is consciously acquired or formed, might more proximally initiate an intentional action that is less proximally initiated by an unconscious urge.)

Recall that Libet himself says that "conscious volitional control may operate . . . to select and control ['the volitional process'], either by permitting or triggering the final motor outcome of the unconsciously initiated process or by vetoing the progression to actual motor activation" (1985, p. 529; also see 1999, p. 54). "Triggering" is a kind of initiating. In "triggering the final motor outcome," the acquisition of a proximal intention would be initiating an action in a more direct way than does an urge that initiated the process that issued in the intention. According to one view of things, when proximal action-desires help to initiate overt actions they do so by helping to produce pertinent proximal intentions the formation or acquisition of which directly initiates actions.[17] What Libet says about triggering here coheres with this.

Nothing warrants Libet's claim that, starting around −550 ms, type II RPs are correlated with decisions or intentions rather than with, for example, urges strong enough to issue pretty regularly in related intentions and actions. Moreover, that, in certain settings, (roughly) proximal urges to do things arise unconsciously—urges on which the agent may or may not act about half a second after they arise—is no cause for worry about free will. Even if one grants Libet much more than his critics tend to grant him, as I have done, it can be shown that his data fall well short of providing good grounds for accepting his main theses.[18]

5   Further Testing

I have argued that the "urge" hypothesis about what the type II RPs indicate in Libet's studies is less implausible than the "decision" or "intention" hypothesis. Is there an independent way to test these hypotheses—that is, to gather evidence about whether it is (roughly) proximal urges that emerge around −550 ms in Libet's studies or instead decisions or intentions?[19] One line of thought runs as follows: (1) all overt intentional actions are caused by decisions (or intentions). (2) The type II RPs, which emerge around −550 ms, are correlated with causes of the flexing actions (because they regularly precede the onset of muscle motion). So (3) these RPs indicate that decisions are made (or intentions acquired) at −550 ms. I have shown that this line of thought is unpersuasive. A lot can happen in a causal process that runs for 550 ms, including a subject's moving from having an unconscious roughly proximal urge to flex to consciously deciding to flex "now" or to consciously acquiring a proximal intention to flex. One can reply that, even so, (3) *might* be true. And, of course, I can run through my argumentation about the veto and related matters again to remind the imaginary respondent why (3) is improbable. But what about a test?

If makings of proximal decisions to flex or acquisitions of proximal intentions to flex (or the physical events that realize these things) cause muscle motion, how long does it take them to do that? Does it take about 550 ms? Might reaction time experiments show that 550 ms is too long a time for this?

Some caution is in order here. Lüder Deeke has distinguished among three kinds of decision: decisions about what to do, decisions about how to do something, and decisions about when to do something (1996, pp. 59–60). In typical reaction time experiments, subjects have decided in advance to perform an assigned task—to A, for short—whenever they detect the "go" signal.[20] When they detect the signal, there is no need for a proximal *decision* to A, as Deeke observes (p. 59). (If all decisions are responses to uncertainty about what to do and subjects are not uncertain about what to do when they detect the signal, there is no place here for proximal decisions to A.[21]) However, it is plausible that when they detect the signal, they acquire an *intention* to A now, a proximal intention. That is, it is plausible that the combination of their conditional intention to A when they detect the signal (or the neural realizer of that intention) and their detection of the signal (or the neural realizer of that detection) produces a proximal intention to A. (A familiar example of a conditional intention of this "when" kind is your intention, while stopped at a red light, to start driving again when the light turns green.) The acquisition of this proximal intention (or the neural realization of that event) would then initiate the A-ing.[22] And in at least one reaction time experiment (described shortly) that is very similar to Libet's main experiments, the time between the "go" signal and the onset of muscle motion is much shorter than 550 ms. This is evidence that proximal intentions to flex—as opposed, for example, to (roughly) proximal urges to flex—emerge much closer to the time of the onset of muscle motion than 550 ms. There is no reason, in principle, that it should take people any longer to start flexing their wrists when executing a proximal intention to flex in Libet's studies than it takes them to do this when executing such an intention in a reaction time study.

The line of reasoning that I have just sketched depends on the assumption that, in reaction time studies, a proximal intention to A is at work. An alternative possibility is that the combination of subjects' conditional intentions to A when they detect the signal and their detection of the signal initiates the A-ing without there being any proximal intention to A. Of course, there is a parallel possibility in the case of Libet's subjects. Perhaps the combination of their conditional intentions to flex when they next feel like it—conscious intentions, presumably—together with relevant feelings (namely, conscious proximal urges to flex) initiates a flexing without there being any proximal intentions to flex. (They may treat their initial consciousness of the urge as a "go" signal, as suggested by Keller and Heckhausen (1990, p. 352).) If that possibility is an actuality, then Libet's thesis is false, of course: there is no intention to flex "now" in his subjects and, therefore, no such intention is produced by the brain before the mind is aware of it.[23]

The reaction time study I mentioned is reported on pages 103 and 104 of Haggard and Magno 1999:

Subjects sat at a computer watching a clock hand . . . whose rotation period was 2.56 s. . . . After an unpredictable delay, varying from 2.56 to 8 s, a high-frequency tone . . . was played over a loudspeaker. This served as a warning stimulus for the subsequent reaction. 900 ms after the warning stimulus onset, a second tone . . . was played. [It] served as the go signal. Subjects were instructed to respond as rapidly as possible to the go signal with a right-key press on a computer mouse button. Subjects were instructed not to anticipate the go stimulus and were reprimanded if they responded on catch trials. . . . Reaction times were calculated by examining the EMG signal for the onset of the first sustained burst of muscle activity occurring after the go signal.

"Reaction time" here, then, starts *before* any intention to press "now" is acquired: obviously, it takes some time to detect the signal, and if detection of the signal helps to produce a proximal intention, that takes some time too. Haggard and Magno (ibid., p. 104) report that "the mean of the subjects' median reaction times in the control trials was 231 ms." If a proximal intention to press was acquired, that happened nearer to the time of muscle motion than 231 ms and, therefore, much nearer than the 550 ms that Libet claims is the time proximal intentions to flex are unconsciously acquired in his studies. Notice also how close we are getting to Libet's time W, his subjects' reported time of their initial awareness of something he variously describes as an "intention," "urge," "wanting," "decision," "will," or "wish" to move (−200 to −150 ms). Even without putting a great deal of weight on the exact number designating the mean of the median reaction times, one can fairly observe that if proximal intentions to flex are acquired in Libet's studies, Haggard and Magno's results make it look like a much better bet that they are acquired around time W than that they are acquired around −550 ms.[24] How seriously we should take Libet's subjects' reports of the time of their initial awareness of the urge, intention, or whatever is a controversial question, and I will say nothing about it here.

Patrick Haggard, in his contribution to a recent discussion with Libet, asserts that "conceptual analysis could help" (Haggard and Libet 2001, p. 62). This chapter may be read as a test of his assertion. In my opinion, the result is positive. Attention not only to the data but also to the concepts in terms of which the data are analyzed makes it clear that Libet's striking claims about decisions, intentions, and free will are not justified by his results. Libet asserts that his "discovery that the brain unconsciously initiates the volitional process well before the person becomes aware of an intention or wish to act voluntarily . . . clearly has a profound impact on how we view the nature of free will" (2004, p. 201). Not so. That, in certain settings, (roughly) proximal urges to do things arise unconsciously or issue from causes of which the agent is not conscious—urges on which the agent may or may not subsequently act—is a cause neither for worry nor for enthusiasm about free will.[25]

Notes

1. As I use "consistent" (following standard philosophical practice), to say that p is *consistent* with q is to say that "p and q" is not a contradiction.

2. So if the occurrence of x (at time t_1) indeterministically causes the occurrence of y (at t_2), then a complete description of the universe at t_1 together with a complete statement of the laws of nature does *not* entail that y occurs at t_2. There was at most a high probability that the occurrence of x at t_1 would cause the occurrence of y at t_2.

3. Jing Zhu writes: "Libet's account has received wide acceptance and is becoming the standard story." (2003, p. 62) His supporting references are Freeman 2000, Haggard and Libet 2001, McCrone 1999, Norretranders 1998, and Wegner 2002.

4. In a later article, Libet writes that "the brain has begun the specific preparatory processes for the voluntary act well before the subject is even aware of any wish or intention to act" (1992, p. 263).

5. Some passages in which two or more of these terms are used interchangeably are quoted in sections 3 and 4 below. Libet, Gleason et al. (1983, p. 627) report that "the subject was asked to note and later report the time of appearance of his conscious *awareness of 'wanting' to perform* a given self-initiated movement. The experience was also described as an 'urge' or 'intention' or 'decision' to move, though subjects usually settled for the words 'wanting' or 'urge'."

6. For conceptual discussion of wanting (or desiring), including its connection with motivation and its place in a developed causal theory of action, see Mele 2003.

7. I lack the space here to discuss other philosophical examinations of Libet's work. Recent examinations include Dennett 2003, Rosenthal 2002, and Zhu 2003.

8. I say "appears to" because an author may wish to distinguish an intention to flex one's wrist from an intention to initiate a flexing of one's wrist. I discuss initiation in section 4. For completeness, I observe that if we instead ignore the quotation's first disjunct it makes a claim about when an intention to *prepare* to flex—or to prepare to initiate a flexing of one's wrist—arises.

9. For a more thorough discussion of the experiment, see Libet et al. 1983 or Libet, Gleason et al. 1983.

10. I do not wish to exclude the possibility of such settledness in commissurotomy cases.

11. Another is that they have an intention to prepare to flex, if preparing is understood in such a way that so intending does not entail intending to flex.

12. There is room for disagreement, of course, about just what it means to say that an agent is "conscious of his intention" to A. For the purposes of this chapter, *consciously deciding* to flex now may be regarded as conceptually sufficient for the agent's being conscious of the proximal intention formed in that act of deciding. The agent need not, for example, have a conscious belief that he intends to flex now.

13. Recall that Libet suggests that the activation event occurs between 10 and 90 ms before the onset of muscle motion (1985, p. 537) and later revises the lower limit to 50 ms (2004, pp. 137–138).

14. Libet reports a study in which five subjects are "asked to report the clock time for their awareness of actually moving (M)" (1985, p. 534). The average reported time was −86 ms (p. 533). That is, this time—time M—preceded the beginning of muscle motion by an average of 86 ms. Sue Pockett asked (in correspondence) how this datum bears on the hypotheses I have just identified about when a proximal intention to move might be acquired in Libet's studies. Libet says that the "values for M suggest that it reflects the time of initiation of the final motor cortical output, i.e., the endogenous 'command to move'" (p. 533). This is a reasonable guess. Of course, whether time M (−86 ms) is the average time at which the command *actually* occurs is a separate issue. Even if M "reflects" the time of the command, the reflection might be imperfect. (We *know* that if subject B.D.'s time M—namely, +51 ms (p. 533)—reflects the time of the command, this reflection is imperfect.) Libet's guess implies that time M is closer to the time of this "command" than to the time of the onset of muscle motion. If the command *is* the acquisition of a proximal intention, then, of course, the time of the command is the time at which the proximal intention is acquired. If the acquisition of a proximal intention to move is a *cause* of the command, it occurs earlier than the command. Even if it is assumed that time M is the average time of the "command to move" in these five subjects, this datum also is consistent (see note 1) with the hypotheses I identified about the average time at which Libet's subjects acquire proximal intentions to flex.

15. When does the *action* begin in all this—that is, the person's flexing his wrist or fingers? This is a conceptual question, of course: how one answers it depends on one's answer to the question "What is an action?" Libet identifies "the actual time of the voluntary motor act" with the time "indicated by EMG recorded from the appropriate muscle" (1985, p. 532). I favor an alternative position, but there is no need to disagree with Libet about this for the purposes of this chapter. Following Brand (1984), Frederick Adams and I have defended the thesis that overt intentional actions (i.e., intentional actions that essentially involve peripheral bodily motion) begin in the brain, just after the acquisition of a proximal intention; the action is proximally initiated by the acquisition of the intention (Adams and Mele 1992). (One virtue of this view is that it helps handle certain problems about deviant causal chains; see chapter 2 of Mele 2003.) The relevant intention may be understood, in Libet's words, as an intention "to act now" (1989, p. 183; 1999, p. 54; 2004, p. 148), a proximal intention. (Of course, for Libet, as for me, "now" need not mean "this millisecond.") If I form the intention now to start running now, the action that is my running may begin just after the intention is formed, even though the relevant muscular motions do not begin until milliseconds later.

16. Notice that in addition to "vetoing" urges for actions that are not yet in progress, agents can abort attempts, including attempts at relatively temporally "short" actions. When batting, baseball players often successfully halt the motion of their arms while a swing is in progress. Presumably, they acquire or form an intention to stop swinging while they are in the process of executing an intention to swing. The intention to stop cancels and replaces the intention to swing.

17. See Mele 1992, pp. 71–77, 143–144, 168–170, 176–177, 190–191. Those who view the connection as direct take the view that actions begin in the brain.

18. For example, unlike many critics, I did not challenge Libet's method for timing the relevant conscious experiences.

19. Again, a more cautious formulation of the urge hypothesis is disjunctive and includes the possibilities that what emerges around −550 ms is a (roughly) proximal urge to flex, a pretty reliable relatively proximal causal contributor to such an urge, a (roughly) proximal urge to "prepare" to flex, a simulation of an urge of either kind, and the motor preparedness typically associated with such urges.

20. It should not be assumed that detecting the signal is a conscious event. See Prinz 2003.

21. In a reaction time study in which subjects are instructed to A or B when they detect the signal and not to decide in advance which to do, they may decide between A and B after detecting the signal.

22. Hereafter, the parenthetical clauses should be supplied by the reader. Intentions, in my view, are realized in physical states and events, and their causes are or are realized in physical states and events. I leave it open here that although intentions enter into causal explanations of actions, the causal work is done, not by them (qua intentions), but by their physical realizers. I forgo discussion of the metaphysics of mental causation, but see chapter 2 of Mele 1992.

23. Some researchers have a *nonstandard* conception of intentional action that may encourage them to believe that proximal intentions to flex are present in Libet's subjects but absent in subjects instructed, for example, to flex whenever they hear a tone. The following assertion from Haggard and Clark 2003 is

interesting in this connection: ". . . functional imaging studies of intentional actions typically show activation in the basal ganglia and supplementary motor area . . . while studies of externally triggered actions show activation in the cerebellum and premotor cortex" (pp. 695–696). This assertion implies that "externally triggered actions" are not intentional actions. One study Haggard and Clark cite here compares subjects instructed to raise their right index fingers whenever they wish without waiting more than 4 seconds between raisings with subjects instructed to do this whenever they hear a tone (Jahanshahi et al. 1995). (The tones are separated by no more than 4 seconds.) The first group are said to perform "self-initiated" finger raisings and the second to perform "externally triggered" finger raisings (ibid., p. 913). As I—and most people—understand intentional action, the finger-raising actions of both groups are obviously intentional. But as Haggard and Clark understand intentional action, the finger-raising actions of the second group are not intentional. In the words of Jahanshahi et al., the first group had "the additional requirement of *decision making* about the timing of the movement on each trial, or 'when to do' it" (1995, p. 930, emphasis added); and this is what motivates Haggard and Clark's claim about which finger raisings are intentional and which are not. Now, Haggard and Clark surely would find it odd to say that although the subjects in the second group do not intentionally raise their index fingers, they *intend* to raise them. So they probably are thinking that intentions are coextensive with decisions. If this is their view, then if my earlier claim that not all intentions are acquired in acts of decision making is correct, Haggard and Clark have an unduly restrictive conception of intention—a conception to which their restrictive conception of intentional action might have led them. Researchers with a more standard conception of intentional action will have no problem with the claim that subjects in both groups intentionally raise their index fingers (whether they believe that the second group proximally intend to do so or, instead, that the combination of their conditional intentions to raise their fingers when they detect the signal and their detection of the signal initiates the finger raisings in the absence of proximal intentions to raise them).

24. In a study by Day et al. of eight subjects instructed to flex a wrist when they hear a tone, mean reaction time was 125 ms (1989, p. 653). In their study of five subjects instructed to flex both wrists when they hear a tone, mean reaction time was 93 ms (p. 658). The mean reaction times of both groups of subjects—defined as "the interval from auditory tone to onset of the first antagonist EMG burst" (p. 651)—were much shorter than those of Haggard and Magno's subjects. Day et al.'s subjects, unlike Haggard and Magno's (and Libet's), were not watching a clock.

25. I am grateful to the editors for useful feedback. Parts of this chapter derive from chapter 2 of my in-press book.

References

Adams, F., and Mele, A. 1992. The intention/volition debate. *Canadian Journal of Philosophy* 22: 323–338.

Brand, M. 1984. *Intending and Acting*. MIT Press.

Day, B., J. Rothwell, P. Thompson, A. Maertens de Noordhout, K. Nakashima, K. Shannon, and C. Marsden, 1989. Delay in the execution of voluntary movement by electrical or magnetic brain stimulation in intact man. *Brain* 112: 649–663.

Deecke, L. 1996. Planning, preparation, execution, and imagery of volitional action. *Cognitive Brain Research* 3: 59–64.

Dennett, D. 2003. *Freedom Evolves*. Viking.

Frankfurt, H. 1988. *The Importance of What We Care About*. Cambridge University Press.

Freeman, W. J. 2000. *How Brains Make Up Their Minds*. Columbia University Press.

Gomes, G. 1999. Volition and the readiness potential. *Journal of Consciousness Studies* 6: 59–76.

Haggard, P., and Clark, S. 2003. Intentional action: conscious experience and neural prediction. *Consciousness and Cognition* 12: 695–707.

Haggard, P., and Libet, B. 2001. Conscious intention and brain activity. *Journal of Consciousness Studies* 8: 47–63.

Haggard, P., and Magno E. 1999. Localising awareness of action with transcranial magnetic stimulation. *Experimental Brain Research* 127: 102–107.

Haggard, P., Newman, C., and Magno, E. 1999. On the perceived time of voluntary actions. *British Journal of Psychology* 90: 291–303.

Jahanshahi, M., Jenkins, I. H., Brown, R. Marsden, C. D., Passingham, R., and Brooks, D. 1995. Self-initiated versus externally triggered movements. *Brain* 118: 913–933.

Kane, R. 1996. *The Significance of Free Will*. Oxford University Press.

Keller, I., and Heckhausen, H. 1990. Readiness potentials preceding spontaneous motor acts: voluntary vs. involuntary control. *Electroencephalography and Clinical Neurophysiology* 76: 351–361.

Libet, B. 1985. Unconscious cerebral initiative and the role of conscious will in voluntary action. *Behavioral and Brain Sciences* 8: 529–566.

Libet, B. 1989. The timing of a subjective experience. *Behavioral and Brain Sciences* 12: 183–184.

Libet, B. 1992. The neural time-factor in perception, volition and free will. *Revue de Métaphysique et de Morale* 2: 255–272.

Libet, B. 1999. Do we have free will? *Journal of Consciousness Studies* 6: 47–57.

Libet, B. 2001. Consciousness, free action and the brain. *Journal of Consciousness Studies* 8: 59–65.

Libet, B. 2004. *Mind Time*. Harvard University Press.

Libet, B., Wright, E., and Gleason, C. 1982. Readiness potentials preceding unrestricted "spontaneous" vs. pre-planned voluntary acts. *Electroencephalography and Clinical Neurophysiology* 54: 322–335.

Libet, B., Gleason, C., Wright E., and Pearl, D. 1983. Time of unconscious intention to act in relation to onset of cerebral activity (Readiness-Potential). *Brain* 106: 623–642.

Libet, B., Wright, E., and Curtis, A. 1983. Preparation- or intention-to-act, in relation to pre-event potentials recorded at the vertex. *Electroencephalography and Clinical Neurophysiology* 56: 367–372.

Marcel, A. 2003. The sense of agency: Awareness and ownership of action. In *Agency and Self-Awareness*, ed. J. Roessler and N. Eilan. Clarendon.

McCrone, J. 1999. *Going Inside: A Tour Round the Single Moment of Consciousness*. Faber and Faber.

Mele, A. 1992. *Springs of Action: Understanding Intentional Behavior*. Oxford University Press.

Mele, A. 1997. Strength of motivation and being in control: Learning from Libet. *American Philosophical Quarterly* 34: 319–333.

Mele, A. 2003. *Motivation and Agency*. Oxford University Press.

Mele, A. In press. *Free Will and Luck*. Oxford University Press.

Norretranders, T. 1998. *The User Illusion: Cutting Consciousness Down to Size*. Viking.

Pereboom, D. 2001. *Living without Free Will*. Cambridge University Press.

Prinz, W. 2003. How do we know about our own actions? In *Voluntary Action*, ed. S. Maasen et al. Oxford University Press.

Rosenthal, D. 2002. The timing of conscious states. *Consciousness and Cognition* 11: 215–220.

Smith, M. 2003. Rational capacities. In *Weakness of Will and Practical Irrationality*, ed. S. Stroud and C. Tappolet. Clarendon.

Wegner, D. 2002. *The Illusion of Conscious Will*. MIT Press.

11 Of Windmills and Straw Men: Folk Assumptions of Mind and Action

Bertram F. Malle

Prologue

A few days ago I finally gave in to the belief that it is really my brain that makes decisions, forms intentions, and executes actions and that "I" and my feelings of intending and deciding are at best spectators of the only show in town, the only real causes of behavior. Since then I have let my brain do the deciding and intending as before, but without me, without my trying, without my illusory control. Funny thing is, my brain just didn't do anything. It didn't intend to do the laundry, it didn't bike to the office, it didn't decide to write this overdue chapter. As I saw it, my brain didn't do much at all, except present me with all kinds of thoughts and observations of its own inactivity. So I changed my mind again and rejected the belief that it is really my brain that makes decisions. Since then, I have biked to the office twice, I haven't done the laundry yet, but at least I have started writing this chapter.

1 Common Sense and Folk Assumptions

Ordinary people assume that they have access to their mental states, shape the world with their intentions, and understand the reasons for their actions. In contrast, several scholars have claimed that these folk assumptions are misguided. In this chapter I examine the conceptual and empirical foundations of such skeptical claims.

My analysis focuses on skepticism about awareness of one's own mind and actions and skepticism about intentional agency. In each case, I find that skeptics often misrepresent the folk assumptions about these phenomena and about such key concepts as *intention*, *action*, and *reason*. As a result, scientific discussions about introspection, action explanation, and intentional agency often portray folk psychology in the form of a straw man—not as the complex array of concepts and assumptions that uniquely characterize human beings. Much of the skepticism about folk psychology also resembles a battle against windmills—fighting perceived enemies of the scientific worldview that may, in reality, be no enemies at all.

In everyday parlance, common sense is a good thing; not so in much of psychology. It is common sense to assume that people have beliefs, desires, and intentions, act on their intentions, and thus have control over many of their actions—in fact, it would count as a serious lack of common sense to assume otherwise. But a good number of scientists argue that all or most of these assumptions are mistaken. Relying on their common sense, people seemingly have no idea how the mind works. "There is not the slightest awareness [among people] of the possibility that what appears in personal conscious experience might not be the fundament for everything else." (Maasen, Prinz, and Roth 2003, p. 9) So people are informed that they have no reliable access to their mental states (Nisbett and Wilson 1977), that their brains know that they are going to act before they intend to so act (Libet, Gleason, Wright, and Pearl 1983), and that any impression of controlling their actions is illusory (Wegner 2002).

Each of these revisionist claims has to be examined in its own terms, and I will do so shortly. But first I want to clarify what this talk about "common-sense" or folk assumptions should really mean. Common sense appears to be what ordinary people think, or assume, or are committed to. Of course, there may be quite a bit of variation, across people, across cultures, and across historical times. So what is constant enough to count as a genuine common-sense view? A growing literature in social psychology, developmental psychology, and cognitive science suggests that the core of common sense is a set of concepts and assumptions about the nature of mind and behavior, typically labeled folk concepts and folk-conceptual assumptions (Astington 1991; d'Andrade 1987; Malle, Moses, and Baldwin 2001; Wellman 1990).

The first thing to note about these folk concepts and their relationships is that they are not simply beliefs about some facts in the world (Malle 2005). There are plenty of commonly held cultural beliefs and community opinions that are not folk-conceptual assumptions. What folk concepts do is frame a phenomenon in a certain way—categorize a domain into relevant parts and organize their systematic relationships. The concept of intentionality, for example, shapes the observation of events in such a way that subsequent processing (e.g., explanation, prediction, or moral evaluation) differs quite systematically depending on the perception of a behavior as intentional or unintentional, with significant repercussions in social, legal, and political life (Malle and Knobe 1997; Malle, Moses, and Baldwin 2001).

Because of the strong influence of folk concepts on cognition and social life, scholars who talk about things like intentionality, awareness, and choice must make a fundamental decision: Are they going to talk about these things the way ordinary people do (that is, are they going to use the folk concepts with their normal meaning and reference), or are they introducing technical terms? One would hope that, if the latter, they would just use a new word, but that is not always done. (See Malle and Nelson 2003.) Ultimately, whenever a scientist describes a folk assumption and claims that some evidence shows it to be wrong, the scientist has to adhere to the folk meaning of the relevant concepts, or else the evidence isn't relevant.

The meaning of a folk concept can't just be intuited by any given researcher; it will have to be shown empirically by means of a systematic description and analysis of what ordinary people assume. In the absence of solid data, there is quite some disagreement about what folk psychology's assumptions are, about how folk concepts are defined, and about how they are related to each other (Malle and Knobe 1997). An empirical backing of the initial description and explication of folk concepts is important not just because it is the scientifically rigorous thing to do but also because scholars often underestimate the sophistication and complexity of these concepts.

2 Overview

This chapter examines skeptical or revisionist claims about two key folk assumptions: *awareness* (the assumption that people have awareness of their own mental states, including current thoughts and feelings, and of their reasons and intentions to act), and *intentional agency* (the assumption that a necessary cause of intentional behavior is the agent's conscious intention to act). I will examine skeptical claims mainly from the empirical sciences and will evaluate them both for their target accuracy (whether they actually hit folk assumptions) and for their internal validity. But first I need to clear two preliminary hurdles.

The first hurdle is that the assumptions of awareness and intentional agency aren't always neatly separated (Pacherie, this volume). John Bargh, for example writes: "Conscious intention and behavioral (motor) systems are fundamentally dissociated in the brain. *In other words*, the evidence shows that much if not most of the workings of the motor systems that guide action are opaque to conscious access." (2005, p. 43; emphasis added) I see two distinct questions here: whether intentions do in fact control the organism's motor system (the intentional-agency assumption) and what is or is not available to conscious access (the awareness assumption). Daniel Wegner warns against mingling the issues of awareness and intentional agency when he writes that "questions of how thought or consciousness might cause action" (intentional agency) have "been muddled together with questions of the person's experience of such causation" (awareness) (2005, p. 32). I fear, however, that Wegner may contribute to this muddling by claiming that "conscious will is a cognitive feeling" (p. 31) and that "intention is important not as a cause, but because it is a conscious preview of the action" (p. 28). I do, however, agree with Wegner's programmatic claim that we must separate the question of what the person is aware of (through feeling, experience, or preview) from the question of what is the actual causal role of intentions. (I will return to Wegner's model in section 3.)

The second hurdle is that the assumption of intentional agency is often intertwined with rather metaphysical claims about free will, causality, and mind-body dualism. For example, Patrick Haggard and Sam Clark state that "a modern neuroscientist cannot believe in 'free will' in Descartes' sense: conscious experience must be a consequence of brain activity rather than a cause of it" (2002, p. 705). While trying to eschew Cartesian dualism, this statement still seems to rely on the notion of a purely conscious event that is somehow not encompassed in a complete description of brain activity. Only if such an event exists would we have to label it a separate *consequence* of brain activity. I will try to keep the folk assumptions of awareness and intentional agency separate from questions about mind-body dualism and causality, because folk psychology does not have to be (and probably is not) committed to a particular view on the mind-body relation, as long as there is a *conceptual* and *functional* distinction made between mental and nonmental events. But I will not always succeed; the discussion of intentional agency will drag us into the murky depths of the free will problem, and it is not clear we will emerge unscathed.

3   The Folk Assumption of Awareness

Awareness of Mental States

Ever since introspectionism was discredited as a scientific method in psychology (because science can never be intersubjective if scientists use their own minds to test hypotheses), many have expressed skepticism about the very possibility of introspection. For example, Francis Crick (1979) wrote that "we are deceived at every level by our introspection." More recently, Alison Gopnik (1993) claimed that our experience of "directly perceiving" our own mental states is the mere result of expertise and practice in inferring those mental states from other information, and Bargh suggested that "people do not and cannot have direct access to acts of causal intention and choice" (2005, p. 42). Perhaps the most widely cited analysis of introspection was offered by Richard Nisbett and Tim Wilson (1977), whose analysis will help us sort out what people are aware of and what people *assume* they are aware of. (See also Ross, this volume.)

Nisbett and Wilson typically described their data and their analysis as concerning introspection. In their abstract, for example, they claimed that their review suggests "little or no *introspective* access to higher-order mental processes" (1977, p. 233), and they used the word 'introspection' in several other programmatic phrases. However, Nisbett and Wilson did not question a person's entire capacity to introspect on (i.e., be aware of) ongoing mental states or contents; they questioned specifically human access to *higher-order mental or cognitive processes*—that is, "the processes mediating the effects of a stimulus on a response" (p. 231). What was at issue for them was the accuracy of reporting on "the effects of particular stimuli on higher order, inference-based responses" (p. 233). There is little doubt that Nisbett and Wilson made a good case for at least some of these limitations (White 1988). But can their data and their conclusions inform us about the adequacy of ordinary people's assumption about introspection?

There isn't a solid model of the "folk theory of introspection," but awareness of mental states appears to have at least two defining conditions (d'Andrade 1987; Malle et al. 2000): (a) that the event (state, process) introspected is conscious and (b) that the act of introspection occurs simultaneously with the event. The first condition excludes the misnomer "unconscious introspection," and the second rules out mere memory of conscious processes as a reliable candidate for self-awareness. Thus, people assume awareness of their ongoing conscious perceptions, feelings, thoughts, intentions, and reasons for acting, but not of their unconscious wishes or past emotions. All of Nisbett and Wilson's (1977) reviewed and reported data, however, seem to violate either condition (a) or condition (b). For example, people's documented inability to report on the effects of subtle experimental manipulations (e.g., dissonance inductions, subliminal stimulus presentation, attitude change) should not threaten the folk assumption of mental awareness, because none of these stimulus-induced processes are considered conscious. (In fact, the experimenters take great pains to keep them unconscious.) Many of Nisbett and Wilson's reported and reviewed data also involve memory judgments. But most important, virtually all of the relevant mental processes they consider are or involve *causal judgments* (e.g., why participants offered certain associative responses, why they chose certain stockings, whether specific features of a target person had influenced their overall impression of the person). There is no folk assumption according to which one always knows the causes of one's mental states and behaviors. Here Nisbett and Wilson may show limitations of human causal cognition but not limitations of human introspection.

There is one exception, however: People do assume that they know their intentions and their reasons for action (d'Andrade 1987; Malle 1999; Malle and Knobe 1997, 2001). Here were have not a straw man but an actual folk assumption: Intentional actions are assumed to have privileged status for the actor, and in two ways. First, awareness that one is acting with the intention to so act is a defining feature of the folk concept of intentionality (Malle and Knobe 1997). Second, because intentions are conceptualized as the outcome of a reasoning process that combines relevant beliefs and desires as the *reasons* for acting (Malle and Knobe 2001), the actor is normally aware of her reasons to act. I will return to the role of intentions; here I discuss the awareness of reasons.

Let's be clear about the folk concept of reason. Reasons are agents' mental states whose content they considered and in light of which they formed an intention to act (Malle 1999). Reasons, in this sense, have both explanatory force and causal force—they make intelligible why ("for what reason") the agent acted, and they were the mental states that actually issued in an intention and, subsequently, in an action. Even though reason explanations are most frequently used in the first-person (actor) perspective, people don't reserve reason explanations for that perspective. They feel perfectly comfortable ascribing reasons to others from a third-person perspective, and they even feel comfortable ascribing reasons to whole groups (O'Laughlin and Malle 2002). Moreover, reasons are not the only explanation mode people offer for intentional behavior. An important additional mode comprises CHR (causal history of reason) explanations (Malle 1999), which cite factors that lay in the background of those reasons and brought them about (e.g., context, culture, personality, habits, unconscious mental states). Here are two reason (R) explanations and two CHR explanations for the same action:

Anne invited Ben for dinner because . . . it was her roommate's birthday. (R)

she hadn't seen him in a month. (R)

she is generous. (CHR)

they are friends. (CHR)

The awareness assumption for reasons, then, goes something like this: If actors are honest and undeluded, the reason explanations they give for their actions cite the very reasons for which they acted—the contentful mental states such as beliefs and desires that generated the intention to act. There is no incorrigibility (people can misremember, and observers can muster evidence that proves certain reason claims wrong); but there is privileged access in that actors normally know the reasons for which they acted, because the very action was performed on the grounds of and in light of those reasons.

Nisbett and Wilson presented results from several studies that argue against this sort of privileged access. In perhaps the most famous of these studies, passersby in a department store were asked to evaluate items of clothing (such as nightgowns or stockings) and to choose the one that was of the best quality. The items were all identical, however, except that they were arranged horizontally on a clothing rack. Nisbett and Wilson showed that articles on the left were more likely to be chosen than articles on the right. But "when asked about the reasons for their choices, no subject ever mentioned spontaneously the position of the article" (1977, pp. 243–244). This study is usually taken to show that people can't really explain why they acted, that they don't have any privileged access to the causes of their behavior, and therefore that "it may be quite misleading for social scientists to ask their subjects about the influences on their evaluations, choices, or behavior" (ibid., p. 247).

But here is the problem: In this shopping study actors offered *reason explanations* whereas the researchers expected a causal-history explanation. Nothing in the study shows that actors weren't accurate in their report of their reasons for acting or that they were "unable to tell the experimenter why [they] chose the pair of stockings on the right" (Bayer, Ferguson, and Gollwitzer 2003, p. 100). In fact, it is quite likely that most participants honestly reported their reasons for choosing one or the other stocking: for example, because they like it better, or that it seemed of better quality. At the same time, participants were not aware of certain factors (such as spatial position) that brought about those reasons—that is, they didn't correctly identify the causal history of those reasons. Such a finding obviously does not invalidate the assumption about agents' awareness of their reasons; it only illustrates something that people would readily admit: that they don't have any special knowledge of or access to the causal history of their reasons. In fact, my colleagues and I have demonstrated that the assumption of awareness is one critical feature that distinguishes reason explanations from CHR explanations (Malle 1999; Malle et al. 2000). And just as the two kinds of explanations are complementary in everyday explanations (Malle 2004), they are complementary for explaining participants' actions in Nisbett and Wilson's study. The position of stockings or nightgowns may have unwittingly triggered some people's *belief* that "these look well-made" or a *liking* of their sheen, and the content of these mental states may have been the reasons for the choice of "the best" pair of stockings. People's reasons, if honestly reported, simply were the reasons for which they acted (perhaps trivial reasons appropriate to the trivial choice); and they did have unfettered access to those reasons.

Even though people do seem to know their reasons for acting, they don't know every factor that contributed causally to their actions. Besides position effects, a variety of other stimuli (e.g., concepts, feelings, associations) can be used to subliminally prime people's thinking and thereby influence their choices. (See Bargh 2005 for a review.) But to the extent that the primed behavior in question is intentional, people should still be aware of their intentions and their reasons for acting. We can't conclude that individuals are "not aware of the actual causes of their behavior" (Bargh 2005, p. 38), because causal-history factors are no more "actual" than the reasons that issued in the person's intention to act. We certainly cannot conclude, at least from these experiments, that "the individual's behavior is being 'controlled' by external stimuli, not by his or her own consciously accessible intentions or acts of will" (ibid., p. 38). We can conclude that people weren't aware of stimuli that were carefully designed to be unconscious influences on their behavior; and we can conclude that, in general, people will not be aware of a host of factors that lay in the causal history of their reasons. But none of the experiments reviewed and reported by Nisbett and Wilson (1977) and Bargh (2005) refute the assumption that people are aware of their reasons.

The distinction between reasons and CHR factors is not just of theoretical significance; it has significant social import as well. People have no trouble distinguishing (in practice and judgment) between CHR explanations and reason explanations, and they are very upset when the legal system conflates the two (Wilson 1997). The defendant who wanted to kill the child was not "controlled" by such external stimuli as his abusive childhood, nor were these stimuli the "actual causes" of his behavior. The person decided to kill the child with whatever reasons he had, and for that he is held responsible. One may feel empathy with a criminal who was starved, abused, tortured, or humiliated, but if there was a point at which the person intended to act in a harmful way, the causal history can at best mitigate the blame; it cannot relieve the person of responsibility (Banks, this volume, Kaplan, this volume). Judgments of responsibility rest squarely on the transition of reasons to intentions and actions. Consequently, a compelling threat to folk assumptions of intentional action would have to zero in on this transition; it is what people defend when they hear claims of an "illusion of free will"; it is the raw nerve touched by legal, medical, or political processes that question the unique implications of intentional agency and the unique role of reasons.

But before we take on the heavy issue of agency and free will, we must examine one other skeptical claim about awareness.

Awareness of Action

One might think that, even if there is some doubt about people's awareness of their intentions and reasons, surely there can't be any doubt about people's awareness of their actions. There can indeed. Besides claims that people lack access to their mental states, there are also suggestions in the literature that people lack awareness of their own actions. Bargh (2005) underscores "just how unaware we are of how we move and make movements in space" (p. 45) and that people have "little or no direct conscious access to their actual hand movements" (p. 46). Marc Jeannerod, too, suggests that "normal subjects are poorly aware of their own movements" (2002, p. 312). Now, any movement is an extremely complex neurophysiological process, and no folk psychology would ever assume access to all that. To evaluate the skeptical claims about action awareness we have to draw a few distinctions. One is between visual perception of one's movement and internal access to that movement. Internal access breaks down further into (a) proprioceptive/somatosensory information, (b) information about the motor commands and adjustments during the movement, and (c) awareness of the intended end state of the movement.

The empirical research in the domain of action control provides fairly clear data on these different types of access. (See Blakemore, Wolpert, and Frith 2002 for a review.) People normally have good visual information about their executed movements, but they are not particularly sensitive to variations in this execution as long as the actual movement conforms reasonably well to the intended movement. In a study by Elena Daprati and colleagues (1997), for example, people saw a video display of either their own or another person's hand (both in gloves) performing either the same or different movements (such as stretching a particular finger). When the other person's hand performed a different movement, participants easily recognized the video-displayed hand as either theirs or the other's. When the other person's hand performed the same movement, however, they misjudged the other's hand as theirs in about 30 percent of cases.

People are more sensitive to proprioceptive and somatosensory information. When performing an intentional act, the central nervous system predicts the sensory consequences of that act and compares these predictions to the sensory feedback during and after the movement (Blakemore, Frith, and Wolpert 2001). When the feedback matches the prediction (as in the normal case of self-initiated movement), the CNS attenuates the sensory feedback. This attenuation is one of the key indicators of having acted oneself rather than having been acted on, and it explains why tickling oneself is less noticeable (because it is attenuated) than being tickled by another person (Blakemore, Wolpert, and Frith 2000).

People are not finely attuned to the specific motor commands and adjustments their motor system makes during the execution of a movement. This is not surprising, given the complex physical and physiological structure of most movements. For example, when participants were given false feedback about their drawing motions, their hands still completed the drawing task with appropriate corrections of movement, but the participants themselves were not aware of any deviant movements (Fourneret and Jeannerod 1998). Once again, the match between intended and completed action appears to make explicit feedback about slight movement alterations unnecessary.

Studies on the time perception of self-generated action also address the question of what people are aware of and when. In these studies, participants watch a rotating hand on a clock face and indicate at what time point a certain event occurred (e.g., a tone, an externally induced muscle twitch, a self-initiated action). People's estimates of the time at which they perform a simple action (e.g., pressing a lever) can precede the onset of relevant muscle activity by up to 90 milliseconds (Libet et al. 1983; Haggard, Newman, and Magno 1999). In contrast, perceptions of externally induced events such as tones or transcranial stimulation are typically delayed by 15–80 ms. These findings suggest that action perception is not a reconstructive process (observing oneself → inferring that one acted; see Prinz 2003) but rather a prospective process (predicting one's action on the basis of an intention).

The claim that action perception is prospective appears to be challenged by findings that time estimates for one's own actions are no faster than time estimates for another person's actions (Wohlschläger, Haggard, Gesierich, and Prinz 2003; Wohlschläger, Engbert, and Haggard 2003). However, in these studies, people were asked to estimate "when the lever was depressed," corresponding to the time of action *completion*, not of initiation. Even under these conditions, self-generated actions were pre-dated (unweighted M across five experiments = −8 ms) whereas other-generated actions were post-dated (M = +8 ms). Most important, in the basic design by Wohlschläger and colleagues, each completed lever pressing triggered a tone 250 ms later. It has been shown that immediate consequences of one's intentional actions such as a tone can "pull" the time estimate for the action toward a later point (Haggard, Clark, and Kalogeras 2002), presumably because the action and its reliable effect are perceived as a unit (Heider 1958). When the tone was eliminated, self-generated action estimates sped up (M = −20 ms) whereas other-action estimates stayed the same (M = +5 ms).

The intriguing conclusion from research on action control and chronometric action perception is that people have more access to their movements *before* they occur (via intentions and "predictions" of the system) than during or after. As long as the intended movement and its consequences obtain roughly as expected, little updated information reaches consciousness. From a cybernetic standpoint this makes good sense—an efficient motor system invests heavily in the planning and execution of a movement but provides explicit feedback only if the plan failed. Another way of putting it is that people may not have detailed awareness of their *movements* (the physical motion pattern of their limbs and body) but are perfectly aware of their *actions*—what they are intending to do no matter how it is exactly implemented by the motor system (Jeannerod, this volume).

4 The Folk Assumption of Intentional Agency

Humans consider themselves and others as agents who are capable of intentional action. This is the assumption of intentional agency, perhaps the very core of folk psychology. Intentionality is a complex folk concept that specifies under what conditions people judge a behavior as intentional (or done on purpose). Observational and experimental research suggest that this judgment relies on at least five conditions (Malle and Knobe 1997): An action is considered intentional when the agent had (1) a desire for an outcome, (2) a belief that the action would lead to that outcome, (3) an intention to perform the action, (4) the skill to perform the action,

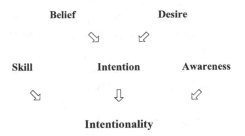

Figure 11.1
The folk concept of intentionality (Malle and Knobe 1997).

and (5) awareness of fulfilling the intention while performing the action (figure 11.1). The folk concept of intentionality thus defines the key ingredients of intentional action and relates them to each other. There is little doubt that the intentionality concept has enormous impact on social perception, self-regulation, communication, and just about all interpersonal, aesthetic, legal, and moral dealings in the social world (Gibbs 1999; Malle and Knobe 1997; Malle, Moses, and Baldwin 2001; Marshall 1968; Shaver 1985). Perhaps the most important function of the intentionality concept is to divide all behavioral events into two different domains that are subsequently processed in distinct ways by such operations as attention, explanation, prediction, or moral evaluation. When explaining behavior, for example, people account for intentional behavior primarily in terms of the agent's reasons, but they account for unintentional behavior in terms of causes (Buss 1978; Heider 1958; Malle 1999). Arguably, these explanation modes correspond to two models of causality. On the one hand, there are causal processes that involve the formation of intentions out of reasons (involving awareness and choice); on the other hand, there are causal processes that are mechanistic, involving no reasons, intention, awareness, or choice (Malle 2001, 2004).

These assumptions about intentional action and its causal structure are, in the eyes of many scholars, deeply mistaken. According to Wegner and Wheatley, "psychological science suggests that all behavior can be ascribed to mechanisms that transcend human agency" (1999, p. 480), and "the real causal mechanism is the marvelously intricate web of causation that is the topic of scientific psychology" (ibid., p. 490). For Prinz, "there appears to be no support for the folk psychology notion that the act follows the will, in the sense that physical action is caused by mental events that precede them" (2003, p. 26).

In the same sprit, the intentional agency assumption is criticized for implying a mystical "free will." Maasen, Prinz, and Roth find a "jargon of free will in everyday language" (2003, p. 8). And this notion of free will is unacceptable because it "requires us to accept local pockets of indeterminism in an otherwise deterministically conceived word view" (ibid.). A massive philosophical debate is caving in on us here, as the tension between free will and the presupposition of determinism is one of the deeply unresolved issues in modern thinking.

Simplifying the task somewhat, I set aside the question of determinism. Even so, understanding what the assumption of free will means is sufficiently challenging. Is the intentional-agency assumption equivalent to a theory of "free will?" Does it at least imply free will? Or does it leave this difficult issue untouched? I am sure that in one way or another ordinary people regard their *actions* as "free," if what is meant by that is having options, considering them and, in their light, forming an intention to act (which is just the intentional-agency assumption restated). Perhaps more narrowly, acting "freely" contrasts with acting under duress or constraints (which may still be intentional, as when I hand over my wallet to the robber who sticks a gun in my side), and of course it contrasts with a whole host of unintentional events—from failed attempts to accidental side effects, unwelcome mental states, and wholly unconscious cognitive processes.

But do people assume that their *will* is free? If 'will' refers to desires (wants, wishes), people don't. Desires are typically caused by internal or external stimuli, and it makes little sense to say that a person "formed" a desire (the same way one can form an intention; see Malle and Knobe 2001). Thus, "free will" can refer to the freedom to form intentions or to make choices—and once more, this interpretation is well covered by the intentional-agency assumption.

Is there anything entailed by the notion of free will that is not already expressed by the intentional-agency assumption? Some people have argued that free will implies a lack of causes, corresponding to the belief "that willfulness somehow springs forth from some special uncaused place" (Bayr et al., p. 100). And of course that would make scientists nervous, because "to choose a spouse, a job, a religious creed—or even to choose to rob a bank—is the peak of a causal chain that runs back to the origin of life and down to the nature of atoms and molecules" (Blakemore 1988, p. 270). However, we need not worry, because an uncaused will directly contradicts the folk concept of intentionality in which the intentional action is caused (among other things, by an intention), the intention is caused (among other things, by the reasons in light of which the agent formed the intention), and reasons are caused (by other mental states, external events, and many other CHR factors). Exactly how an intention is caused by the reasons in light of which it was adopted is a difficult question (and one on which folk psychology is silent), but there is no evidence for the idea that ordinary people consider intentions "uncaused causes."

Another proposal is that "our actions are free as long as they are primarily determined by our conscious, rather than unconscious decisions" (Klein 2002, p. 277). Note that the attribute "free" is applied here to actions, not to a will. But all the better, because such an assumption of consciousness or awareness seems entailed by the folk concept of intentionality, in which the agent is aware of her intention when acting intentionally (Malle and Knobe 1997). We might add that this sort of freedom-as-consciousness also holds for intentions because people assume that agents are aware of their reasons when deciding to act.

In sum, there is no evidence available that *will* is actually a folk concept (such as *intentionality* or *intention*), and the notion of "free will" is at best vague and at worst meaningless. The folk assumption of intentional agency, in contrast, is a clearer and fairer target of scientific skepticism. In the following I discuss three such skeptical proposals that threaten this folk assumption: (1) that intentional actions are not caused by *conscious* states, (2) that intentional actions are not caused by *intentions*, and (3) that actions are not caused by *anything mental*.

No Consciousness

The first thesis is that "the real causes of human action are unconscious" (Wegner and Wheatley 1999, p. 490). Such a thesis would be supported by cases of intentional action that are unambiguously and directly brought about by unconscious processes; this evidence would then contradict the folk assumption that conscious intentions cause intentional action.

Some of the most extensive research on unconscious causes of behavior comes from John Bargh's laboratory. (See Bargh 2005 for a review.) Bargh and his colleagues have shown, for example, that experimental participants who are unconsciously primed with words like 'Florida' and 'retire' walk more slowly after the experiment than a control group, and that people primed with words like 'achieve' do objectively better on a Scrabble-type task. Do these findings threaten the folk assumption of intentional agency? They do not, as long as the behaviors affected by unconscious priming are unintentional. For example, Chartrand and Bargh (1996) showed that classic patterns of impression formation (e.g., clustering of information and better recall for target behavior) can be achieved by subconsciously priming the participant with words related to impression formation (e.g., 'evaluate', 'judge'). However, the participants did not "intentionally form an impression" (the post-experimental interviews make this very clear); rather, certain cognitive effects obtained without the participant actively aiming at those effects. The same consideration applies to "walking slowly" after being primed by 'Florida' and probably even to "trying harder" in the Scrabble task after being primed by 'achieve'. Of course, both "walking" and "solving the task" are intentional actions. But the unconscious priming did not affect the intentional action itself (the agent decided to walk or to solve the task independent of the prime) but rather the way, manner, or style in which the action was performed—aspects that typically are not within the scope of the agent's intention (Nahmias 2002; Norman and Shallice 1986). Along the same lines, intentional actions come with motor command adjustments in response to subtle changes in the environment and with electrochemical processes at the motor synapses. All of these are unconscious; none of them are performed intentionally.[1]

Thus, we have to find cases in which it was itself an intentional action that was influenced by unconscious priming. A case discussed earlier is Nisbett and Wilson's (1977) shopping study, in which more people chose the "best" item (clearly an intentional action) under the apparent unconscious influence of physical position. However, I have argued that this position effect illustrates the operation of a causal-history factor (which typically operates outside consciousness) and is thus perfectly compatible with the interpretation that people acted on their intentions and reasons.

A more compelling case to consider is a study in which people primed with words such as 'rude' and 'impolite' were more likely than control participants to interrupt an ongoing conversation and ask for the next experimental task (Bargh, Chen, and Burrows 1996). The act of interrupting is normally intentional, and the priming exerted an unconscious influence on the action. But what is the relationship between the priming and this intention? The participants' intention was neither absent nor unconscious, and we can be sure that all of them had reasons to interrupt (or not interrupt, as was the case for a third of them). The priming effect may have disinhibited and thereby strengthened their desire reason ("I want to ask them") or provided a belief reason ("They are rude to ignore me"), thus again serving as CHR factors. Or the priming may have facilitated the execution of the relevant intention—for example, by weakening feelings of reluctance, doubt, and anxiety. In this case, the priming was an "enabling factor" (Malle 1999)—a process that is seen as helping the agent turn an intention into action. (A less complex enabling factor explanation would be "She finished her exam in just 30 minutes because she had one of those new calculators.") The folk theory of intentional action thus leaves room for causal contributions outside the reason → intention chain, in the form of causal-history factors and enabling factors, both of which can operate in a nonconscious, nonintentional manner. To the extent that the above studies manipulated these factors but left the intention intact, the studies do not invalidate the folk assumption of intentional agency.

How about cases in which the agent forms "implementation intentions" (Gollwitzer 1999)? For example: "When the light turns green, I will slam the pedal to show this guy who has the faster car." Here an intention is formed well in advance of the action, but the intention is a conditional one: The agent commits to a proximal intention (Mele 2003) to act if and when a suitable environmental stimulus is present. Is the implemented action one that is both intentional and caused by unconscious processes? One way to handle this case is to say that the primary cause of the action is the proximal intention and the rest are just enabling factors (parallel to the guitarist who forms a conscious decision to play "Asturias" but then relies on unconscious motor programs to implement the action). This may be a logically acceptable defense of the folk assumption, but it doesn't seem entirely satisfactory.

Perhaps it is necessary to clarify what happens at the time the action is performed—what the agent's state of mind is at the moment the stimulus triggers the action. Gollwitzer (1999) suggests that no conscious intention is necessary at that time; what initiates the action is an automatic goal activation, with external stimuli acting as "direct elicitors of goal-directed action" (Gollwitzer and Moskowitz 1996, p. 370). Currently there is no decisive evidence for the claim that agents are in fact not conscious of the action initiation. But even if we grant the absence of a moment of conscious choice, there has to be at least a proximal intention to *continue* what one is doing if the behavior in question should count as intentional. The previously established stimulus-goal association may initiate a behavior without the agent's conscious awareness. However, for that behavior to be considered intentional (or to *become* intentional) the agent must at some point gain awareness of it and approve it. There are probably a number of behaviors that are initiated unconsciously and then subjected to the agent's (conscious) decision to either continue or halt. (Detected action slips are the classic case of halted behaviors of this sort.) If, however, the agent remains entirely unaware of the behavior throughout its implementation, people are unlikely to consider this an intentional action. That would apply, for example, to the case of implementation intentions preventing automatic stereotype activation (Moskowitz, Gollwitzer, Wasel, and Schaal 1999), an arguably unintentional behavior.

In sum, there are few, if any, cases that unambiguously show an intentional action that is primarily or solely caused by unconscious processes. The best candidates are behaviors triggered by the joint operation of implementation intentions and environmental stimuli, but even here doubts remain that make these behaviors unlikely to topple the folk assumption of intentional agency. After all, the behaviors in question have as a necessary requirement a prior conscious intention, and the issue is merely how the intended action is implemented. Whichever way one comes down on the issue of implementation intentions, there is currently no justification for concluding that intentional actions are in general or primarily caused by unconscious processes.

No Intentions

Perhaps the no-consciousness thesis already grants too much to folk psychology. Why accept the assumption that an *intention* causes an action in the first place? The alternative thesis is that intentional actions are caused by processes other than the agent's intention—either because no intention was present or because it was present but not causally active. This thesis has been forcefully argued by Daniel Wegner and his colleagues (Wegner 2002, 2005; Wegner and Wheatley 1999), so the evidence he presents serves as a good starting point.

Wegner's arguments against intentions as the primary causes of action are part of his theory of apparent mental causation, which tries to account for the "experience of conscious will." What Wegner calls the experience will[2] is the folk notion that one's own conscious intention is the primary cause of one's action. This notion, Wegner counters, is an illusion. His theory claims that "people perceive that they are intending and understand behavior as intended or unintended—but that they do not really intend" (2003, p. 10). The experience of intention (conscious will) is merely a preview of action. When an agent perceives the conjunction between an intention and an action, it gives rise to the experience of will but it does not reveal the genuine causes of action. "The impression that a thought has caused an action rests on a causal inference that is always open to question." (Wegner and Wheatley 1999, p. 482) However, Wegner's Humean skepticism about mental causality does not provide strong grounds for rejecting the folk notion of intentional agency.

First, skepticism about inferences of causality may convince us that we are sometimes wrong in inferring causality from a mere conjunction of events, but that should not prevent us from generally trusting such causal inferences in everyday experiences and in scientific experiments. If no perception of causal conjunction between two events could ever reveal true causality, no psychological experiments could ever give us proof that something other than intentions causes action. Second, everything we know from the scientific study of intentional action (see the preceding section) suggests that intentions do play a primary causal role in this process—not just as illusory previews but as efficacious causes. So people can't be that far off in their perception of intention-action conjunctions.

But there is more ammunition. Wegner (2003) and Wegner and Wheatley (1999) discuss a host of phenomena that are intended to show the dissociation between perceived and actual mental causes and thus the questionable status of intention as an actual cause. In one set of phenomena, the agent does not experience the action as willed even though her will is causally involved. Such things as table-turning, Ouija-board spelling, water dowsing, and pendulum divining are depicted as "circumstances that can produce actions with all the signs of voluntariness—but that nonetheless feel unwilled" (Wegner and Wheatley 1999, p. 482). But what is meant by 'voluntariness' here? Surely these activities are not considered intentional actions. Unless the agents are actively trying to deceive others (e.g., a water diviner intending to turn his wrists subtly but denying that he did so intentionally), they wouldn't consider their behaviors "willed," because they did not intend to bring them about. The same can be said about cases cited by Pockett, who refers to unusual experiences of being controlled or having "anarchic" hands as "apparently purposeful movements . . . made in the absence of any sense of volition" (2004, p.

27). I don't believe we can consider these behaviors relevant to the intentional-agency assumption, given that the agent does not even feel he or she has performed them (let alone performed them intentionally). There is no denying the existence of behaviors that people perform unintentionally or unconsciously and that they subsequently fail to "own" (even though they at least partially caused them; see Wegner, Fuller, and Sparro 2003). But precisely because they are not considered intentional (by the agent and other ordinary folks), they don't threaten the intentional-agency assumption.

The cases we should be after are ones in which the agent has an intention (or rather the mere *perception* of an intention), acts in accordance with the intention, and believes to have acted intentionally, but in reality some other causal process brought about the action. In this case, the agent truly has the illusion of having acted intentionally. A candidate for such a case is an experiment by Wegner and Wheatley designed to show that participants can "experience willful action when in fact they have done nothing" (1999, p. 487).

Wegner and Wheatley's experiment involved a participant and a confederate sitting across from each other and jointly operating a small board that controlled the pointer on a computer screen. Throughout, the participants heard music and words over headphones (whereas the confederate received movement instructions). The pair were instructed to jointly move the pointer across a picture of 50 "tiny toys." Every 30 seconds or so (signaled by a 10-second stretch of music), the pair had to "make a stop" and each person rated the extent to which he or she "allowed the stop to happen" (0 percent) or "intended to make the stop" (100 percent). On some trials ("unforced stops"), the participant was presented with the word for one of the objects 2 seconds into the music window (when they were to make a stop), and the confederate allowed the participant to direct the pointer on those trials. On other trials ("forced stops"), the participant also heard a target word but the confederate was instructed to subtly try to direct the pointer to that object. The hypothesis was that if (1) a target word was presented in advance and (2) the stop occurred on the corresponding target object, participants would think about the object, connect that thought to the apparently corresponding action, and have the illusion of having intended to stop the pointer on that object.

One would like to see three results co-occurring in the critical trials of this experiment: (a) participants experienced "conscious will" (an intention, in folk terminology) in advance of the stop, (b) they felt they performed the relevant stopping action intentionally, and (c) this action was in fact caused by something else (the confederate). But the results are inconclusive on all three counts.

Regarding (a), there was no measure of prior intention (or "will"), only a post-action measure of "having intended to make the stop." Thus, whatever results we find, they could be accounted for by confabulations after the fact instead of (illusory) online perceptions of mind-action connection. Indirect evidence also leaves the issue of prior intentions unclear. On the one hand, post-experiment interviews appeared to suggest that "participants often searched for items onscreen that they had heard named over the headphones" (p. 489), suggesting that they might have had some vague intention toward those objects. On the other hand, Wegner and Wheatley report that in the unforced stop trials participants did not actually move the pointer any closer to the target objects whose words they had heard than to other target objects, suggesting that they had not formed an intention to move the pointer to those targets.

Regarding (b), it is not clear whether people considered the stopping behavior really an intentional action. The forced stops were rated right in the middle between "intended" and "allowed" (M = 52 percent), and so were the unforced stops (M = 56 percent). The latter number is remarkable, because in these trials (if the confederate followed instructions) the participant alone moved the pointer. The effect of the critical manipulation (presenting participants with words naming the target objects and having the confederate move the pointer to those objects) increased ratings to 62 percent. Such a number instills frail confidence in the interpretation that people "reported having performed this movement intentionally" (p. 489). This confidence is further weakened when we consider the wording of the intentionality measure: "intended to make the stop"—not "intended to make the stop *on this particular object.*" Even if we presume that people felt (mildly) they had intended the action in question, it is not clear whether their rating endorsed an intention to merely stop or stop at that time or whether it actually endorsed an intention to stop *on this object.*

Regarding (c), the experiment does not securely rule out the possibility that participants actually contributed to the critical actions of stopping on the target objects in the "forced stop" trials. One problem is that only those "forced stop" trials were analyzed in which the confederate actually succeeded in moving the pointer to the target object. But why did the confederate succeed on some trials and not on others? Could the participant have in fact contributed to the joint movement on the "success" trials by allowing to approach the target object or perhaps even co-directing the pointer toward it, whereas in the failed (and excluded) cases the participant was aiming at something else?

In sum, this experiment does not convincingly support the thesis that intentions are experienced by agents but do not actually bring about intentional behavior. In light of the current difficulties with evidence in support of the no-intention thesis, some skeptics might turn to a more radical thesis: that actions aren't caused by mental states at all but are simply products of brain processes that agents can neither control nor have access to.

No Mental States

The third skeptical position emphasizes that there is no such thing as "mind" or "consciousness" as distinct from matter and physical processes. Proponents of this view typically cite neuroscience experiments designed to demonstrate that intentional action is directly caused and controlled by brain processes and that intentions (or rather experiences of intentions) are too late in the causal chain or entirely left out of the loop.

In one such experiment, trans-magnetic stimulation (TMS) was shown to influence participants' decisions to use their right hand rather than their left (Ammon and Gandevia 1990). These decisions were intentional ones, which participants experienced as quite natural, and they were unaware that the TMS had influenced those decisions. However, we cannot conclude very much from these data, because they are entirely consistent with the notion that TMS triggered an idea or preference or desire (not an intention) and that the person took this preliminary motivational state into account when deciding to act one way or another. If participants were experiencing their actions as intentional but were unable to *not* make the movement they were preparing, then we would have a rather striking result that might show a direct causal link between brain stimulation (of an intention) and intentional action.

It is quite possible, in contrast, to create direct causal connections between brain states and *unintentional* behavior. For example, Itzhak Fried and his colleagues found that electrical stimulation in the anterior part of the human supplementary motor area (SMA) reliably elicited laughter in one particular patient (Fried, Wilson, MacDonald, and Behnke 1998). In an earlier study, Fried et al. (1991) found that electrical stimulation of the SMA in epilepsy patients could elicit a whole range of motor responses (e.g., flexing hip, elevating arm, continuous vowel vocalization), but there were no indications that these responses were experienced as intentional actions.

Perhaps the most frequently cited research challenging the folk assumption of intentional agency is the study by Benjamin Libet and colleagues (1983). Participants flexed their fingers at a roughly self-chosen time and read (from a rotating clock display) the time W at which they initially became aware of wanting to perform the movement and, in a separate set of trials, the time M at which they actually moved. In addition to these subjective time estimates, the researchers recorded EEG patterns, and in particular a so-called readiness potential (RP), an "indicator of cerebral activity" (p. 636). The main finding was that the RP markedly preceded the (estimated) time W at which participants became aware of their wanting to perform the movement, which itself preceded the time M of actually moving. This finding is taken by many scholars as standing "in apparent contradiction to the traditional Cartesian concept of free will" (Wohlschläger 2003, p. 586).

Many scholars have written about this study—see, for example, the commentaries on Libet's 1985 article in *Behavioral and Brain Sciences* and the special issue (volume 11, number 2) of *Consciousness and Cognition*. I will make only two points here. The first point is that the folk concept of intentionality distinguishes clearly between desires and intentions (Malle and Knobe 2001), and so must we when interpreting Libet's data. Desires can be caused by all kinds of external or internal events, most of them unconscious and out of the person's control. Intentions, in contrast, are the output of a reasoning process that takes desires and beliefs as inputs and comes with a characteristic commitment to act. Mele (2003, in press, and in this volume) argues cogently for interpreting the early RP as the emergence of an urge or desire, not the brain correlate of an intention or decision. Note that the participants implemented a general action plan: to wait for a full revolution of the clock (2.56 s) and thereafter flex the finger anytime they felt like doing so. Thus, they had to somehow decide *when* to flex the finger and presumably waited for any kind of "notion" to do it *very soon*. It is quite plausible that the emergence of the RP coincides with such a notion or desire. Whether the reported moment of awareness (*W*) reflects the conscious registering of this desire or the commitment to *act now* (an intention) is unclear. But nothing in the original data suggests that the RP indicates the brain correlate of a decision, and Libet's (1985) later "veto" studies directly contradict the interpretation of RP as an intention (Mele 2003, pp. 182–189).[3]

The second point I want to make is that, despite its problems, Libet's timing paradigm is ingenuous and eminently worth pursuing. Valid timing, however, depends on valid instructions, and valid instructions must direct people's attention to the mental states they themselves distinguish within their folk theory of mind and action. The time *W* at which one should feel an initial "urge" or "intention" or "desire" to flex a finger seems like a rather muddled state to me, and we now know enough about the folk conceptualization of mental states (especially those preceding action) that we can sharpen such instructions. It would seem prudent, for example, to invite the participant to make choices between pairs of items (e.g., objects, colors, or sounds) from a larger pool, with each trial presenting a different pair (hence, a new decision situation). Upon seeing each pair of items, the participant estimates the moment (D) at which one item feels slightly more desirable than the other (but there is still uncertainty) and then the moment (I) at which the person is committed to actually picking one item. In some trials, moreover, the participant should hold back the choice action (H) but sustain the intention, and then finally make the choice. With the best brain imaging and chronometric techniques currently available we should be able to examine physical correlates and timing of awareness of these distinct mental states.

Summary

Consistent with folk psychology, experiments in psychology and neuroscience show that urges, desires, and other motivational states are often caused unconsciously—by the brain, the physical environment, or an experimenter. There is no evidence, however, that rules out conscious intentions as being formed on the basis of these motivational states and causing intentional action. In fact, quite a bit of research on action control assigns a critical role to intentions as functional states that organize and call upon lower-level motor commands and to which feedback about action effects is compared to asses the success of the action. What we are left with is the deep question of what these intentions are made of (Pacherie, this volume). I have no trouble thinking of intentions as real organismic states that have functional attributes, characteristic patterns of emergence (i.e., contentful reasoning from beliefs and desires), and characteristic patterns of consequences (i.e., motor commands, afferent predictions, etc.). Somehow, of course, they have to be implemented in the brain, but that is only slightly more puzzling than the fact that my solid desk here is somehow implemented in terms of tiny physical particles. I cannot write on these particles, they are not dirty or pretty, and I can't own them or sell them. Similarly, I can't form a brain state, I can only form an intention, and no single brain state will cause my action of ending this paragraph. Sure, this is all puzzling, but I can't endorse giving up the perfectly reasonable language and folk-conceptual framework of mind and action just because its physical implementation is unclear.

Epilogue: If Mind Cannot Cause Matter . . .

Earlier I cited Haggard and Clark's dictum that "conscious experience must be a consequence of brain activity rather than a cause of it" (2002, p. 705). This quote reflects a trend among other scholars who are perfectly comfortable with consciousness or mental states as results of neurological events but not as causes of such events. For example, Wegner (2005, p. 20) argues against the notion that "a person (or some other inner agent such as 'consciousness' or 'the will') is a legitimate cause of the person's observed thought or behavior." Instead, "the operation of controlled mental processes is part of the mental mechanism that gives rise to a sense of conscious will and the agent self in the person" (ibid.). But if an entity or a process is suspect as a cause of X, should it not equally be suspect as a result of X? What sort of causal interaction are we to imagine that logically guarantees a causal one-way street? In fact, if we adopt some form of identity theory, according to which consciousness, intentions, or mental states don't exist separate from brain states, then necessarily the mental states (qua brain states) can be causes and effects of other brain states. If, alternatively, we adopt a model according to which mental states are conceptually distinct from brain states (e.g., are properties of brain states), I can see no justification for admitting them as effects but not causes of brain states. Once causal interaction exists at all, it should logically be possible in both directions.

Acknowledgments

This chapter benefited from discussions with Scott Frey and from comments on an early draft from Al Mele, Tim Bayne, and the editors of the volume.

Notes

1. It would also be odd to say that the adjustments were performed "unintentionally," just as it would be odd to say that my dopamine reuptake inhibition was done unintentionally. We apply the terms unintentional and intentional to behaviors that can in principle be intentional; those that cannot may be labeled "nonintentional" or "involuntary."

2. For discussions of the ambiguities in Wegner's concept of experience of conscious will, see the chapter by Bayne in this volume and Nahmias 2002.

3. A parallel case is the card task described by Bechara, Damasio, Tranel, and Damasio (1997), in which participants take cards from two decks, one of which (the "bad" one) offers on average more punishment than the other. The researchers found an affective-physiological marker of "warning" about the bad deck that emerged before the participant become conscious of which deck is bad. Once more, this finding is compatible with folk assumptions, as a feeling (or desire or fear or preference) can emerge out of unconscious processes but then feeds into the active decision process (i.e., forming an intention to take from the "good" deck).

References

Ammon, K., and Gandevia, S. C. 1990. Transcranial magnetic stimulation can influence the selection of motor programmes. *Journal of Neurology, Neurosurgery and Psychiatry* 53: 705–707.

Bargh, J. A. 2005. Bypassing the will: Towards demystifying behavioral priming effects. In *The New Unconscious*, ed. R. Hassin et al. Oxford University Press.

Bargh, J. A., Chen, M., and Burrows, L. 1996. Automaticity of social behavior: Direct effects of trait construct and stereotype activation on action. *Journal of Personality and Social Psychology* 71: 230–244.

Bargh, J. A., Gollwitzer, P. M., Chai, A. L., Barndollar, K., and Troetschel, R. 2001. Automated will: Nonconscious activation and pursuit of behavioral goals. *Journal of Personality and Social Psychology* 81: 1014–1027.

Bayer, U. C., Ferguson, M. J., and Gollwitzer, P. M. 2003. Voluntary action from the perspective of social-personality psychology. In *Voluntary Action*, ed. S. Maasen et al. Oxford University Press.

Bechara, A., Damasio, H., Tranel, D., and Damasio, A. R. 1997. Deciding advantageously before knowing the advantageous strategy. *Science* 275, no. 5304: 1293–1294.

Blakemore, C. 1988. *The Mind Machine*. BBC Books.

Blakemore, S.-J., Frith, C. D., and Wolpert, D. W. 2001. The cerebellum is involved in predicting the sensory consequences of action. *Neuroreport* 12: 1879–1885.

Blakemore, S.-J., Wolpert, D. M., and Frith, C. D. 2000. Why can't you tickle yourself? *Neuroreport* 11, no. 11: R11–R16.

Blakemore, S.-J., Wolpert, D. M., and Frith, C. D. 2002. Abnormalities in the awareness of action. *Trends in Cognitive Sciences* 6: 237–242.

Brandstätter, V., Lengfelder, A., and Gollwitzer, P. M. 2001. Implementation intentions and efficient action initiation. *Journal of Personality and Social Psychology* 81: 946–960.

Buss, A. R. 1978. Causes and reasons in attribution theory: A conceptual critique. *Journal of Personality and Social Psychology* 36: 1311–1321.

Castiello, U., Paulignan, Y., and Jeannerod, M. 1991. Temporal dissociation of motor responses and subjective awareness: A study in normal subjects. *Brain* 114: 2639–2655.

Chartrand, T. L., and Bargh, J. A. 1996. Automatic activation of impression formation and memorization goals: Nonconscious goal priming reproduces the effects of explicit task instructions. *Journal of Personality and Social Psychology* 71: 464–478.

Crick, F. H. C. 1979. Thinking about the brain. *Scientific American* 241: 181–188.

D'Andrade, R. 1987. A folk model of the mind. In *Cultural Models in Language and Thought*, ed. D. Holland and N. Quinn. Cambridge University Press.

Daprati, E., Franck, N., Georgieff, N., Proust, J., Pacherie, E., Dalery, J., and Jeannerod, M. 1997. Looking for the agent: An investigation into consciousness of action and self-consciousness in schizophrenic patients. *Cognition* 65: 71–86.

Fourneret, P., and Jeannerod, M. 1998. Limited conscious monitoring of motor performance in normal subjects. *Neuropsychologia* 36: 1133–1140.

Fried, I., Wilson, C. L., MacDonald, K. A., and Behnke, E. J. 1998. Electric current stimulates laughter. *Nature* 391, no. 6668: 650.

Fried, I., Katz, A., McCarthy, G., Sass, K. J., Williamson, P., Spencer, S. S., and Spencer, D. D. 1991. Functional organisation of human supplementary motor cortex studied by electrical-stimulation. *Journal of Neuroscience* 11: 3656–3666.

Gibbs, R. 1999. *Intentions in the Experience of Meaning*. Cambridge University Press.

Gollwitzer, P. M. 1999. Implementation intentions: Strong effects of simple plans. *American Psychologist* 54: 493–503.

Gollwitzer, P. M., and Moskowitz, G. B. 1996. Goal effects on action and cognition. In *Social Psychology*, ed. E. Higgins and A. Kruglanski. Guilford.

Gopnik, A. 1993. How we know our minds: The illusion of first-person knowledge. *Behavioral and Brain Sciences* 16: 1–14.

Haggard, P., and Clark, S. 2003. Intentional action: Conscious experience and neural prediction. *Consciousness and Cognition* 12: 695–707.

Haggard, P., Clark, S., and Kalogeras, J. 2002. Voluntary action and conscious awareness. *Nature Neuroscience* 5: 382–385.

Haggard, P., Newman, C., and Magno, E. 1999. On the perceived time of voluntary actions. *British Journal of Psychology* 90: 291–303.

Heider, F. 1958. *The Psychology of Interpersonal Relations*. Wiley.

Jeannerod, M. 2002. Naturalization of mental states and personal identity. In *The Languages of the Brain*, ed. A. Galaburda et al. Harvard University Press.

Klein, S. A. 2002. Libet's research on the timing of conscious intention to act: A commentary. *Consciousness and Cognition* 11: 273–279.

Libet, B. 1985. Unconscious cerebral initiative and the role of conscious will in voluntary action. *Behavioral and Brain Sciences* 8: 529–566.

Libet, B., Gleason, C. A., Wright, E. W., and Pearl, D. K. 1983. Time of conscious intention to act in relation to onset of cerebral activity (readiness potential): The unconscious initiation of a freely voluntary act. *Brain* 106: 623–642.

Maasen, S. Prinz, W., and Roth, G., eds. *Voluntary Action: Brains, Minds, and Sociality*. Oxford University Press.

Malle, B. F. 1999. How people explain behavior: A new theoretical framework. *Personality and Social Psychology Review* 3: 23–48.

Malle, B. F. 2001. Folk explanations of intentional action. In *Intentions and Intentionality: Foundations of Social Cognition*, ed. B. Malle et al. MIT Press.

Malle, B. F. 2004. *How the Mind Explains Behavior: Folk Explanations, Meaning, and Social Interaction*. MIT Press.

Malle, B. F. 2005. Folk theory of mind: Conceptual foundations of human social cognition. In *The New Unconscious*, ed. R. Hassin et al. Oxford University Press.

Malle, B. F., and Knobe, J. 1997. The folk concept of intentionality. *Journal of Experimental Social Psychology* 33: 101–121.

Malle, B. F., and Knobe, J. 2001. The distinction between desire and intention: A folk-conceptual analysis. In *Intentions and Intentionality*, ed. B. Malle et al. MIT Press.

Malle, B. F., and Nelson, S. E. 2003. Judging *mens rea*: The tension between folk concepts and legal concepts of intentionality. *Behavioral Sciences and the Law* 21: 563–580.

Malle, B. F., Knobe, J., O'Laughlin, M. J., Pearce, G. E., and Nelson, S. E. 2000. Conceptual structure and social functions of behavior explanations: Beyond person-situation attributions. *Journal of Personality and Social Psychology* 79: 309–326.

Malle, B. F., Moses, L. J., and Baldwin, D. A., eds. 2001. *Intentions and Intentionality: Foundations of Social Cognition*. MIT Press.

Marshall, J. 1968. *Intention in Law and Society*. Funk and Wagnalls.

Mele, A. R. 2003. *Motivation and Agency*. Oxford University Press.

Mele, A. R. In press. Decisions, intentions, urges, and free will: Why Libet has not shown what he says he has. In *Explanation and Causation: Topics in Contemporary Philosophy*, ed. J. Campbell et al. MIT Press.

Moskowitz, G. B., Gollwitzer, P. M., Wasel, W., and Schaal, B. 1999. Preconscious control of stereotype activation through chronic egalitarian goals. *Journal of Personality and Social Psychology* 77: 167–184.

Nahmias, E. 2002. When consciousness matters: A critical review of Daniel Wegner's *The Illusion of Conscious Will. Philosophical Psychology* 15: 527–542.

Norman, D. A., and Shallice, T. 1986. Attention to action: Willed and automatic control of behavior. In *Consciousness and Self-Regulation*, volume 4, ed. R. Davidson et al. Plenum.

Nisbett, R. E., and Wilson, T. D. 1977. Telling more than we know: Verbal reports on mental processes. *Psychological Review* 84: 231–259.

O'Laughlin, M., and Malle, B. F. 2002. How people explain actions performed by groups and individuals. *Journal of Personality and Social Psychology* 82: 33–48.

Pockett, S. 2004. Does consciousness cause behaviour? *Journal of Consciousness Studies* 11: 23–40.

Prinz, W. 2003. How do we know about our own actions? In *Voluntary Action: Brains, Minds, and Sociality*, ed. S. Maasen et al. Oxford University Press.

Rosenthal, D. M. 2002. The timing of conscious states. *Consciousness and Cognition* 11: 215–220.

Searle, J. R. 1983. *Intentionality: An Essay in the Philosophy of Mind*. Cambridge University Press.

Shaver, K. G. 1985. *The Attribution of Blame*. Springer-Verlag.

Wegner, D. M. 2002. *The Illusion of Conscious Will*. MIT Press.

Wegner, D. M. 2003. The mind's self-portrait. *Annals of the New York Academy of Sciences* 1001: 1–14.

Wegner, D. M. 2005. Who is the controller of controlled processes? In *The New Unconscious*, ed. R. Hassin et al. Oxford University Press.

Wegner, D. M., and Wheatley, T. P. 1999. Apparent mental causation: Sources of the experience of will. *American Psychologist* 54: 480–492.

Wegner, D. M., Fuller, V., and Sparrow, B. 2003. Clever hands: Uncontrolled intelligence in facilitated communication. *Journal of Personality and Social Psychology* 85: 1–15.

Wellman, H. 1990. *The Child's Theory of Mind*. MIT Press.

White, P. A. 1988. Knowing more about what we can tell: "Introspective access" and causal report accuracy 10 years later. *British Journal of Psychology* 79: 13–45.

Wilson, J. Q. 1997. *Moral Judgment: Does the Abuse Excuse Threaten Our Legal System?* HarperCollins.

Wohlschläger, A., Engbert, K., and Haggard, P. 2003. Intentionality as a constituting condition for the own self—and other selves. *Consciousness and Cognition* 12: 708–716.

Wohlschläger, A., Haggard, P., Gesierich, B., and Prinz, W. 2003. The perceived onset time of self- and other-generated actions. *Psychological Science* 14: 586–591.

III LAW AND PUBLIC POLICY

12 Does Consciousness Cause Misbehavior?

William P. Banks

Neuroscience and psychology seem to tread closer each year (or day) to the scientific understanding of volition, and along with it, to the understanding of the freedom or constraint of the will, conscience, and moral resolve. The advances depend, as is generally the case in science, on generating and testing theoretical models against data. By their nature, scientific models are prediction machines. They do their work by mechanistic application of their postulates. They do not contain or assume anything like human awareness or consciousness. Assuming consciousness as part of a model is contraindicated for many reasons, high among them being the need to model consciousness itself for it to be a proper part of the model. Without explicit details of operation, consciousness would be a black box inserted in the works, presumably to improve predictions. To put an unexplained center of conscious judgment and decision making into a model is, simply, cheating. There are other reasons, as well, why consciousness is not used as part of a scientific model (Banks, 1993, discusses some; see also, Banks, 1996, on qualia in scientific models of the brain).

The lack of consciousness in a model is not a fault. However, when science begin to address such issues as moral judgment, consciousness is brought into the picture. This is because only *conscious* acts are categorized as right or wrong, moral or immoral. A person who executes some act solely unconsciously, without awareness, is not making a moral choice and would not be judged as harshly as if it were a conscious act. In no other domain of science is there such a need. A model of how one's brain signals a finger to move can be developed without invoking consciousness. When that finger makes the same motion to cause a rifle to shoot someone, we need to know about the person's conscious intent to consider questions about guilt or innocence. A scientific model of action, if it is to cover moral action, thus seems to need to have consciousness in its explanatory domain.

There are alternative ways to handle conscious intent. For example, it could be a social fiction. Actions would be declared conscious or not on the basis of criteria that are supported by the dominant folk model. This approach has its attractions (see Banks, 1993, for my take on it). Prinz (this volume) would probably point out that the need for actions to be conscious to be morally judged is a requirement of society, not a fact of biology. However, my intention here is to cover conscious intention as a problem in neurobiology, as Searle, (2001) put it. If we can see how consciousness is related to volition, then it might be possible to apply better analytic power to the social constructions—which are just as "natural" as the neurophysiological ones, only with a different history.

1   Mental Causation and Freedom of the Will

There are two related questions here: the question of volition (Do we have free will?) and the question of conscious efficacy (Can an idea move a muscle?). Normally the question of the freedom of the will is seen as the only pertinent one for legal and moral judgments, but freedom would be irrelevant if an idea could not move a muscle—that is, if consciously made decisions could not affect action.

Consciousness is an unavoidable part of the picture. Free will seems pointless if it is not *conscious* free will. We are not interested in unconscious freedom of the will, if there is such a thing, or unconscious volition. Even if it could be decisively shown that unconscious intentions exist, traditional thinking about responsibility would not be much affected. From a legal or a moral standpoint, it is the conscious intention that counts in assigning blame or praise, and it is the conscious intention that the court or the moralizer tries to infer. Purportedly nonconscious factors are at best ancillary. They could be mitigating factors, and they sometimes are in a court of law, but they are the main basis for judgment only in cases of outright insanity that overwhelms rationality and makes it impossible for the defendant to distinguish right from wrong.

Unconscious mental causation seems to be in the domain of normal science (if we can even call it "mental" if it is unconscious; see Searle 1997). All sorts of actions can operate unconsciously—even skilled actions and higher cognitive functions such as using memory, selecting the correct words as we speak, or intelligently scanning a scene for an object. Explaining these actions and behaviors is a fairly straightforward theoretical endeavor in psychology—as long as we do not mention consciousness along the way. Hypotheses are generated and tested against neurophysiological and behavioral data, experiments are run, measurements are made, predictions are tested, and so on. The proposed mechanism operates according to its constitutive laws and structure, and there is no need to mention consciousness. Indeed, it is difficult to see how to add it as a causative component to these models. The same sort of theorizing has been applied to processes that have an indisputable conscious aspect. In very few cases is there any mention of consciousness, and never (as far as I know) is there a causal role for it. The question may be asked whether these models of conscious processes can have something about consciousness in them. One reply is that it would have to be shown that the physiological events being modeled operate as they do by virtue of being conscious, in addition to whatever other properties they may have. To add consciousness to a model, it would have to be shown that consciousness somehow *does* something in the model. This is rather difficult to prove, much less model, but its denial leaves consciousness as epiphenomenal in the domains being modeled.

Even if theorists believe (as I do) that conscious states are completely material, there is an utter lack of theoretical principles that relate them to material processes. Again we ask: How can an idea move a muscle? Ideas have no mass and no solid parts that could connect to a neuron or a muscle fiber. The notion that an idea could move a muscle is an absurdity, yet we are certain that we can go from a conscious idea to an action at any moment, just by lifting a finger. It seems a solid fact, but how do we do it? How does a thought lead to an action?

2 The Results of Libet et al. (1983)

The questions of conscious volition and conscious efficacy were forced upon the scientific and philosophical community by the groundbreaking experiment of Libet et al. (1983). They have become unavoidable scientific issues. Libet et al. found that the conscious decision to make a simple motion comes at least 350 milliseconds *after* the brain activity known to lead up to the motion has begun. The measure of this brain activity is termed the *readiness potential* (RP). Other experiments have found an even longer nonconscious period before the subjectively reported time of decision. The clear implication of this finding is that the conscious decision was not the cause of the action; rather, the action was initiated by unconscious processes, and some time later it was claimed as a conscious decision. This may be a single case, but if there is even one unambiguous case where an act was unconsciously initiated before a conscious decision to act in that way was reported, our concepts of conscious control of our behavior must be rethought.

The idea that consciousness is not quite the master of the ship has a long history in philosophy, psychology, and literature, but this is the first (and so far the only) direct neurophysiological evidence for it. Most people take the philosophical arguments and psychological evidence with interest but ultimately cum grano salis. However, electrical brain recordings are *science* and therefore definitive support for the position. Thus, the findings of Libet et al. have had and will continue to have an impact disproportionate to their scope.

These findings have been challenged on many fronts. Banks and Pockett (in press) have attempted an exhaustive review of the challenges. In brief, the results have been replicated in several labs, and possible errors or physiological delays in reporting cannot account for the results. In fact, many of the possible systematic errors or artifacts would work to reduce the measured effect, not create it as some sort of artifact.

Some of the criticisms focus on the meaning of clock times ascribed to conscious events. These we found significant in that they illustrate the importance of pre-scientific (folk-model) assumptions about what mental events are and how they relate to clock time. Some interpretations of the findings seem to treat ideas as things (with extension in time rather than space) and mental events as interactions of the ideas in real time that corresponds to clock time. By this intuitive model, thoughts and conscious decisions would be locked to physical time. Dennett and Kinsbourne (1992), Haggard and Clark (1999), Durgin and Sternberg (2002), Christie and Barresi (2002), Nijhawan (1994), and Watanabe et al. (2002) have reported a number of different findings that show that apparent sequencing and relative timing of events can differ from their order as presented. However, even if there is time-shifting in the perceptual ordering of events, it is not large enough to change the fact that the onset of the preparatory brain activity is recorded well before the participants indicate that they decided to act.

Mele's interpretation of Libet's findings (in this volume and in a work still in press) is that the moment of onset of the RP coincides with an unconscious *urge* to move, and the decision to act comes later. The urge is nonconscious but also non-specific. The actual decision to move occurs at exactly the point indicated by participants and is the cause of the specific action. Thus, by this account, conscious efficacy is not challenged, and the sense of willing the action is not simply a tardy acknowledgment of a process already begun unconsciously. The action itself issues from a conscious command.

Whereas this argument is speculative (and how can an urge be nonconscious?), a similar proposal by Trevena and Miller (2002) is testable. They had their participants choose unsystematically to move either the left or the right hand on each trial and report when they had made that decision. In their study this report came very shortly after the onset of the lateralized RP (the LRP) for moving the chosen hand. The argument is that the two-hand choice measures the time of the conscious decision, and this decision comes very close to the time of the motion, supporting the hypothesis of conscious control of action.

This result is not decisive, because in Trevena and Miller's data the mean LRP still started before the decision. Before this study, Haggard and Eimer (1999) used a different technique to determine whether the RP or the LRP was the better correlate with the reported decision to move. They found that the LRP was the better predictor. They also found the LRP to precede the reported instant of decision by 454 ms—a larger nonconscious interval than found by Trevena and Miller, and long enough to be beyond the range of the potential artifacts discussed by Banks and Pockett. The results indicate that the LRP is a better choice than the RP as a measure of the unconscious precursor of the action, but it is still unconscious. If Mele's argument were to be modified to assert that the LRP marks only a more *specific* unconscious "urge," we would be headed to a battle over labels rather than substance. However, Pacherie's three-level analysis of volition (this volume) could provide a principled basis for moving this argument from semantics to substance.

The familiar account of the Libet paradigm is that the RP is part of a process that culminates in the prescribed motion, with a conscious decision reported along the way. This account assumes that the process that generates the RP (or LRP) is both necessary and sufficient to generate the response, and the conscious decision is neither. These claims of necessity and sufficiency have not been tested in any of the research on the finding of Libet et al. The standard account fails if these assumptions are not supportable.

A test of the necessity of the RP would determine whether any motions followed conscious decisions *without* a preceding RP. Because the RP can be imaged only in averages over many trials, there could be a subset of trials mixed in with the majority that do not have an RP before the decision to act. More precise measuring that allowed imaging of single trials could decide this issue. There may also be statistical techniques that could test whether blocks of trials contain some cases with no RP before the reported decision. Without a test of the association of the RP with the response the RP cannot be accepted (or rejected) as necessary for the action. The claim that the conscious decision does the real work (sometimes following a noncausal RP) cannot be rejected.

Sufficiency of the RP-generating process is the other crucial gap. The most common story here is that the unconscious process as measured by the RP is sufficient in and of itself to initiate the action—and the conscious decision is an ineffective latecomer, along for the ride. For this to be verified, we need an absence of cases in which RP potentials are found but do not eventuate in the response. It is possible that robust RPs crop up frequently during the critical interval, but only when the conscious decision is reported is there a response. In this case the unconscious process would clearly not be a sufficient cause of the action. We do not detect the ineffective RPs because recording RPs requires back-averaging from the response. The RPs that do not eventuate in a response would therefore not be discovered. That is not a reason to conclude that they do not exist.

One test of sufficiency is possible if the LRP is indeed the critical readiness potential. An LRP is detected by the difference between left-hemisphere and right-hemisphere motor cortex EEGs. Back-averaging from times at which the EEG difference passes a threshold voltage would determine whether there are LRPs with no response. If this procedure finds LRPs or RP-LRP sequences that do not eventuate in an action, the RP is shown not to be sufficient for the action. This finding, coupled with a finding that the RP was necessary for the action to take place, would imply that the RP plus something else is needed. That something else could be the conscious decision to act, or it could be another process, as yet unknown.

Another source of evidence on sufficiency of the RP is the fact that participants sometimes reported their decision after the response had already been made. Perhaps more tellingly, they were sometimes surprised by a response they did not consciously decide to make. Either of these observations support the conclusion that the process generating the RP was causally sufficient to cause the action, but they are essentially anecdotal. Systematic research to determine the frequency of these reports and the conditions that lead to them is needed. It is possible that with more attentive participants, every response would follow a decision to act.

It is surprising that, with so much interest in the findings of Libet et al. in both scientific and philosophic quarters, the lack of evidence on the necessity and sufficiency of unconscious activity measured by the RP has not been seen as an issue. In the absence of the needed research, I will go along with the crowd and act as though the RP were necessary and sufficient for the action. If the tests show either assumption to be false, the conclusions customarily based on the results of Libet et al. would be wrong. However, the most likely outcome, eventually, is a broadening of our understanding of the full range of neural processes responsible for the actions and phenomenology in the paradigm. These concerns about sufficiency and necessity would be superseded by more basic questions.

3   Volition, Free Will, and Responsibility

It is not possible to discuss free will without first deciding how we define it. The philosophical positions on freedom of the will fall into two broad classifications: *incompatibilism* and *compatibilism*. Incompatibilism is the consequence of assuming a definition of freedom of the will that is inconsistent with causal determinism. By this definition, free action is entirely original with the actor. No historical, biological, or cultural factors, and no pressures in the current environment determine the action. These factors may set up the playing field for the decision (the "decision space"), but the decision itself is independently, freely, and exclusively willed by the actor. In the parlance of responsibility and blame, if I do something bad, the buck stops with me—the decision cannot be predicted from or blamed on any previous conditions on the planet. For many, this is the only true definition of free will.

This definition creates a basic contradiction. A free action, being causally free of the physical world, would be an exception to determinism and would not be reconcilable with the concept of a causally self-contained universe. If everything is determined by antecedent events, including my actions and thoughts, there is no room for this kind of free will. One version of incompatibilism solves the contradiction by denying free will altogether; this position is sometimes discussed as a consequence of hard determinism. The sense that we have free will is itself causally determined, perhaps by genetics or brain structure, and is simply not a correct intuition. Simply put, free will is an illusion.

The other version of incompatibilism, termed *libertarianism*, attempts to save the same concept of free will within a deterministic world. If all events, including our actions, can in principle be predicted adequately from an earlier physical state of affairs, there does not seem to be room for an influence of freedom as defined. One resolution is to assume that willing obeys its own set of principles and is not part of the physical order. Libertarian free will would by this account depend upon a "mental" substance that is undetermined and separate from physical nature. The modern version of this resolution is attributed to Descartes, who formulated what is termed *substance dualism*. Matter, in the causally closed and complete physical world is one substance; spirit or mind is the other. This does create a resolution, though superficially and at the considerable cost of many intractable problems. Dualism cannot be accepted as a scientific hypothesis because by definition it does not allow causal explanations.

An approach to saving the libertarian position without dualism is to deny that the physical world is deterministic. Quantum theory, which is nondeterministic and does not require any supernatural substance, has some vigorous advocates (Hameroff 1998; Hameroff and Penrose 1995; Kane 1996; Penrose 1989; Penrose et al. 2000). There are strong arguments against this approach (Grush and Churchland 1996; Spier and Thomas 1998; Stenger 1995). My own view is that the quantum approach is a version of what Strawson (1962) termed "the obscure and panicky metaphysics of libertarianism," although here it is dressed in the language of physicalism.

If quantum theory is invoked to allow freedom in a deterministic world, it does so by allowing unpredictability of actions. There is a logical error behind the equation of unpredictability with freedom. The implicit argument is that, because free actions are unpredictable, any factor that causes unpredictability enables libertarian free will. This is the error of the undistributed middle.

However, even if we accept the hypothesis that quantum events are the source of ultimate freedom, we have a hollow solution. If our actions depend on unpredictable events at a subatomic level, these actions come from a source not available to consciousness, and the criterion that free actions be conscious is not maintained. Furthermore, ultimate personal agency in any meaningful sense is missing if the action does not come from the felt, willed, personally owned act. Action might as well emerge from some murky web of causes as from the lurch of an electron.

The attempts to use quantum theory to save libertarian freedom are myopic. They focus on the narrow issues around predictability and determinism without effectively confronting the larger issues that make free will important in the first place.

Despite heroic efforts of persuasion from the quantuam-theoretic camp, we are simply not made more free by the introduction of a bit of pure randomness. A random process in decisions or actions would just be a nuisance. Further, the theory that free will hinges on a random, nonconscious process does not support the connection between freedom and responsibility that is often given as a reason for clinging to a libertarian concept of free will.

A functional argument for quantum theory is that a bit of unpredictability is useful in tricking predators or prey. If that were so, this functionality would not be confined to humans. Any species that faces such an environment would be likely to develop free will if unpredictability is adaptive. It may seem odd to suggest that dogs, cats, and cows have free will, but it is not a philosophical argument against quantum-theoretic freedom. However, it is an argument that quantum-theoretic freedom does not itself confer ownership of actions and all the aspects of responsible action, unless I have sorely underestimated the moral dimension of dogs, cats, and cows, not to mention fish.

There are still more arguments for libertarian free will, but these are reverse arguments—they have the form that libertarian free will *must* exist for other reasons. One of these reasons is the fear that the underpinnings of morality would be lost if we abandoned a belief in libertarian free will. I consider this a dictatorial argument. That is, it is argued that we must, for the good of society, enforce a doctrine that cannot be supported through science or reason. It would be better to find other reasons to support morality, if this support is even needed. All the materialists and non-libertarians I know continue to act like good citizens.

Another argument of the reverse type comes from what Clark (1999) calls "fear of mechanism." This has several forms, but it amounts to a fear that our very souls will be dethroned by scientific explanation. On one account it would be that our thoughts are "nothing but" neural events. The "nothing but" trope adds nothing to a scientific explanation. It is "nothing but" rhetoric and it is surprising that anyone finds this tacked-on statement to be the least bit substantive.

The other fear may be of metaphysical reduction. Aside from the "nothing but" (we are "nothing but" a bunch of atoms, etc.) issue, it is a fear that the causes of our actions go right through us, and the explanations go right through in the other direction. Responsibility does not reside in the person but the causes of behavior. This fear derives from the widespread assumption that volition, behavior, character, and even subjective experience can be reduced to structural, neural, and biochemical events, which are in turn reduced to genetics and determining experiences. Genetics is then reduced to chemistry, which is reduced to physics, to particle physics, and ultimately to the Grand Unifying Theory. The assumption is that the science of it has not all been worked out yet (the degree to which it has not been worked out is greatly underestimated), but the project will be completed eventually because the existing world is completely reducible to previous states and science is the way to find the mechanisms. This presumed reduction is a fiction, but it seems to be part of the folk theory of science—and for some a mistaken reason to reject science. (See Van Fraassen 1980 for an interesting argument; see also Fodor 2000.) This fiction is not restricted to the non-academic public. E. O. Wilson's *Consilience* (1998) is a testament of belief in it.

Yet another reverse argument comes from a recognition that the metaphysical dualism required by our intuitive models of volition (Bloom 2004; Clarke and Cohen 2004) is inconsistent with determinism and must be saved. Common sense would be all wrong if there was no free will. More likely, for most people it is not even a matter for discussion. There is no fear of mechanism, only discomfort at the idea, quickly rejected, that mind and matter are not different substances with different rules, and with consciousness and freedom in the one substance and scientific determinism in the other.

Clarke and Cohen (2004) find another reverse argument. This is that punishment solely for the sake of retribution depends on the assumption of libertarian freedom. In other words, to justify the sense that retribution is right and fair, it is thought that we need to possess transcendental freedom. I personally have never understood this or any other justification of retributive punishment (other than as an expression of anger), but to some it is a powerful one. It does help me understand why members of some avowedly dualistic religions are both "pro-life" and in favor of capital punishment. In both cases they see a soul that is either to be rescued or to deserve the harshest retribution. Why a theory of freedom justifies any particular form of punishment remains, however, an open question.

These arguments will probably not suffice to persuade anyone in disagreement with my opinion that libertarian freedom is not part of an analysis of action. There continue to be philosophical arguments for libertarianism and continuing, valiant attempts to save it. (See the chapter by Ross in this volume.) In my view the only meaningful form of libertarian freedom is along the lines of Kant's noumenal self. In such a formulation, ideas are related by reasoning, not physical or neurobiological causes, and freedom of the will is in a world of reason isolated from physical determinism. Agency derived from this source would express the person's inner, autonomous self and be uncaused by any worldly factors. This, of course, requires a dualistic metaphysics (Kantian, not Cartesian, in this case) and is unacceptable. Still, it is miles ahead of anything derived from quantum indeterminacy.

Finally, I need to recognize another dictatorial argument, this one *against* libertarian free will. The argument is that because the world is a closed, deterministic physical system, there is no room for libertarian free will. Therefore, we must find positions on volition that do not involve free will. There may even be some anxiety associated with the idea that the world is not deterministic—and hence unpredictable, open to the possibility of the supernatural, and in violation of a faith we live by. Yes, determinism qualifies as a matter of faith. It is not itself a testable scientific hypothesis. Macroscopic determinism falls apart at the quantum level, but there are still (probabilistic) laws in quantum theory, and the indeterminacy averages out, so to speak, when we consider most of the interesting objects of study—brains, neurons, hormones, etc. We need this faith to do our work, but it is nonetheless a faith and the source of a dictatorial position regarding volition.

The alternative to libertarian free will is termed *compatibilism*. It is not a single theory, but rather the concept that volition, along with other mental faculties, is part of the physical causal order and is in principle predictable from antecedent states. The critical difference is the definition of free will. Compatibilist freedom is a lack of restraints on our willed actions, even if the willing itself is determined by antecedent states. Volition is part of the natural order, even though most of our actions feel free.

We may rightly ask, then, why we feel free when our actions are determined by past events. One reason is that we have no access to most of the predetermining factors. Our genetic makeup and the structure of our brains are opaque to introspection. As for cultural and historical determinants, we are probably aware of some and not of others, and we can at best theorize about their effects on us. If our culture, language, political system, and so forth are taken as the "way things are" then we typically do not feel constrained by them, even though they powerfully influence our mental lives and determine much of what we do.

The compatibilist has a good response to a recurring argument for libertarian free will. This is that the sense we have of free will is perception of a truth. (See, for example, Libet 1999.) This argument reminds me of Descartes' "clear and distinct" criterion. It is not a very good argument. It assumes the infallibility of intuition.

The compatibilist has a better reason for the feeling of freedom: the causes of behavior have become encoded in the structure of our personal self, and thus in our goals, plans, desires, temperament, morals, and all aspects of our character. When we act in a manner consistent with our self we are acting freely because we are acting self-consistently. We are doing what we want to do, never mind that the wanting itself is causally determined. This sounds something like a Kantian self, without the transcendental freedom.

Of course there are times when we feel unfree because of inner conflicts or inhibitions. There is no guarantee that a consistent, entirely coherent and unified personality will emerge from the many different and conflicting influences and genetic dispositions that formed us. This is the area in which counseling, psychotherapy, and self-forming actions come into play. Self-forming actions are associated with libertarian views (Kane 1996, 2002), but they should belong to compatibilism as well. Among the various influences in a conflicted but self-reflective mind, some will aim toward resolution and a healthy and creative self. One's resilience is itself a product of determining external factors, but they are complex and largely unavailable to introspection or an outside observer. Questions of how we face internal conflict, what mental or personal effort is and how it works, and what mental pain is are all psychological questions and do not require a libertarian theory of freedom.

Two novels, *Brave New World* and *Walden II*, come to mind here. If our sense of freedom comes from being what we are, why not stage-manage the events that determine what we are so there are no conflicts? In *Brave New World* we have an object lesson in how technology can create a dystopia—or so it seems to us, not having been raised properly. Walden II is supposedly a utopia, where people feel the most free, but it is often seen as a dystopia—again, by people not raised properly. The irony is that our perspective on these societies is a result of our relatively unmanaged personal histories, which led to our metaphysical assumptions and to our conflicts, neuroses, futile hopes, and unattainable goals. As a compatibilist, I must say: this is the way it is. Live with it. It is exactly this situation that the libertarian finds unacceptable.

When we speak of the self as a product of antecedent events, there are two different matters to consider. One is our introspective feeling of freedom, discussed above. The other is the nature of the causal relations. How much can we explain? The idea that behavior and mental events can be completely reduced to neural or environmental events is a fantasy, or for some a groundless fear. The successful scientific explanations in this area are limited to specific abilities and functions and rarely have the form of a reduction to, say, a neural or biochemical level. Many scientific findings in psychology are correlational and incomplete, rather than causal and rigorous. For example, it has been known for some time that dopamine antagonists are effective in reducing delusions and hallucinations for some schizophrenics. There is no model here, only a finding and a number of theories. Clearly this is an illustration that there are effects that cross from the one level to the other, but it is not a reduction. The successes in psychological modeling and computer simulation are entirely at a functional level. There is no reduction whatsoever.

A misplaced confidence in ontological reduction may be an impediment to understanding compatibilism. If it is assumed that there is a reductive hierarchy in nature, then compatibilism seems to put psychological properties at an artificial stopping place. Why not go to the neural level or lower? The simple reason is that it's like saying chemistry is an artificial stopping place on the way to physics. It is clear that chemistry is not going to be reduced wholesale to physics, and if it were chemists would continue to do their work at the chemical level. Reduction of psychology to neuroscience (or environment, nature and nurture, etc.) is just as unlikely.

If large-scale reduction is out of the picture, there is still the possibility that some antecedent states (and linking theoretical concepts) predict some psychological states. Is volitional origination in the person threatened by these smaller-scale causal links? I argue that even in these cases we can stop with the person. Here is an analogy that may illustrate my position concretely. Suppose we are preparing to cut down a tree. We know that the tree grew from a seed and has many properties that are predictable from its DNA, the nature of cellulose, the microstructure of wood, the soil and water conditions, the amount of sunlight it received, as well as the physics of water, the evolution of the vegetable kingdom, the evolutionary history of chlorophyll and leaves, evolution of size, and the cosmological history of the Earth. We do not care about any of that. We are interested only in whether the saw is sharp enough, how much the tree weighs, where it will fall, and so on. In other words, we deal with the product of the putative causal chain. The product is what is real; the causal chain is an elaborate and mostly unverified construction.

By the same token we act on the basis of the "product"—who we are—and deal with others in the same way. Consider the response often made when a person is asked to do something that violates his or her principles. Responses such as "I'm not that sort of person" and "I could never do a thing like that" are revealing. These locutions relate the proposed action to the properties of one's self. The proposed actions may in fact be neither illegal nor immoral. They are simply a part of the way we are constituted. Just as in the case of the tree, we don't refer to a causal history; we deal with what is before us, with what we are. I don't know why I could "never do a thing like that." I just won't do it—it's not *me*.

Greene and Cohen (2004) propose that the person acts as a kind of "bottleneck" between antecedent events and actions. This is essentially the proposal above, and is in the spirit of Strawson's influential 1962 essay on freedom and responsibility. The great range of determining causes become encoded in the person (the self). These causes do not directly determine behavior but act indirectly through reasoning, memory, desire, etc. Action can come from causal properties that stop with the self. The "bottleneck" is not a passive channel, but a location of emergent properties. Searle (1992) gives a good illustration of emergence. If we make a wheel out of plastic, some properties of the wheel—density, tensile strength, etc.—are derived from the properties of the plastic, but the fact that it rolls when put on a hill cannot be so predicted. Rolling is a consequence of the shape, not the material.

A promise at the beginning of this chapter was to propose an approach to consciously initiated actions that did not stumble on dualist assumptions. Here is a neurological story: Brain processes that are not conscious may initiate a chain of events that leads to an action. The local history of these processes might include a need or demand from the limbic system, and the response of prefrontal and cingulate areas to the subsequent input from limbic connections. This activity, in turn, would result in plans that require access to memories, norms of propriety probably encoded in prefrontal cortex, action sequences encoded in SMA (supplementary motor areas) and pre-motor cortex, and other areas. (For an outline of some critical areas, see figure 1.2 in chapter 1 of the present volume.) Motor commands would involve primary motor cortex and various feedforward and feedback control mechanisms.

Where is consciousness, the sense of control, and ownership of action in this fanciful story? First, the actions feel free and owned by us because they are generated by us, and in their formation rely on information that is also part of our sense of self. Whether or not the actions are explainable from a lower level, the "shape" of the self, like the wheel, is not. Volition becomes personal when derived from the formed character of the self.

There are some specific mechanisms that contribute greatly to the sense of ownership. The completed feedback loops and verified efference copies confer a visceral sense of ownership. (See the chapters by Pockett and Jeannerod in the present volume.) They link actions to the self-generated plans and thus unite the actions with the sense of self. This is a neural system that confers ownership by verifying personal origination of the action. Gray (1995 and in press) has organized the psychological and neurophysiological evidence into a theory of how conscious contents about volition are the products of such processes. Verified feedback and feedforward is also a source of ownership of action. The disconnect between action and control mechanisms in schizophrenia seems responsible for feelings that one's actions are under the control of others, that thoughts are "inserted" by others, and that hallucinatory "voices" are not recognized as one's own productions. (See, for example, Spence and Frith 1999; also see Jeannerod in this volume.)

So, do ideas move muscles? I put this question in such a crude form for a reason. It is so crude as to be a joke, a sarcastic expression of the stark failure of attempts to see into the shadow between the idea and the act. The best answer I know is that formulated by Pacherie in this volume. Conscious ideas belong to an elaborate structure that supports volition. The ideas that form our awareness of action do not themselves move muscles. They "move" not muscles but other ideas that are unconscious and eventually engage action systems, entirely impenetrable to introspection. We have no idea *how* we move muscles because of this impenetrability. We are aware of the general aspects of the action and the goal, but have neither the need nor the ability to see further into the process. Action in this formulation has just the sort of transparency that perception has. The muscles just move when we want them to, with the same immediacy with which perceptual objects appear, even though they require enormous amounts of unconscious processing.

The unconscious neural events do more than carry through the execution in a straight line from the "idea." They operate with feedforward and feedback mechanisms to track the motion. These mechanisms may result in conscious attention to the action, especially when difficulties are encountered. The monitoring mechanisms also seem to be partly responsible for ownership of an action—the stamp that makes it "mine." Essential aspects of feedback may not simply manage deliberate action (as in Jeannerod's and Pockett's contributions to this volume) but go beyond the immediate corrections of action and draw on constraints encoded in the brain structures that support the self. Actions would then be evaluated for the harm they might do or evaluated against norms of ethical behavior. Personal ownership would seem a natural outcome of such a process.

4   Perception of Volition

Wegner (2002; see also Wegner and Wheatley 1999) and many others have concluded that our sense of agency and free will is an illusion. Their evidence comes from experiments in which cues to volition were absent or cleverly manipulated. Ferguson and Bargh (2004), Festinger (1957), Ross and Nisbett (1991), and Nisbett and Wilson (1979) are among those who have reported illusions of volition, intention, or responsibility for action. In all these cases the participant reports on his or her reason for making a certain action or choice. The results show that people take responsibility for things they had no control over, they miss cases where they were responsible for an event, and they freely confabulate reasons, intentions, goals, and preferences when asked their reasons for actions. These self-reports are a variety of introspection. They are judgments of one's internal states on the basis of internal and external cues, memory, and expectations. These introspections are best treated as fallible interpretations of available evidence. These interpretations are normally useful in helping us function. A clever experientalist can, however, cause them to be quite wrong.

As Ross notes in this volume, one argument for free will is the introspective evidence that we have free will. Ross argues that the best way of evaluating these claims is through research on introspection. The nature of introspection is also vital to understanding reports of casual efficacy. I do not think this is correct. First, it is not plausible to consider introspection to be a direct window on the working of the mind. The concept of "privileged access" in this sense is not credible; it is much like an introspective version of naïve realism. There is sufficient research on seemingly direct introspective reports to show that basic feelings like pain and emotions are interpretations. Chapman and Nakamura (1999) and Gustafson (1995) review research showing that the "raw feel" of pain so often given by philosophers as an example of pure sensation is not so raw after all, but an interpretation of sensory and situational evidence.

My conjecture is that introspection amounts to a problem-solving process, much like active perception of the physical world. It never occurs to us that our perceptions are anything but direct registration of objects in the world. Perception is quick, and we don't see it at work. But even when perception is not so quick we are not aware of the complex mechanisms that support it. Likewise, we sometimes feel simply *angry*, and as far as we are concerned that is a brute, elemental fact. It is quick and seemingly authoritative. Further introspection rarely changes the feeling, even though the anger has demonstrable situational influences (reviewed in Mandler 1984).

Because hypotheses need to be generated in order to be tested, introspection can be very theory-laden and subject to all sorts of cultural and scientific biases (Clark 1999). If I believe in spirit possession I may be sincere in my introspective conclusion that my aberrant and disturbing behavior was caused by a wicked spirit that slipped into my mind and took over (Yi 2000). If I think a felt stimulus is an indicator of something that may harm me, I will honestly feel it as painful even though the same stimulus causes no pain if it is thought to be harmless (Chapman and Nakamura 1999). If I have a deep belief in free will, I am likely to find evidence for it introspectively, not because I am distorting the evidence but because that is my best hypothesis to explain certain introspections. A compatibilist would probably remark on how free she feels when she acts in accord with her predispositions.

By the argument I make here, the experiments like Wegner's that are taken to demonstrate "the illusion of conscious will" are better described as situations that create illusions of volition. It could be put this way: imagine a volition "detector" that continually gathers evidence about our intentions, our actions, and the feedback information that confirms our ownership. This is an extremely important aspect of normal behavior in social life. Clever experimentalists create illusions of volition much like visual illusions, and for the same reason. In volition we (Westerners) carry the hypothesis that we are agents; with absent or distorted evidence we have no other hypothesis for our actions and come up with the "illusory" accounts of our willing. This no more supports the claim that conscious will is an illusion than visual illusions support the claim that visual perception is illusory.

However, the research on illusions of volition are valuable for other reasons than exposing our folly. It is a maxim that one of the best windows into the operation of a mechanism is its behavior when it fails, and this is the proper use of these data. Our sense of willing is an interpretation, normally useful, but sometimes mistaken, like any perception. Paradigms like Wegner's should be considered as tools to understanding how volition works rather than demonstrations that conscious will is illusory.

These considerations are relevant to our everyday concepts of volition, which in turn affect our moral and legal judgments. They do not seem to be part of folk wisdom. What effect would these ideas have if they were generally accepted to be true?

5 Folk Models of Volition and the Law

Malle (2004) has undertaken a comprehensive and much-needed empirical analysis of folk models of volition. The schema he has worked out elegantly summarizes the model as having the folk-defined concepts of belief and desire leading to intention. Intention plus ability and awareness lead to intentionality, which is here the mental state that leads to taking an action in relation to an object.

Malle concludes that free will does not appear to be part of the folk model. I disagree. He may have come to this conclusion because his participants were not interrogated about the specific issues that define free will. The model could perfectly well have carried the assumption that choices are made freely, and that freedom is necessary for choices to be morally judged. I would argue that people generally have a concept of freedom that is essentially libertarian. Greene and Cohen (2004) make the case that legal principles depend on a libertarian theory of freedom to establish guilt and justify retributive punishment. Gunther (2003) also makes a case on the basis of German law that libertarian assumptions are among the principles behind legal reasoning.

Malle (this volume) has more recently contributed a refined analysis of how free will is handled in the folk model of volition. He does not find evidence for a concept of "will" or "free will" to put in the model. He argues that the notion of freedom violates the folk-theoretic concept of intentionality, in which the action results from an intention. The intention is in turn caused by a set of reasons, conditions, mental states, personal traits, and so on. If folk models were internally consistent, this would be a strong argument against having both free will and causes of intentions in the model, but I do not think consistency is a strong suit of folk models. Further, I think there are several facts to deal with if freedom is not considered part of the model. For example, Gunther (2003) shows that freedom is implicitly assumed in jurisprudence, which generally reflects folk-model "common sense." Consider also the argument in the everyday moral sphere that the man is guilty because "he could have done something other than what he did." This seems to reflect a belief in a kind of absolute freedom of action. In fact, this is one argument used to support libertarian freedom (Kane 1996), but perhaps it could be interpreted differently in folk intuitions. My own opinion is that the reason we feel free in our actions is precisely that we are not aware of most of the causes of our behavior, and that for this reason it is possible for us to think of acts—ours and others'—as freely willed.

The law, just as folk theory (see Gunther 2003 for a discussion of the contradictory ideas that are incorporated in culture, and of course folk theories), can contain separate principles that are philosophically inconsistent. Thus there is a mixture of libertarian and compatibilist thinking in judging guilt and punishment. The idea of prison as a "correctional" institution is compatibilist notion. The next step from the compatibilist perspective would be to replace punishment with rehabilitation programs, even psychotherapy. There are several examples of this approach. In some states drug offenders are required to complete treatment programs as a condition of probation. Sexual offenders and spousal abusers are in some jurisdictions put into treatment programs, often while they are serving jail time. The ultimate compatibilist (and hard determinist) position would replace punishment altogether with some form of treatment. The only function of incarceration would be to protect the public from the offenders until they can be released as productive members of society.

The libertarian position is linked to retributive punishment. This is punishment that is not aimed to reform but to deliver "just deserts" to bad people. The libertarian judgment of compatibilist programs is that these programs are dangerously "soft on crime." Punishment has side benefits of protecting society and creating a reward structure that discourages criminal activity, but these are not the main reasons. The distinction between the two versions of freedom comes to a crux with capital punishment. To the compatibilist it makes no sense at all. The only purpose can be to assure permanent protection from the offender, and that can be accomplished more cheaply and with less fuss by sentences of life without possibility of parole. To the libertarian death is the only right and fitting punishment for certain crimes.

Greene and Cohen conclude that neuroscience research challenging freedom of the will would have little immediate influence on legal decision making. The significant effect, they conclude, will be on the underlying folk theory that yields the intuitions that drive legal decision making. The law reflects what is commonly understood to be the case, and common knowledge (folk theories) about everything from physics to religion is involved. The effects of scientific knowledge are slow and uncertain, but over time they can create a sea change in the common understanding of volition, responsibility, even metaphysics, and thus the law. These are the sort of changes that caused people to stop prosecuting women for witchcraft, to cease believing that some individuals are capable of putting the "evil eye" on others, and so on. These are seen as superstitions now, but at the time they had enough credibility to lead to torture and execution. Will the concept of libertarian free will be categorized as a superstition in a generation or two? If so, what will the consequence be?

It is possible that jurisprudence would be little changed if belief in libertarian freedom were abandoned. Freedom of action is only one of the components of judgments of guilt. In a court of law it is likely to be in the background. Being forced to commit a crime is, however, a constraint on freedom that could reduce one's culpability. Outside of such special circumstances we are all free or unfree in the same sense. We do not normally take a measure of a person based on whether he or she possesses free will, as we would on intelligence, creativity, or athletic ability, in which there are known individual differences. Individual differences that are more relevant are rationality and intent. The rationality criterion leads to questions such as "Did the person understand the consequences of the action?" and "Was the person able to see that is was wrong?" Greene and Cohen (2004) emphasize rationality. Intent is equally important. The example from Aristotle could not be clearer. If I shoot an arrow, miss my target, and kill another person I did not see, this is an accident. I would feel terrible about it, but I would not be convicted of murder. Now I shoot my arrow carelessly, with no intent to hit any specific person, but in a direction that I know exposes people to danger. I did not intend to hit anyone, but I lacked the intent to avoid harm (or the reasoning ability to see the consequences). There is some culpability there, and likely legal consequences. Finally, I aim at a man with the intent to kill him, and I do. That is murder. In the present volume, Kaplan discusses the role of intent in responsibility.

For both intention and rationality, psychology and neuroscience have something to say. Scientific evidence is now adduced in court along with traditional forms of evidence to show that a person was out of control (could not restrain an urge, as in a crime of passion) As for rationality, a person may be argued to be less culpable because of mental retardation or a state of diminished capacity. The US Supreme Court recently handed down an opinion that mentally retarded individuals cannot be subject to the death penalty because of their presumed lack of reasoning ability. Another recent judgment was that capital punishment can be applied only to those above the age of 18, also in part because of a presumed immature ability to reason clearly.

If psychological science continues to make discoveries in areas of the nervous system involved in reasoning, planning, and emotion, one consequence could be that sophisticated tests could be used to determine reasoning ability and intent, just as IQ tests are used now to determine if a defendant is mentally deficient. This is not in itself a bad outcome. The better we can measure the psychological traits germane to a legal case, the better justice will be served. On the other hand, this will bring psychology and neuroscience further into the courtroom, again not a bad thing in itself. An unintended consequence could be, over years and decades, a gradual psychologizing of the legal process. How far would it go? Might defendants be given subtle implicit tests of guilty knowledge? For example, EEG measures can be used to tell whether a defendant has previously seen certain objects from the crime scene. This test could obviously be an indicator of guilt. What I am getting to is that these approaches get more and more invasive as we literally get deeper into the brain and individual psychology. There are obvious concerns here. Now suppose these techniques in the hands of authoritarian governments, or our own democratic government gone paranoid in, say, a war on terrorism. A single clause in the next Patriot Act, or the one after that, could open the door to the effective loss of privacy. The good news here is that torture will be unnecessary. The bad news is that the Orwellian concept of thought crimes can be applied practically.

Consider some extremes. The ultimate application of compatibilist (and hard determinist) ideas could be procedures like the Ludovici treatment in *A Clockwork Orange*. The idea is that offenders have got something wrong in their wiring and they need to be "fixed." There have been proposals to use brain surgery to correct violent behavior and "chemical castration" for sexual offenders. Where would this stop? Once punishment is dissociated from guilt and replaced with socially beneficial "treatment" we could imagine brain scans and DNA tests to catch and treat offenders before they offend. Because social criteria define what is criminal and what is not, the legal system could possibly reach out to fix people who have unhealthy political beliefs and politically incorrect ideas and actions (as in the Stalin-era mental hospitals, where dissidents were sometimes given therapeutic prefrontal lobotomies).

Greene and Cohen express the hope that the changes in folk concepts resulting from neuroscience will lead to a more "progressive, consequentialist approach to the criminal law." I hope so as well. Kaplan (this volume) has a more pessimistic view. I think that what saves us from the extremes of a ruthless social program of "correction" is the conviction that individual human rights are supremely important, possibly more so than social order. In highly collectivistic and authoritarian societies, or any society in a panic over some threat, these extremes are on the table as suitable options.

No one can predict the effects of scientific conclusions about will and freedom on the law and folk wisdom over the next century. There are many uses of science in legal settings, and these sometimes take time to be established, as for example, when DNA tests were finally recognized as valid sources of evidence. One good effect of a scientifically aware folk wisdom would be the general recognition by jurors and lawmakers that the science behind forensics needs to be understood and taken seriously. A bad effect would be to have technology supplant moral decisions, with the idea that sociopaths and potential criminals could be removed for therapy before they have a chance to do harm.

These are modest conclusions. More broadly, one might expect scientific findings to tip the balance in treatment of convicted offenders from retribution to rehabilitation. However, there are many other factors at work. Despite the great recent advances in neuroscience and the seeming increase in public interest in findings related to brain and behavior, the legal system in the United States has apparently taken a retributive turn. In California, for example, a "three strikes" law has been in effect since March 1994, the third strike leading to a lifetime of imprisonment. Petty crimes sometimes constitute the third strike that puts an offender away for life, but a recent ballot initiative to require the third strike be a violent offense was turned down by the voters. It is somewhat surprising that the increase in the understanding of physiological foundations of behavior has not led to a trend toward compatibilist theories of volition. I have always assumed that compatibilist thinking tends toward treatment, even therapy, rather than punishment. The connection between neuroscientific knowledge and compatibilism could be weaker than I thought, or perhaps compatibilist thinking does not reduce the tendency to endorse retributive punishment.

We come to the question I began with: "Does consciousness cause misbehavior?" This question encompasses the full range of questions raised in this paper. To answer it we need to know how we consciously make a finger move in the first place and what complications—neural, social, personal—are involved when the finger triggers a pistol pointed at a person. Because concepts of responsibility depend on consciousness of action we need to know more about the relationship between consciousness and volition. Further, following Prinz (this volume), I think that the need for conscious control to confer responsibility has influenced the concept of consciousness itself. As for an idea moving a muscle, this concept is a caricature of a fiction. It is not, however, too far from our intuitions. I wiggle a finger to show that I can move at will and experience what seems a direct translation from thought to action. The apparent directness of motion comes from the inaccessibility of all the processes that lead to the conscious intention and that follow it. By this, ideas move muscles but only as a monitoring function that is itself part of an elaborate neural apparatus supporting action. The apparent direct connection from idea to action is analogous to the apparent transparency of perception. It's the way it looks to us, not the way it happens.

I think a compatibilist view like Strawson's (1962) gives something like the freedom vainly sought in libertarian theories, and I hope it is durable. I worry about a time when we do not think consciousness causes misbehavior because we come to think that the arguments over free will are "nothing but" theology, that freedom of the will is a superstition, the human mind is indeed "nothing but" a bunch of neurons, and technology is the answer to crime. These are part of the pessimistic view Strawson (1962) wished to avoid. It is fitting to close with a quote from his article that connects volition with our personal mental constitution, not a set of arbitrary causes:

What is wrong is to forget that these practices, and their reception, the reactions to them, really are expressions of our moral attitudes and not merely devices we calculatingly employ for regulative purposes. Our practices do not merely exploit our natures, they express them.

Acknowledgments

This research and writing was supported by a Sontag grant. I thank Peter Ross for his invaluable comments on this article.

References

Baars, B. J. 1997. *In the Theater of Consciousness: The Workspace of the Mind*. Oxford University Press.

Banks, W. P., and Pockett, S. In press. Libet's work on the neuroscience of free will. In *The Blackwell Companion to Consciousness*, ed. M. Velmans. Blackwell.

Bloom, P. 2004. *Descartes' Baby: How the Science of Child Development Explains What Makes Us Human*. Basic Books.

Chalmers, D. 1995. *The Conscious Mind: In Search of a Fundamental Theory*. Oxford University Press.

Chapman, C. R., and Nakamura, Y. 1999. A passion of the soul: An introduction to pain for consciousness researchers. *Consciousness and Cognition* 8, no. 4: 391–422.

Christie, J., and Barresi, J. 2002. Using illusory line motion to differentiate misrepresentation (Stalinesque) and misremembering (Orwellian) accounts of consciousness. *Consciousness and Cognition* 11, no. 2: 347–365.

Clark, T. W. 1999. Fear of mechanism: A compatibilist critique of *The Volitional Brain*. *Journal of Consciousness Studies* 6, no. 8–9: 279–293

Davidson, D. 1980. *Essays on Actions and Events*. Clarendon.

Dennett, D. 1991. *Consciousness Explained*. Little, Brown.

Dennett, D., and Kinsbourne, M. 1992. Time and the observer: The where and when of consciousness in the brain. *Behavioral and Brain Sciences* 15: 183–247

Durgin, F. H., and Sternberg, S. 2002. The time of consciousness and vice versa. *Consciousness and Cognition* 11, no. 2: 284–290.

Ferguson, M. J., and Bargh, J. A. 2004. How social perception can automatically influence behavior. *Trends in Cognitive Sciences* 8, no. 1: 33–39.

Festinger, L. 1957. *Theory of Cognitive Dissonance*. Stanford University Press.

Fodor, J. 2000. "Special sciences." In *Readings in the Philosophy of Science*, ed. T. Schick Jr. Mayfield.

Freud, S. 1954. *Psychopathology of Everyday Life*. E. Benn.

Gazzaniga, M. S. 1998. *The Mind's Past*. University of California Press.

Gray, J. A. 1995. The contents of consciousness: A neuropsychological conjecture. *Behavioral and Brain Sciences* 18, no. 4: 659–722.

Greene, J. D., and Cohen, J. D. 2004. For the law, neuroscience changes nothing and everything. *Philosophical Transactions of the Royal Society of London* B 359: 1775–1785.

Greene, J. D., Sommerville, R. B., Nystrom, L. E., Darley, J. M., and Cohen, J. D. 2001. An fMRI investigation of emotional engagement in moral judgment. *Science* 293, no. 5537: 2105–2108.

Grush, R., and Chuchland, P. S. 1995. Gaps in Penrose's toilings. *Journal of Consciousness Studies* 2, no. 1: 10–29.

Gunther, K. 2003. Voluntary action and criminal responsibility. In *Voluntary Action*, ed. S. Maasen et al. Oxford University Press.

Gustafson, D. 1995. Belief in pain. *Consciousness and Cognition* 4, no. 3: 323–345.

Haggard, P., and Clark, S. 2003. Intentional action: Conscious experience and neural prediction. *Consciousness and Cognition* 12, no. 4: 695–707.

Haggard, P., and Eimer, M. 1999. On the relation between brain potentials and awareness of voluntary movements. *Experimental Brain Research* 126: 128–133.

Hameroff, S., and Penrose, R. 1995. Orchestrated reduction of quantum coherence in brain microtubules: A model for consciousness. In *Scale in conscious experience*, ed. J. King and K. Pribram. Erlbaum.

Illes, J., Kirschen, M. P., and Gabrieli, J. D. E. 2003. From neuroimaging to neuroethics. *Nature Neuroscience* 6, no. 3: 205.

Kane, Robert. 1996. *The Significance of Free Will*. Oxford University Press.

Kane, Robert. 2002. Some neglected pathways in the free will labyrinth. In *The Oxford Handbook of Free Will*, ed. R. Kane. Oxford University Press.

Libet, B. 1994. A testable field theory of mind-brain interaction. *Journal of Consciousness Studies* 1, no. 1: 119–126.

Libet, B. 1999. Do we have free will? *Journal of Consciousness Studies* 6: 47–57.

Libet, B. 2002. The timing of mental events: Libet's experimental findings and their implications. *Consciousness and Cognition* 11, no. 2: 291–299.

Libet, B., Gleason, C. A., Wright, E. W., and Pearl, D. K. 1983. Time of conscious intention to act in relation to onset of cerebral activity (readiness-potential). *Brain* 106: 623–642.

Malle, B. F. 2004. *How the Mind Explains Behavior: Folk Explanations, Meaning, and Social Interaction*. MIT Press.

Mandler, G. 2003. Emotion. In *Handbook of Psychology: History of psychology,* volume 1, ed. D. Freedheim. Wiley.

McDowell, J. 1985. Functionalism and anomalous monism. In *Actions and Events*, ed. E. LePore and B. McLaughlin. Blackwell.

Nijhawan, R. 1994. Motion extrapolation in catching. *Nature* 370: 256–257.

Nisbett, R. E., and Wilson, T. D. 1977. Telling more than we know: Verbal reports on mental processes. *Psychological Review* 84: 231–259.

Ross, L., and Nisbett, R. E. 1991. *The Person and the Situation: Perspectives of Social Psychology*. McGraw-Hill.

Schacter, S., and Singer, J. 1962. Cognitive, social and physiological determinants of emotional states. *Psychological Review* 69: 379–399.

Searle, J. 1992. *The Rediscovery of the Mind*. MIT Press.

Searle, J. R. 1997. *The Mystery of Consciousness*. New York Review of Books.

Seife, C. 2004. Quantum information theory: A general surrenders the field, but black hole battle rages on. *Science* 305, no. 5686: 934–936.

Skinner, B. F. 1971. *Beyond Freedom and Dignity*. Knopf.

Spence, S. A., and Frith, C. D. 1999. Towards a functional anatomy of volition. *Journal of Consciousness Studies* 6, no. 8–9: 11–29.

Spier, E., and Thomas, A. 1998. A quantum of consciousness? A glance at a physical theory for a mind. *Trends in Cognitive Sciences* 2: 124–125.

Stenger, V. J. 1995. *The Unconscious Quantum: Metaphysics in Modern Physics and Cosmology*. Prometheus Books.

Strawson, P. F. 1962. Freedom and resentment. *Proceedings of the British Academy* 48: 1–25.

Trevena, J. A., and Miller, J. 2002. Cortical movement preparation before and after a conscious decision to move. *Consciousness and Cognition* 11: 162–190.

Van Fraassen, B. C. 1980. *The Scientific Image*. Clarendon.

Watanabe, K., Nijhawan, R., and Shimojo, S. 2002. Shifts in perceived position of flashed stimuli by illusory object motion. *Vision Research* 42, no. 24: 2545–2650.

Wegner, D. M. 2002. *The Illusion of Conscious Will*. MIT Press.

Wegner, D. M., and Wheatley, T. P. 1999. Apparent mental causation: Sources of the experience of will. *American Psychologist* 54: 480–492.

Wilson, E. O. 1998. *Consilience: The Unity of Knowledge*. Knopf.

Yi, K. 2000. Shin-byung (divine illness) in a Korean woman. *Culture, Medicine and Psychiatry* 24, no. 4: 471–486.

13 Free Will as a Social Institution

Wolfgang Prinz

Does consciousness cause behavior? In this chapter I examine this question in the domain of voluntary action and free will. Though the chapter begins and concludes with broad perspectives on conscious experience and consciousness (Prinz 2003), the bulk of the argument will focus on issues of volition and free will (Prinz 2004). Free will serves as an example to illustrate how I conceive of conscious experience and its causal role for behavior in general. My message is twofold: consciousness is not a brute fact of nature but a matter of social construction. Still, conscious experience plays a causal role in the control of behavior.

1 Conscious Experience

What does "conscious experience" really mean? Let me first say what I do *not* mean when I use this term. I do not refer to consciousness as a state in which a person can be more conscious or less conscious or even unconscious. This notion of consciousness describes the *disposition* to produce conscious mental contents. Theories of this disposition may specify the conditions under which consciousness comes and goes, without telling us anything about what is responsible for the conscious nature of these contents.

This brings me to what I do mean and what I wish to explicate here: the conscious nature of mental contents. We cannot be conscious in a pure or empty form. It is always *specific contents* of which we are aware, and it is only through our awareness of these contents that we recognize that we are conscious. Thus, like people who can be in conscious or unconscious states, mental contents can be conscious or non-conscious. Depending on our theoretical tastes, we then use such labels as *unconscious* or *preconscious* mental contents, or those that are *inaccessible to conscious experience*.

How, then, is conscious experience possible, and what exactly is its conscious component? When answering this question, I shall follow a characterization given by Brentano (1870/1924). Brentano uses an extremely simple example to discuss the nature of what he calls mental acts. He raises the question of what actually happens when we hear a tone. What is responsible for the conscious nature of the act of hearing a tone? According to Brentano, there are two contents interwoven in this mental act: the tone that we hear and the fact that we hear it. However, these two mental contents are not represented in the same way. The tone is the primary object of hearing; we can observe it directly in the mental act. Hearing itself is a secondary object of the mental act. Brentano says that it cannot be observed directly, but attains consciousness in another, indirect form: "We can observe the tones that we hear, but we cannot observe the hearing of the tones. This is because it is only in the hearing of the tones that the hearing itself is also assessed." (ibid., p. 181)

That is as far as Brentano goes. However, if we want an exhaustive characterization of the structure of mental acts, we have to go one step further: If it is true that hearing the tone contains not only the tone itself but also, implicitly, its hearing, then the subject hearing it must also be contained in the act in another encapsulation. Just as a tone is hardly conceivable without a hearing directed toward it, a hearing is hardly conceivable without a mental self, or a subject who hears. Accordingly, conscious mental acts are characterized by what is sometimes termed "me-ness" (Kihlstrom 1997). This may be called the implicit presence of the mental self in mental acts.

What sort of explanations do we then need in order to finally say that we *understand*, conclusively, how the conscious nature of mental contents arises? If it is true that the relationship of mental contents to an implicitly present self forms the decisive foundation for the formation of their conscious nature, then the problem of explanation shifts from consciousness to self—that is, to the issue of the formation of the mental self and its implicit representation in mental acts.

Therefore, we need theories that explain the role of the implicitly present mental self. An understanding of this role would simultaneously mean an understanding of how the conscious nature of mental contents arises. Because the quality of conscious awareness does not merely arise when the condition of the implicit presence of the self is fulfilled but also consists in precisely this condition being met, it would then become possible to understand not only—in correlational terms—under which conditions conscious mental contents emerge but also—in foundational terms—why they acquire a conscious quality as opposed to some other quality.

This distinction addresses one of the major problems faced by research into what some have termed the neural correlates of consciousness (Metzinger 2000): Even if we had an exact and comprehensive account of the neural correlates of consciousness, we would still be far from understanding why these neural processes bring forth precisely this particular quality, and not some other. And, vice versa, we would be just as uncertain why certain neural processes bring forth the quality of conscious awareness while others do not. Theories on the relation between brain functions and consciousness offer, at best, correlational relations that help us to know how the brain sustains conscious experience, but not foundational relations that help us to understand those relationships.

To address these issues I will pursue two lines of argument: a narrow one and a broad one. The narrow one is concerned with the role of the mental self in voluntary action and free will. The broad one, to which I will return at the end of the chapter, is concerned with an evolutionary scenario for the emergence of mental selves and their foundational role for the formation of conscious experience.

2 Free Will

Asking a psychologist to discuss free will is like asking a zoologist to lecture on unicorns: neither phenomenon belongs to the science where the expert is at home. Expositions on unicorns are arguably better suited to the human sciences than the natural sciences, for while they have no natural history, these creatures do have a cultural story to tell. Studies in cultural history may reveal how unicorns were initially fabricated, why the notion of them has persevered, and just what people get out of continuing to believe in them.

In this chapter I will think of free will as scholars of the human sciences think of unicorns. I will discuss freedom of will in terms of empirical facts and psychological theories; more important, I will treat the notion of free will as a product of collective endeavor—not the unicorn itself, as it were, but the notion of a unicorn. I will address these questions: Why do people feel free in their choices and believe that they are free, although they may not be? Under what conditions do healthy minds develop intuitions of free will? What psychological, social, and cultural effects do these intuitions encourage? These issues go beyond the isolated study of cognitive and volitional functions to explore how the functions themselves are (individually and collectively) constituted through mutual perception and attribution. They include, for instance, how functions of free will are seen in social psychology, developmental psychology, evolutionary psychology, and psychohistory.

I shall proceed in four steps. First, I shall confront our quotidian intuition of free will with maxims of scientific psychology, concluding that the two are not particularly compatible. Second, I shall examine psychological mechanisms and cultural conditions that favor the emergence of free will intuitions. Third, I shall look at the psychological benefits and social functions supported by our intuitions of free will. Finally, to resolve the contradiction between denying and praising free will, I shall consider cultural facts and artifacts.

Denying Free Will

The Idiom of Agency and Intuitions of Free Will: Psychological Explanation of Actions

We spend a large portion of our lives thinking about behavior—deliberating over our own actions and ruminating over those of others. Thinking about behavior is not only an individual pastime, it is also one of our favorite social hobbies. Everyday conversation consists in large measure of communicative exchanges about who does what when, why people do what they do, and what we think about the whole business.

The list of mental states that may be seen as the cause of some particular behavior spans many different options, each invoking its own distinct explanation of the behavior in question. In simple cases we explain behavior by identifying an intention to attain a specific goal. Here we have the prototypical case for acting voluntarily: We assume that a person plans an action and then executes it in order to accomplish certain objectives. We say that John washes his car because he believes that doing so will impress his rich aunt. Of course, positing a mental state as the cause of subsequent behavior does not account for how the action proceeded. But it can specify why a certain behavior occurred at all. The assumption of antecedent mental states does not indicate how an action happens; it indicates what a specific action was for. If we were to inquire why the person did what she did, she would give us reasons.

Other explanations for behavior use the logic of causes instead of reasons. If you smashed a vase in rage, common opinion holds that you did not do so for any particular reason, but that nevertheless your action was caused. A mental state of anger is understood as causative of destructive behavior, but not as a reason for it. Such acts have no goal that performing them may attain.

Habitual behavior is different from voluntary action, too. If you ask people during their morning grooming routine just why they are now brushing their teeth, the answer will normally not include any immediate reason or cause. Explanations for this type of behavior normally assume that the original causal mental states occurred long ago: at one time reasons were present (namely when the person acquired the habit at issue), but they faded as the habit gradually took hold. The reasons have not disappeared entirely and can be recalled. You know why you brush your teeth, but you don't state your reasons every time you do it.

In the following I shall concentrate on prototypical voluntary behavior and the jargon used in quotidian speech to describe it. Voluntary acts happen because agents want to achieve certain goals and believe that performing certain acts will get them there.

Free Will Vernacular: Morally Evaluating Action

Everyday talk about behavior usually revolves not only around the explanation of action but also around evaluation and justification; we want to know the reason for an action, how to evaluate it, and, finally, whether or not it is justified. On one level we judge the actions themselves, and their consequences. But on another level we also judge the person responsible for that action. We hold people responsible for their behavior and we justify doing so by assuming that they are free in their decisions to act. These underlying convictions permeate our everyday phrases for describing the freedom of will. They are so familiar that they hardly need explanation. We simply assume that, in almost all walks of life, we could act other than we actually do—if only we wanted to. We understand our actual behavior to be an outcome of voluntary decision. While our decisions are also invariably shaped by a number of circumstances, of which we are more or less aware, we believe that ultimate responsibility for the final decision rests with each person individually. We are ourselves the authors of our decisions and actions. We all experience this authorship and freedom and attribute it to each other. This is at the core of what I call our intuition of free will.

One important consequence of our free will vernacular is that we sometimes waive further explanation. For instance, when a court judge asks a defendant why he did a certain thing, the accused often details causes and reasons apparently beyond his own control. In other words: A defendant will say that under the circumstances he had no choice but to do as he did, thus turning over the causal responsibility for the actions in question to the circumstances that prevailed. Now, a judge may or may not accept certain factors as influential. When she accepts explanatory reasons and causes that regress further and further back into the past of the defendant she forgoes the option of attributing both the action and the consequences for it to that person—and personal responsibility evaporates into thin air. In order to attribute personal responsibility, a judge must interrupt the chain of causes at some point and dispense with further explanation.

Thus, talk of free will has two sides. On the one hand, we use it to describe fundamental psychological facts, that is, to describe the personal experience of free will intuitions that seem so blindingly self-evident. On the other, the permission it grants to waive further explanation serves an essentially moral (or even legal) purpose, namely, that of ascribing outcomes of behavior to individual persons. What should we think of this shorthand? Hen or egg—which came first? Is free will a basic fact of human mental constitution issuing welcome social by-products? Or is it a social device serving to collectively regulate individual behavior? Do psychological facts precede social institutions—or dare we suggest that social functions actually produce psychological facts?

Science and Our Intuition of Free Will

How does the notion of free will line up with maxims of scientific psychology? We must be careful to distinguish between the empirical fact that we experience an intuition of free will and the theoretical construct of free will itself.

The empirical fact is a phenomenon like any other that can be explored and explained using tools of psychology. No problem. But guidelines for psychological explanation falter when we switch from viewing free will as an empirical phenomenon to thinking of it as a theoretical construct, by believing *that we feel free, because we are free*. We run up against two standards of science: first, that we must distinguish between perception and reality; and second, that we must posit causal closure and thoroughgoing determinism.

Perception and Reality

Psychology has a long history of confusing observational facts with theoretical constructs. Cognition, attention, will, feelings—in the past all these phenomena were mistakenly promoted up from the ranks of mere observational facts to be seen as explanatory constructs. This promotion happened—and still occurs in some areas of research—because of a deep and stubborn misconception about the status of introspection.

A widespread but false construal says that the way we could perceive psychological events in our minds (introspection) is entirely different from the way we perceive material events in the world. As concerns the *perception of material events in the world*, more than a century of experimental research has opened our eyes to the fact that human perception involves *realistic constructivism*—a term meant to characterize the supposed relationship between perception and reality (in a somewhat paradoxical phrase, though). The working model underlying research in perception is realistic inasmuch as it relies on the notion that contents of perception refer to genuinely existing circumstances in the real world. But at the same time it is constructivist because it assumes that contents of perception result from constructive procedures in which perceptual systems process input data according to certain categories, using its own means of representation. Among other elements, these constructive processes include the following:

Selective representation Only a small quantity of all input data actually gets processed, and only a small amount of what gets processed later actually becomes conscious representation.

Content focus Perceptual representations include contents only. Underlying constructive processes are not themselves represented.

Categorical transformation Perceptual contents get organized into categories; they present the outcome of an interaction between current input data and stored knowledge.

There are also other significant elements, but for present purposes these three suffice to illustrate that what we perceive is not reality as it is in and of itself, but the result of construal: Human perception is highly selective, significantly transformed, and shaped to suit certain categories.

In contrast, widespread opinion holds that our *perception of psychological events in our minds* is not a normal perceptual process at all but, rather, a sui generis mental activity in which a thinking subject is aware of its own mental goings-on. The perception of mental events is supposedly not a process of representation and transformation, and therefore it makes little sense to question how perceived contents relate to genuine facts. The perception of mental events is considered an immediate awareness of genuine facts—with no room for error. Percepts and reality are one and the same. This makes it seem legitimate to view mental phenomena, as they present themselves to us, as theoretical constructs. Accordingly, it seems legitimate to conclude that we *feel free* because apparently we *are free*. The observation of feeling free implies the theoretical fact of being free.

Is this convincing? Is introspection privileged access? We have little evidence for it. On the contrary, upon close examination we find that what we do know suggests that our perception of our own mental events is equally construed, transformed, and selectively focused. We must distinguish between reality and our perception of reality for both material events in the world and psychological events in our minds.

For instance, studies on insightful thought indicate that when people think they are unable to note the actual nature of their thought processes. At best, persons can report their individual thoughts; occasionally they can also reconstruct the direction their thoughts took leading up to a certain insight. But they know nothing about the thought-producing process. Here we must rely on theory to identify what the person experienced (and can report) as a selective output produced by submental mechanisms to which experience has no access. Trying to recall a name one has forgotten is also a good example. When we try to remember a certain name, we often experience a disquieting mental state of being altogether unable to retrieve it, or of faintly fathoming some fraction of it. And then, suddenly, the entire name emerges, seemingly from nowhere, and that is all a person can report when asked about what just took place. But theory tells us that more was involved. Once again, theory says that the phenomena accessible at the subjective level are products of events at the subpersonal level, namely, mechanisms executing a search procedure, scavenging that person's stock of knowledge. The same holds for comprehending written text: Try to watch yourself while reading and you will only notice whether or not you understand the text. The practicing reader never knows how understanding a text works; the theoretician does.

Our own perception of mental events provides only an inconsistent and incomplete picture of the underlying processes at work. It is a highly selective, content-focused representation of products created by mechanisms which are themselves imperceptible. We are not actually aware of mental processes themselves, we are aware of individual mental states that may reveal something about the underlying processes that caused them. It is not only perfectly respectable but necessary that we inquire how our perception of mental events relates to the reality of the underlying functional machinery. Whatever introspection about the nature of mental events may tell us, it is itself a product of selective representation, content focus, and categorical transformation. Thus, the fact that we *feel free* says nothing whatsoever about whether the events underlying that feeling are voluntary or determined.

Indeterminism and Waiving Explanation

Freedom of will is conceptually incompatible with scientific explanation in that it compels us to accept local gaps of indeterminism in an otherwise deterministic worldview. While we are accustomed to various sorts of indeterminism—or at least a lack of determinability—in certain areas such as quantum physics and chaos theory, indeterminism in the area of mental events is more radical than mere breaks in causal chains: Here it implies a kind of determinism deprived of causal antecedents, something that we may call *autonomous authorship*. This authorship is attributed to an autonomous subject deciding on her own—a kind of unmoved mover, as it were. Attempts to reconcile freedom of will with quantum physics and the non-determinability of chaotic systems are doomed to failure because free will is not simply the absence of causal determination. The concept of free will is more sophisticated. It demands that we view subjects as the autonomous authors of their actions, equipped with a will and in a position to decide freely.

From a scientific point of view, waiving explanation is unfathomable; it is not compatible with an enlightened and critical scientific stance. Accepting the tenets of indeterminism would require that we surrender our practice of explanation. In lieu of that there is only one possible conclusion: that scientific psychology has no room for a theoretical construct called the freedom of will. A psychologist must be intellectually committed to denying free will if his work is to be deemed scientifically sound.

Explaining Free Will

Adhering, then, to the practices of scientific psychology, the legitimate task to tackle is that of explaining our intuition of free will as a psychological fact. Where do our intuitions of free will come from? Why do subjects feel free although in fact they are not? Obviously, in order to answer these questions we need a theory that clearly distinguishes the functional reality of subpersonal volitional mechanisms from a phenomenal awareness of personal choices based on free will. We must make a distinction if we want to have it both ways: a perception of free will within a world that is deterministic.

Typically, intuitions of free will emerge in situations that involve deciding to act in some way. It even seems that these intuitions are, by their very nature, linked to decisions involving action. Why do intuitions of free will not surface to guide our thoughts, fantasies, moods, and feelings—at least not to the extent that they accompany voluntary decisions related to action? Answering this question leads us to the second essential condition under which intuitions of free will emerge: the active part played by the self. While decisions about actions constitute the occasions on which intuitions of free will are articulated, the subjects to whom we attribute the underlying freedom are persons. A decision is not in and of itself free; the *self*, we say, is free to make a decision. *We* experience freedom—*we* make decisions, *we* are free to make those decisions, and *we* could decide and do otherwise. Surely we may be confronted with an interplay of motives, interests, and preferences that may influence our choice. Yet in the end our self, being aware of all these forces acting upon it, seems to decide on its own what to do. However, we might also see it the other way around: If the ability to make decisions on one's own is a constitutive feature of a self, then explaining our intuition of free will is tantamount to explaining the role of the self.

What sort of theory could accommodate a thorough distinction between subpersonal causal processes that produce decisions on the one hand and personal awareness of agency, where decisions appear to be the outcome of individual choice, on the other? The very question presupposes that the subpersonal production of decision processes is "real," whereas how this reality appears to the individual would have to count as "a perception" of something—at least initially. Thinking of those perceptions as belonging to reality will be considered later in the chapter.

Action-Decisions: Subpersonal Mechanisms

Various fields in psychology explore the events and mechanisms that produce action-decisions. Motivation psychology, social psychology, evolutionary psychology, and the psychology of economics all investigate the phenomenon of decision production, meaning that we must deal with a wide range of applicable yet mutually incompatible theoretical taxonomies. Nevertheless, I would like to outline a few lines of convergence among them. Most theories agree that decision making has at least three ingredients, which I will call *preferences*, *action-knowledge*, and *situation evaluation*. Explaining this without excessive details will require the use of mentalist terms. Nonetheless, the processes outlined can be conceptualized as subpersonal mechanisms.

The first ingredient is systems of representation with ordered *preferences* (e.g., drives, needs, motives, and interests). These systems represent hierarchies of objectives, and they do so on various time scales, from very long-term (at most, life-long) preferential dispositions to short-term and current sets of needs. Current needs are embedded in long-term dispositions but are not entirely determined by them. The reverse is also true: Long-term dispositions develop out of current needs but are not entirely determined by them. Research in this area is focused not only on the general principles underpinning the design of the preference system but also on individual differences, including the configuration and origin of preferences and preference assignment at varying scales of time, the dynamics of reciprocal effects among scales of time, and, last but not least, how preference arrangements are altered through learning and interaction.

The second ingredient is representational systems for *action-knowledge*. By this I mean knowledge about how action is related to the effects it brings about. This knowledge is organized in a way that makes it accessible and allows it to be used in two ways: from actions to effects and from effects to actions. Both uses are elements of action planning. Forward-directed models provide information about possible effects of certain actions. The other way around, inverse models provide information about possible actions appropriate for achieving certain goals (intended effects). Action-knowledge must also be organized along various time scales, corresponding to how long an action-effect relationship may last: from a fraction of a second to years. Research in this field also focuses on how knowledge of actions originates, how it is organized, and how it is changed through learning. It also addresses the difficult question of whether and how declared knowledge about actions can be exploited for procedural action control.

Third, and finally, action-decisions require *situation evaluation*, i.e., procedures and algorithms that provide running evaluations of prevailing circumstances in terms of current goals and behavioral options. These procedures guarantee that the current situation, in which an agent is involved, gets represented in a format that is commensurate with the agent's representational systems for preferences and action-knowledge. This guarantees not only that the current situation can be continually evaluated in terms of upcoming decisions, but also that future decisions can be enriched with additional, and more specific, options tailored to the circumstances. A central research concern here is how perception and memory processes are organized to support running updates for the representation of circumstances for various periods of time.

Different theories combine these ingredients in various ways. But no matter how the process itself may be conceptualized in detail, the decisive fact is that decisions for action are a combined product of preferences, knowledge about action, and evaluations of circumstances. There is no room left for any personal agent actually making a decision; decisions happen on their own.

Self: Personal Perception

What should we think of the constitutive role of the self in our intuitions of free will? Is it a nice illusion, produced by vain self-deceit? Our answer depends on our concept of what we call the self. What is subjectivity? What is real about our perception of being or having a self? In the following I shall distinguish roughly between two concepts of subjectivity: a naturalist one and a constructivist one.

Naturalism The classical view includes concepts of subjectivity saying that the self is a natural organ of the soul. This organ is the bearer of subjectivity, personality, and individuality. Like other organs of the body, it is a naturally given feature of the mind developed prior to and independent of experience. Experience does not cause the self to exist, it merely influences its individual unfolding.

I would like to call the basic notion underlying this concept *self-naturalism*, meaning that the self is the naturally given, intrinsic central organ of the mind. The self coordinates and controls the activity of other psychological and mental functions. It permeates every aspect of mental life; we find it in thought, in feelings, in volition—and in every other psychological function. This intuition is deeply rooted in our quotidian psychological notions. Thus, it is not surprising to find this type of self-naturalistic intuition—in various guises—playing prominent parts even in science, and in psychological as well as in philosophical theories. The doctrine of privileged access to one's own psychological events, a concept that surfaces frequently in both disciplines, is the epistemological flip side of the ontological doctrine of self-naturalism.

Constructivism Constructivist theories of subjectivity believe that the self is not a natural organ of the mind/soul, but rather an acquired knowledge structure that subserves specific functions. The idea here is that the self itself is a mental content. The representational structures that support it develop parallel to and in interaction with other representational structures. In other words, the self evolves along with other structures involved in action-related decisions.

The basic intuition supporting this concept is what I would like to call *self-constructivism*: A self is based on knowledge organized in a special way, but its relationship to other representational structures is not predetermined, it is influenced through the learning and socialization events that create patterns of knowledge. Thus, wherever the self appears to play a central or controlling part in mental life, we must ask how this particular role evolved (on the time scales of evolution, development, and learning) and what benefits it offers. This view says, then, that the configuration and the role of the mental self are not given from the outset; they are generated secondarily. The history of the self thus becomes an object of developmental, historical, and/or evolutionary reconstruction (or, perhaps, deconstruction, as some would claim).

Self-Deceit?

Let us now return to the question of what to think of the personal interpretation of those outcomes of subpersonal processes that are constitutive of our intuition of free will. Should we think of them as dangerous deceits, as nice illusions, or as useful fictions? As I said, the answer depends on how we view the mental self. If we adhere to the naturalistic concept, we must conclude that the feeling of free will is an illusion. Trying to accommodate both notions—namely, that on the one hand decisions can be entirely explained by underlying subpersonal mechanisms while on the other hand the self is an independent, natural organ of the mind—entails that any self-ascription of decisions must involve self-deception. We fool ourselves in thinking that we are autonomous authors of decisions to act.

If, in contrast, we adhere to the constructivist concept, the notion of illusion becomes meaningless, because there is no independent, natural self ascribing things to itself that do not belong to it. Instead, the diagnosis here is that patterns of knowledge which bear the self are arranged in such a way that preferences, action-knowledge, and the evaluation of circumstances are intimately and reciprocally linked. The self surfaces to serve the function of an author of decisions to act, and this authorship is its proper function—the specific function for which it is made.

Attribution Discourse

Since naturalism is mainstream, the burden of proof is on the constructivist side. If the mental self is not the prespecified organ emerging from a natural architecture of the mind, how does it get produced and fabricated? By no means should this construction be considered the heroic deed of a single individual. Instead, we must see the mental self as being socially constituted as a part of discourse about subjectivity and consciousness. This happens within a culturally standardized scheme of interpretation that guides the socialization of individuals and, among other things, attributes to them a mental configuration centered around a self.

Discourse about attribution permeates everyday life at several levels. We negotiate attribution most directly in face-to-face interaction within our micro-social realms, without necessarily using verbal communication. More complex systems of attribution are at work within linguistically bound discourse at the macro-social level: predominantly, for instance, when using psychological common sense, that set of quotidian psychological constructs employed by cultures and linguistic communities for explaining the behavior of human agents. Thus, modern folk psychology is based on the idea of a subject having at his or her core an explicit, constant self. Discourse about morals and rights are no less relevant when they identify the self as an autonomous source of decisions to act.

Now, when agents in social groups organize their mutual interaction and communication at the micro and macro levels in such a way that each agent expects each of the others to also have a self, every one of the agents—new arrivals, too—is confronted with a broad discursive situation that already provides a role for him in the shape of a self. Awareness of foreign ascriptions to oneself induces self-ascriptions, and the agent becomes accustomed to the role of a self ascribed to him by others. A person thinks of himself as others think of him.

These micro and macro social interactions are supported by, inter alia, *narrative discourses* of various kinds. Fictional stories in books and movies are packed with talk about willing and behaving. We tell stories to our children in order to explain to them just what we mean by 'person' and how thought is related to behavior. We thereby provide them with two tools. One is the explicit semantics of the culture in which they live—its customs, practices, values, standards, myths, and legends. The other is the implicit syntax of its folk psychology, which specifies how human agents function, what they think and do, how their thinking is related to their doing, and how they are rewarded or punished for their behavior—be it in heaven or on earth.

In Praise of Free Will

Attribution discourse offers an answer to the question of how living beings come to understand themselves as subjects, as authors of cognition and action, governed by intuitions of free will. According to this, free will—as the Cambridge philosopher Martin Kusch puts it (1997, 1999)—is a *social institution*, made by people and for people. Like most other social institutions, it builds on compelling intuitions that are shared and communicated among individuals. Intuitions of free will emerge if and when individuals learn, in social discourse, to develop a self as a source of action-decisions and actions. And since this self is created predominantly for the purpose of establishing authorship for action and thought, it makes little sense to question whether that authorship is an illusion, for there exists no self before or beyond mental authorship.

Now, we may ask just what a social institution of autonomous selves equipped with intuitions of free will is good for. What does it offer individuals psychologically? How does it help them forge a social and political community?

Psychological Effects

The psychological effects that the ascription of a self has for an individual depends on the role one attributes to the personal interpretation of subpersonal processes that constitute decision making. Thus far, for the sake of simplicity, I have described the subpersonal processes as being something real and the personal processes of interpretation as providing a perceptual representation of that reality. At this point we must abandon simplicity, because nothing would be worse than to conclude, in reverse, that only so-called reality is effective, while its perception is epiphenomenal and inefficacious. Like every other social institution, autonomous selves are not fictions; they are real—*real as artifacts* (Kusch 1997, p. 18). The reality of the artifact is in this case expressed by the fact that the personal perception of subpersonal processes must itself also be supported by subpersonal representational processes—processes consisting of elements similar to all the other representational processes.

This means that personal perception, too, can only develop out of underlying subpersonal processes. If so there is no reason whatsoever to view them as less real and efficacious than the outcomes of the subpersonal decision-making events to which they refer. This is the way institutional facts become functional in individuals and causally efficacious for their behavior. Attribution discourse ensures that institutional notions such as *self*, *will*, and *free will* get implemented in individual knowledge structures at the level of personal intuitions and at the level of subpersonal representations. Thus, peoples' intuitions of self and the workings of will and free will have the same causal potential to affect behavior as their intuitions about the workings of other things and events in their environment.

Still, what exactly are these intuitions about self, will and free will good for? What effect do they have and on what kind of behavior do they make an impact? An initially plausible idea would be that the self creates its own systems for preferences, action-knowledge, and evaluation, and that these are superimposed upon given structures. But this would mean doubling entities without necessity, thus violating Occam's Razor. When we deny such duplication, what remains is *procedural changes*—alterations in the algorithms that operate on those contents and result in an elaboration of the decision-making processes.

The decisive procedural effect of the system of self is probably to slow down the subpersonal decision-producing system, which is itself designed to be quick and efficient. Delaying decisions to act provides an opportunity for elaboration and increases the depth of processing in the representational systems relevant to a certain decision. It allows an expansion of the information base provided for making a decision, and this additional information may modify the eventual decision itself (*explication*). In-depth processing may also activate additional processing and evaluation procedures, that further influence the final decision (*deliberation*). This somewhat cumbersome analysis of representations boils down to simple maxims that we have been told all our lives, so often, in fact, that we give the advice ourselves: take your time, think carefully, know what you really want, study your options, and so on.

Explication and deliberation may influence decisions, but their power is limited. They can only act on the information existing within a person's representational system—one's own preferences, knowledge, and evaluations of circumstances. However, competent language users are in a position to break down the solipsistic closure of this system through *communication* and *argumentation*. When individuals communicate about and argue for the products of their (initially private) explications and deliberations, they establish reciprocal suggestions for modifying decision behavior, and these are not only related to aspects of procedure; they also include changing the contents that are foundational to the decisions. Communicative exchange, therefore, may have the effect that elaboration initially related to procedures also influences the content of a decision.

Social Functions

Authorship and intuitions of free will not only influence the psychological dispositions of individuals, they also alter the shape of the collective in which those individuals see themselves as a community. It is probably not off the mark to propose that this is its true achievement –perhaps even its genuine psycho-historical raison d'être.

For one thing, authorship and intuitions of free will influence *discourses and institutions that regulate behavior*—namely morals and rights. As we saw above, one central achievement of our talk of free will is that it allows us to attribute action and its consequences to the people who act. We make people responsible for what they do. The attestation of free will terminates any otherwise lengthy regress in explanation. Though we may accept that all kinds of circumstances contributed to some behavior, we do not assume that an individual was helplessly commanded by them. The individual could have done otherwise, and therefore he must claim responsibility for the deed. Responsibility is the price of freedom. The vernacular of free will, then, identifies, both within discourse and in the institutions regulating behavior, a source that issues decisions to act. It leaves little room for justifying behavior by citing external authorities or circumstances. It identifies as the source of decisions the same instance that gets sanctioned or rewarded: the person, the agent.

And finally, talk of free will acts back on *discourse and institutions for political development of will*. To the extent that agents in social collectives mutually ascribe autonomy and responsibility for their action-decisions to one another, they will also come to apply these ascriptions to the collective itself and its political development of will. When this happens, authoritarian leadership becomes obsolete—and with it the discourse and the institutions that legitimized and guaranteed it. Paternalism gets replaced by mechanisms of collective will development, as evidenced in many epochs and cultures and at various levels within a social system. In the extreme case of modern Western democracies, these mechanisms are carried by the ideology of the social contract between equal and autonomous individuals and embodied in democratic forms of will development at various levels of society. The idea of democracy is thus founded on the notion of personal autonomy and free will. If we cherish one, we must praise the other.

Real Artifacts

In the end, do we or don't we have free will? Confoundingly, the answer must be "Yes and no." In actuality we don't, but in practice we do.

When we don't know the answer to a difficult question, it can help to answer an easier question first. Do humans have wheels? Answer: In actuality they don't, but in practice they do. Humans don't naturally have wheels. But they have invented wheels and built them into all sorts of vehicles. When using these vehicles, they effectively do have wheels. Do humans have rights and obligations? Answer: In actuality they don't, but in practice they do. Humans don't naturally have rights and obligations. But they have invented rights and obligations and introduced them into all sorts of regulations pertaining to action. In relying on these regulations, humans effectively do have rights and obligations. And now the hard question: Do humans have free will? Answer: In actuality they don't, but in practice they do. Naturally they don't have free will. But they have invented free will and inserted it into all sorts of theories to account for their actions. In relying on these theories, humans effectively do have free will.

Human beings have free will in the same sense that they have wheels or rights and obligations. Wheels, rights, and free will are artifacts that people fashion for themselves and integrate in their sense of self. For those reliant upon them, these artifacts are by no means fictitious; they are just as real as the natural environment we inhabit, and they govern an agent's scope of action with the same inexorable logic.

3   A Stone Age Tale

How might selves have emerged in evolution, or perhaps in human evolution, or perhaps in early human history? If it is true that mental selves are construed through attribution discourse, how, then, might such discourse have emerged in the first place? Answers to these questions must take the form of psycho-historical scenarios explaining how mental selves came about and what advantages were associated with their emergence. Modules for such scenarios have been presented by Dennett (1990, 1992), Donald (2001), Edelmann (1989), Jaynes (1976), Metzinger (1993, 2003), and Mithen (1996). The following scenario is built from some of these modules.

Let us look back to the Stone Age for a moment and try to imagine how the development of autonomous selves may have started. For this we posit an intelligent proto-human with the capacity to evaluate behaviorally relevant implications of a current situation and to convert that knowledge into appropriate action. Imagine that such evaluation depends on complex algorithms that developed over the course of lengthy learning processes, and that additional algorithms guarantee that the outcomes of those evaluations are compared to current priorities and transformed into decisions to act. As complex as these calculations may be, they are subject to one essential restriction: They evaluate only those options that are related to the prevailing situation. Processes related to remembering past or planning future events are irrelevant; this way of being is entirely chained to the present.

Dual Representation

How can our proto-human escape this imprisonment and achieve what Edelmann (1989) calls "freedom from the present"? It must develop the ability to generate representations of things or circumstances that are not present in the current situation. Generating such representations has two sides. On the one hand, it allows representational decoupling of the individual from the current actual situation. On the other hand, this decoupling cannot be complete, since the normal perception of the current surrounding situation has to continue to function. A simultaneous processing of represented and experienced contents requires a processing architecture that allows represented information to be processed up front, while current perceptual information continues to be processed in the background. I call this ability *dual representation.*

Naturally, we do not know when, where, by what means, or how often evolution brought forth mental processing arrangements enabling dual representation. But we can be certain that the ability became advantageous to survival when animals started living in groups that relied on symbolic communication, because under such circumstances individuals are able to become recipients of communications or messages related to things lying beyond the presently perceived horizon. Subjects can understand symbolic messages only when they are in a position to generate representations. However, they must be able to do so without risking their lives, i.e. without losing contact with their present environment. The design of their mental system must therefore allow for dual representation. Dual representation is thus a prerequisite for symbolic communication to function. And our species, whose evolutionary career is entirely founded on symbolic communication, must possess a highly efficient system of dual representation.

Dual representation and symbolic communication enhance the cognitive potential of human beings in many ways. One of them is to develop a notion of self.

Attributing Authorship

Up to this point we have only been considering representations that are induced by receiving verbal messages, i.e., ideas resulting from causes external to the subject. But as soon as a system of dual representation is instated, there is also room for generating internally induced representations—memories, fantasies, plans, and so forth. For the sake of brevity I shall call these kinds of internally induced representations *thoughts*.

Thoughts are comparable to messages; both refer to things that are not present in the current situation. However, there is one important feature that distinguishes internally induced thoughts from externally induced representations. Verbally induced representations are always accompanied by a perception of an act of communication, i.e. by a perception of the person who is the author of the message, whereas when internally induced thoughts occur we have no awareness of an immediate author at work producing them. How can we link those thoughts to the immediate situation?

In these cases we generally assume that the principle of personal authorship applies. Yet this principle can be construed in a number of different ways. One might think that the thoughts can be traced back to invisible authors or authorities, such as the voices of gods, priests, and kings. Another, historically more modern assumption is to locate the source of thoughts in one's own body and to trace them back to an independent, personal subject bound to the body of the agent: the mental self. In both cases the author of the thoughts is not a component of those thoughts; it remains external, related to the thoughts by authorship.

Now, when explaining volition, this idea can also be applied to thoughts concerning action, such as goals and action plans. This hypothetical extension of our attribution scenario leads us to posit selves that not only act as cognitive authors, producing mental contents, but also act as dynamic authors, making decisions and setting behavior into motion. The solutions available for attributing authorship remain the same—except that here social and political implications of the attribution process become increasingly conspicuous. Since goals guide action, the question of where those goals originate becomes more than simply an interesting riddle regarding attribution. Goal origins are of considerable social and political importance because they specify where we believe the causes lie that make people behave as they do. The ancient notion placed authorship of acts and objectives in the hands of invisible personal authorities, external, obedience-demanding forces that somehow told the agent what to do. The modern solution holds that authorship lies within the personal self, substituting autonomy for subservience.

Conclusion

This scenario says that the mental self is a device for solving an attribution problem: the self is construed as the author of internally induced representations. The scenario is built on two principles: dual representation and attribution to persons. Dual representation forms part of the natural history of human cognition and action, whereas attribution to persons concerns the cultural history. Understanding the emergence of mental selves requires both natural and cultural conditions to be met.

We are now in a position to come back to the question from which we started: How can consciousness cause behavior? The answer I now propose is simply this: Consciousness matters. It matters because it reflects functional facts that are relevant to the control of behavior. Conscious awareness is not just a particular quality that may, under some conditions, color certain kinds of representational facts. Rather, it is the manifestation of a particular representational fact—the act of inculcating the mental self in the operative mechanisms used for representing and controlling the environment. This inculcation has far-reaching consequences for the individual and for social control of human conduct. It provides efficient procedures for elaborating the action-decisions of individuals and for communicating about action-decisions within a collective. Individual self-control and mutual social control both depend on collectively constituted conscious experience and could not do without it.

Acknowledgments

This chapter is derived from manuscripts translated by Cynthia Klohr and Jonathan Harrow. I thank Cheryce Kramer for numerous critical comments, questions, and suggestions that helped to shape the final version.

References

Brentano, F. 1874. *Psychologie vom empirischen Standpunkt*, volume 1 (Meiner, 1924).

Dennett, D. C. 1990. The Origin of Selves. Report 14/1990, Research Group on Cognition and the Brain, ZiF, University of Bielefeld, Germany.

Dennet, D. C. 1992. The self as the center of narrative gravity. In *Self and Consciousness: Multiple Perspectives*, ed. F. Kessel et al. Erlbaum.

Donald, M. W. 2001. *A Mind So Rare: The Evolution of Human Consciousness*. Norton.

Edelman, G. M. 1989. *The Remembered Present: A Biological Theory of Consciousness*. Basic Books.

Jaynes, J. 1976. *The Origin of Consciousness in the Breakdown of the Bicameral Mind*. Houghton Mifflin.

Kihlstrom, J. 1997. Consciousness and me-ness. In *Scientific Approaches to Consciousness*, ed. J. Cohen and J. Schooler. Erlbaum.

Kusch, M. 1997. The sociophilosophy of folk psychology. *Studies in the History and Philosophy of Science* 28: 1–25.

Kusch, M. 1999. *Psychological Knowledge: A Social History and Philosophy*. Routledge.

Luhmann, N. 1984. *Soziale Systeme. Grundriss einer allgemeinen Theorie*. Suhrkamp.

Metzinger, T. 1993. *Subjekt und Selbstmodell. Die Perspektive phänomenalen Bewußtseins vor dem Hintergrund einer naturalistischen Theorie mentaler Repräsentationen*. Mentis.

Metzinger, T., ed. 2000. *Neural Correlates of Consciousness: Empirical and Conceptual Questions*. MIT Press.

Metzinger, T. 2003. *Being No One: The Self-Model Theory of Subjectivity*. MIT Press.

Mithen, S. 1996. *The Prehistory of Mind: A Search for the Origins of Art, Religion, and Science.* Thames and Hudson.

Prinz, W. 2003. Emerging selves: Representational foundations of subjectivity. *Consciousness and Cognition* 12: 515–528.

Prinz, W. 2004. Kritik des freien Willens: Bemerkungen über eine soziale Institution. *Psychologische Rundschau* 55, no. 4: 198–206.

14 Truth and/or Consequences: Neuroscience and Criminal Responsibility

Leonard V. Kaplan

1 Approaching Responsibility through Academic Law

What challenges does the new neuroscience literature present for criminal jurisprudence? In this chapter I caution that neuroscience has such powerful rhetorical strength that its claims will be likely to have impact beyond what it purports to prove. Defense lawyers will certainly attempt to use on behalf of their clients any findings of the new brain research that might be said to negate or diminish the attribution of responsibility. Claims that the behavior of defendants such as addicts was caused by brain pathology are perhaps the least objectionable application, one unlikely to prevail because of cultural repulsion with addictions to drugs and alcohol generally. But the use of such data to undercut contemporary notions of human agency presents a more clear danger.

The new brain research could well augment tendencies that have been part of Western culture from both Athens (philosophy) and Jerusalem (theology) toward the public control of deviant behavior based on character and/or perceived social dangerousness regardless of demonstrable criminal intention. Perhaps my fear, it will be argued, is an over reaction- a psycho-socially hysterical reading of culture as tending toward a dystopian Brave New World, or more bounded, a Clockwork Orange legal application. What I intend here is an abbreviated description of fragments of the Western heritage leading to the contemporary notion of the autonomous self, with its assumption of human agency. This same history, I claim, can just as well support visions of individuals as socially contingent and incapable of real choice. The law generally assumes autonomy, but I think it instructive for neuroscientists to attend to potential abuses that might accompany the appropriation of the new findings. What may well be at stake is a shifting understanding of fundamental ascriptions of responsibility.

What models of attributing criminal fault are now in place? Are present theoretical models so effective that a change in models of fault attribution would represent bad policy or social consequence? Why do I think that neuroscience poses a social threat? In this chapter I respond to these questions. I will very briefly outline the genealogies from philosophy and theology that have informed the contemporary view of the attribution of criminal culpability. I will point to the fact that invariably both Athens and Jerusalem present models that are in conflict with themselves and each other in supporting very different and conflicting representations of philosophical anthropology.

What is the most obvious threat posed by the new neuroscience to criminal jurisprudence? Though many brain research findings have potential for altering legal processes, my concern here is with the potential critique of consciousness and thereby of intent as central to any attribution of criminal fault. The most radical reading of brain research with respect to criminal culpability would negate consciousness and intent as predicate for fault based on agency. If consciousness and the sense of controlled intent within it are posited as not only epiphenomenal but also illusory with respect to prediction and control of social dangerousness, might such a view undermine notions of personal development toward autonomy as an actual possibility?

The ideal of individual autonomy as the endpoint of human potential is socially fashioned and has developed over considerable time to become the model of the self in liberal political culture. It has become a shibboleth in criminal law that attending to how a society deals with its criminals indicates much about the society. Jurisprudential models of attributing fault do not merely mirror social ascriptions but feedback models of human anthropology. Autonomy as a possible state and as a model of aspiration may come under increased attack. Whatever one's philosophic view of human individuality, circumscribing autonomy has political consequences beyond the epistemological, consequences that are perilous for individual *political* freedom. But isn't autonomy so robust an assumption in criminal justice that any neuroscience findings tending to undermine that assumption will be constrained to very specific criminal justice ascriptions (as well as to therapeutic applications)? I think not.

If autonomy as a model is a political idea beyond any philosophic controversy about determinism and compatibilism, it has not always been so. Certainly, Western theology has not always presumed individuals to be autonomous. Philosophy as well assumed that if autonomy was possible it was not necessarily so for everyone. Pre-enlightenment sentiments are still alive within even liberal cultures. Indeed, liberal culture itself is uncomfortable for its own reasons with the myth of autonomy. We may be at a significant conjuncture where politics, law and neuroscience are enlisted into pernicious practices in the public control of deviant behavior.

Minimally, the new brain research may well reinforce tendencies in political modalities of social control adding to present practices of preventive detention. We now separate certain sex offenders from other convicts and hold them, under the guise of treatment, indeterminately. We may well extend this category to violent criminality. The legal concern here has been reflected in significant numbers of academic essays but with little effect. My own experience in Wisconsin and in England suggests that even when honest and intelligent bureaucrats attempt to police politicians who want to extend categories of preventive detention beyond sexual criminals, the line may be difficult to hold. The English recently have considered preventive detention for the criminally violent. We are seeing in the world's culture, both within and external to liberal states, lapses in or redefinitions of the rule of law with respect to political crime, i.e., terrorism. Reduction of criminal disposition to brain structure and function, even if fraudulent, could look antiseptic and therapeutic compared to some of the state sponsored terror that has recently been on the world's radar.

Sexual offenders do not have interest groups or populations of concerned citizens arguing for their cause. We, in fact, care little for most criminals, generally overrepresented by minorities, whom we now warehouse. The competing philosophies of punishment, whether based on retribution, deterrence or recent attempts at fused models are little more than rationalization for practices that ignore theory for the removal of what is seen as criminal waste. Political dissidents have never been socially popular, at least until martyred. So extending preventive detention based on any seemingly predictive diagnostic would be easily rationalized, I fear.

Let me present some personal history. When I started to consider the subject of criminal responsibility as a young law professor in the middle 1960s and the early 1970s, several factors could enter into a sense that agency was flawed and that therefore attribution was unfair. Minority, age, duress, mistake of law or fact and insanity were received terms to understand or negotiate responsibility attribution. But we also contested what was called the ghetto defense. Statistics, as I remember them, pointed to the fact that 18 out of 20 black males in the Watts ghetto of Los Angeles were likely to have a criminal arrest record before the age of 18.

Did these statistics demonstrate a biological propensity of those living in the ghetto toward criminality? Would the brains of these adolescents light up differently from other aggressive criminals? The ghetto defense did not hold up, not because it was somehow wrong, but because it did not conform to the ideology of human autonomy operative at that point in criminal jurisprudence. It would have indicted the culture and excused crime intolerably. Would neuroscience research mitigate or negate culpability for this class of offender, given that the class is still very much a part of social reality? Public defenders and law professors concerned with ghetto criminality were already attacking notions of individual autonomy as a strategy toward reforms in the war on poverty, which as usual was lost. Their efforts were forgotten in the new neo-liberal milieu. The point here is that reformers have reason to critique assumptions about generalizing autonomy to everyone.

In the 1960s law professors were already committed to looking beyond law to related disciplines to understand the problems that the law had to resolve. Sociology, anthropology, linguistics and finally economics were significantly appropriated. Like many legal theorists of my generation who have approached questions of criminal responsibility, I looked to psychoanalysis. Many who work in the criminal law area had to publish on insanity. But we were already approaching insanity as a concept after the cultural integration of psychoanalysis. Freud, of course, taught us that even reason was more often than not the outcome of irrational processes. This story is well known and for many Freud has been repudiated. But whatever one thinks of the psychoanalytic legacy, it left a very definite mark. I can characterize this as presenting a potential conceptual catastrophe for solving the matter of criminal fault.

Most so-called normal people had some irrational core, the prevailing narrative went. Further—and here was the brilliant move—the discerning analyst could reveal an underlying reason in the form of unconscious motivations that prompted even sometimes crazy behaviors and certainly many self-destructive behaviors by what seemed normal actors. Reason itself was relativized and recognized as often in the service of irrational forces. Of course, philosophy and theology each had proponents of this view from the beginning of those disciplines. Arguably psychoanalysis as a cultural feature helped undermine notions of reason and certainly changed the boundaries of what was considered normality and pathology.

Of interest is the fact that psychoanalysis in the United States was presuming to understand and treat criminality even when Freud himself had long since become a therapeutic nihilist. Institutional practice and the practitioners who earn a living from that practice do not change so quickly when the researchers go away or declare bankruptcy. Texts and what counts as knowledge frequently outlast their original context and can readily turn to something very different from the original intent of the author or the theoretical claims. The search for originality in modernity attracts scholars and practitioners to whatever is new and promising. Those who need that base for a living are not always well motivated or even competent. This has certainly been a problem in the introduction of forensic psychiatry in the courtroom. There is no reason to believe that those who become the forensic experts for courtroom neuroscience application will over time be any better than other forensic professionals.

With Freud, most legal commentators have argued that even if motivation was blocked or dynamically unconscious, attribution of criminal culpability would and should be unchanged from folk notions. Freud would in any event be a compatibilist, the position probably most prominent among philosophers of mind arguing that determinism is compatible with generally holding a subject to agency, i.e. morally or criminally responsible. Famously, Freud was concerned that he was looked on as a story teller and not a scientist. His significant public award was, after all, the Goethe prize for literature. Nevertheless, for good and perhaps bad, Freud set the standard for understanding human motivation over the last one hundred years in Western culture.

Freud's position was that we have unconscious psychological motivations that deceive us about their meanings. Where the libertarian Sartre argued for radical human freedom and found bad faith, Freud also famously argued for at least some minimal human capacity for self-transformation. Where id was, ego shall be. Of course, ego was itself partially and necessarily unconscious, but that did not make it any the less capable of controlling the competing forces of lust, aggression etc. or the self-lacerating forces of the too-constricted superego, which represented the internalized demands of culture and law. But the articulated independent variable for criminal blame was predicted for the most part on intent, not on motivation. No doubt trial lawyers played on jury sympathy by stressing motivational reasons for sympathy to the offender. For all his reductionism, Freud posited a mind that had to be considered separately from brain mechanisms.

Still, the issue for criminal culpability rested on finding *conscious* intent, not motive. Psychoanalysis affected everyday discourse by normalizing notions of unconscious intent, even if few could make conceptual sense of what that might mean. But the law itself by definition could conflate intention with motivation. In self-defense, for example, intent is conflated with motivation.

I should mention here that one reason psychoanalysis failed with respect to establishing boundaries for insanity as against agency in criminal jurisprudence is that psychoanalysis could not and did not seek to establish a boundary between the normal and the pathological. My sense is that the insanity defense is designed to draw a line around the most obvious crazy people, thereby affirming the agency of all but those few. Psychoanalysis made that line very difficult to draw. Psychoanalysis as cultural backdrop may also have contributed to underlying cultural assumptions that have generally doubted the hegemonic notion of human agency.

2 The Epiphenomenality of Consciousness and Legal Excusing Conditions

What does it mean to ask whether consciousness is epiphenomenal? If the question implies that all human behavior is reducible to brain and other biological interactions, negating psychology as a human (narcissistic) illusion, then I resist the presupposition. I posit that mind is still a category that is not reducible to brain, but for criminal jurisprudence is and should remain independent in any ascription of blame and consequent punishment or alternative disposition. But whatever I want to think I must acknowledge that legal excusing conditions have been offered, sometimes successfully circumventing insanity and suggesting something other than intention or insanity can mitigate criminal culpability.

We have with diminished responsibility and certain other recent defenses what I would call the operation of the dialectics of sympathy. Diminished responsibility in American criminal jurisprudence presents conceptual problems that may be logically irresolvable because the concept lacks logical coherence within itself. I understand the concept as a safety valve, i.e., a concept based on inchoate sentiments of justice that allows the jury or judge absent the jury to escape either/or determinants and grade a particular behavior somewhat less than the definition of the proscribed act would seem to dictate. We favor some for attributes or conditions surrounding the proscribed behaviors which would generally fall within the general proscription. The continued cultural distaste with which the insanity defense as escape concept has met from *McNaughton* on has prompted lawyers necessarily and sometimes successfully to create new excusing categories.

Recent history in the criminal jurisprudence of the United States has witnessed a proliferation of disorders and syndromes which seem almost to have been designed for the legal purpose of reducing criminal liability. Post traumatic stress disorder, which has significant biological markers and other clinical indicia is one prominent such entity. Battered women's syndrome itself an example of the more general post traumatic stress disorder has been offered in homicide cases to mitigate a wife's killing of her abusing husband. The cultural conditions for sympathy are not always so easy to adduce, nor are the conceptual boundaries for ascription of reduced fault or excuse always so clear. Less successful attempts have been made to mitigate or excuse criminal behavior because it is *caused* by post partum depression, post menstrual stress, gambling addiction, etc.

Biological correlates with the mitigating or excusing state are most likely present but not necessarily sufficiently distinctive to differentiate biological cause with human reason—the preferred category for criminal jurisprudence. The law in practice does not develop with logical consistency. Over 100 years ago Holmes admonished us that experience invariably trumped logic in the legal process. History defeats logic in his formulation. A question remains: to what extent are legal processes amenable to alteration through reasoned discourse and what constitutes adequate reason? I know of no historian or political philosopher who can more than speculate on historical and cultural tendencies.

3   Classical Philosophy and Responsibility: The Greeks Christianized R (Like) Us?

Western philosophy and theology have provided both conceptual means for rationalizing the ascription of responsibility and the background for understanding differing notions of human anthropology. The various genealogies that have been shaped by theology and philosophy are not always consistent or coherent. The influences of the respective, sometimes fragmented traditions are speculative and not readily readable. Moreover, I am reading this history as a law professor. This means I am reading even the fragments that I am adducing here with a policy goal in mind.

The changing Western narrative on responsibility is one place where genealogy does makes sense. I here suggest several lines of thought that should be considered in understanding the potential implications of the new brain research for jurisprudence and more particularly criminal jurisprudence. Specifically, I want to draw attention to the influences that Western theology and philosophy have had, and may continue to assert, even if perversely.

Philosophical Notions of Responsibility

The philosophers (Athens) contributed concepts and models of personhood, and human agency. They considered such issues as the constitution of character, the definition of the passions and their place with respect to rationality and the nature of control, including the voluntary and involuntary aspects of human potential. This might be called philosophy of mind. A central premise from both Athens and Jerusalem is that punishment should be constrained to fault and fault required agency. Philosophically, retribution was not merely vengeance dressed up, or at least so it can be argued. Punishment also was a state institution that had to clarify social obligation and reflect back certain measures for actual everyday possible conformity. Punishment and its relationship to agency marks the political influence.

Philosophy of mind, political philosophy of state and law, and philosophical anthropology are for both Athens and Jerusalem of a piece. Our science, philosophy, and religion are not integrated into a social whole. This disciplinary division has the power of division of labor but it also makes the relative responsibility of the uses for knowledge problematic. This factor or tendency has to do with the view of human potential, in higher blown Monty Python terms the meaning of life, the likelihood of human achievement. I am speculating that under enlightenment notions of rationality and human agency lies another tradition, one that in the Middle Ages may have been called demonic. We do not name this underlying misanthropic, anti rational tendency to war, greed, and self-righteousness. Let's just call it social psychology.

So we must consider the individual, the institutions of governance implied in punishment or some other social control mechanism like preventive detention and the more speculative question of what the answer to ascription and disposition means to general social understanding. A further simple point should be made, and it is one that examining Athens and Jerusalem makes clear. Philosophy and the theologies of revelation set high standards for the constituent cultures affirmed generally in lip service only. The same is true for us. All the theorizing about the person, mind and brain, the social self and the autonomous self, the nature of retributive theory as opposed to deterrence theory means little in the face of punishment practice in the United States where warehousing and the death penalty are general practice in the face of science and philosophy that would determine significantly different practices.

The Greeks contributed criteria for conceptual intelligibility. But they also recognized and depicted a deeply tragic view of human limitation even before the philosophers altered the Greek worldview. As much as Greek philosophy attempted to transplant the tragedy of the poets with the clarity and fearlessness of the conceptually crisp, tragic poetry did not leave the scene.

Aristotle, though reasonably optimistic about the reach of reason, ordered his version of the mind by asserting more complexity without surprisingly, adding more coherence. He emphasized the continual strife that the psyche had to deal with in ordering various passions and needs to reach any sense of harmony. But even the parts of mind that were allegedly governed by reason were potentially open to the irrational. A. W. Price points out that Aristotle emphasized conflict as central to intra psychic life. A weak individual could want something and know it was not good, deliberate and still pursue it. Another because of passion might fail to recognize or deliberate at all:

I believe that his very notion of practical judgment contains an irresoluble tension: judgment that involves all-in evaluation must be intimately related to the totality of an agent's desires; and yet, if it is to be judgment, it must achieve a reflective distance from them that frees it from dependence upon their fluctuating intensities. Practicality cannot, without equivocation, be at once a feature of the *content* of practical judgment, and a matter of its *effect*. . . . Aristotle is a philosopher of common sense who unfailingly leads us into intellectual territory where common sense is no longer a competent guide. (Price 1995)

Contemporary criminal jurisprudence generally requires little in the form of deliberation to establish even specific intent in those crimes that provide a specific intent element. The very model of deliberation that Aristotle offers as exemplary marks little of what most people do even with respect to major decisions. Most of us read deliberation into any action that seems purposive or otherwise intelligible. Price is right that Aristotle's theory of the working of the conditions and working of deliberation and self-reflection remains obscure. But it also remains a model for human aspiration.

The philosophers contested the tragic view of the poets and raised expectations about the purposeful nature of existence and about human reason to tame the irrational toward the achievement of the good. So they talk in terms of mechanism, for example when Aristotle theorizes about what moves the psyche in mechanistic terms and then talks in more phenomenological language about the conditions of practical deliberation for right human action.

But while I call Aristotle's causal language in *De Anima* to account for the movement of psyche to action mechanistic, the time frame that Jonathan Israel (2001) calls the "crisis of the European mind" saw as insufficiently scientific, i.e., not mechanistic enough to fit the new Cartesian worldview. Aristotle was ultimately appropriated by the Christian cultural settlement into a rationalized scholasticism that provided sufficient cultural connectivity to ensure hierarchical stability for church and state. Progress, itself an ideological term, is not linear. Aristotle's science became dogma, as can the complex thought of any great thinker. Any mode of thinking can become anathema or perversion to its original impulse.

Characteristic ingredients of this common Aristotelian legacy included the idea that all knowledge comes initially from the senses, and that the human mind—as Locke concurred later, in opposition to Descartes—is first a "tabula rasa," and the key notion that all things are constituted of matter and form, the later emanating from the soul or essence of things so that bodies and souls cannot be separate entities in themselves, a concept resulting in the celebrated doctrine of substantial forms. This concept of innate propensities in turn shaped scientific procedures by giving priority to classifying things according to their "qualities" and then explaining the specific responses and characteristics of individual things in terms of primary group properties. Behavior and function consequently arise, and are determined by, the soul or essence of things rather than mechanistically. Hence there is conceptual but no observable or measurable dividing line between the "natural" and the "supernatural," a distinction which could only be clearly made following the rise of the mechanistic world-view.

The philosophers set the standards of rationality for blame and the conditions for punishment that would mitigate or excuse an actor's agency. They grappled with the same kind of problems we have. How to assess will, control, choice, volition, etc? Their solutions are still with us (along with those of theology). But as said it is by no means clear that they worked out the problems they bequeathed to us any more than have we. Further we have not always been so clear about what they did claim. From what I can determine, we still have not sorted out the proper translations of Aristotelian conditions of fault attribution (Zaibert 2003). Notably, we may confuse intent and the unintentional with Aristotle's use of volition and non-volition. Intent as intent is likely not an Aristotelian category. Confusion may be the result of translation but it may also be that Aristotle himself did not resolve the structure and nature of mind and its relationship to biology. Kyron Huigens (2003) argues that Aristotle had no concept of intent, rather one of character. Huigens argues that the way out of the old philosophic tension between retributive and deterrence theories of punishment is to recognize that the place that intent takes in punishment theory for modernity had been within notions of (bad) character and that at least in an implicit sense we still make ascriptions of fault on character and not intent. His resolution is worthy but there are classic cases where we create rules of evidence and institutional procedures to in fact negate the very human predilection to ascribe fault to character and not intent. So we no longer allow jurors to serve if they know an alleged offender, exactly for fear that character will be the prevailing factor and not whatever the particular mens rea required by the definition of the charge. Further, defense lawyers are often at pains to admit the defendant is a generally bad person but did not intend the act in the particular case.

However, in one sense I do not think that the conceptualization of criminal fault has changed much since Aristotle codified his understanding of moral development in the Nicomachean Ethics. Richard Sorabji (1992) warns we must be aware of the intentional and mistaken misreading of predicate philosophers as we discover them in us. Sorabji argues that Brentano found intentionality as an Aristotelian concept, but to get to this interpretation he proceeded through "a long history of distortions" encompassing medieval and early Western philosophy. With this caution and with the understanding that intention differs from intentionality—the consciousness of something in Brentano's formulation, Aristotle's philosophy still seems to fit folk common sense. He seemingly gave us the notion that a person could reflect, deliberate, weigh alternatives and based on empirical assessments he could then make refined prudent judgments.

Now this model was generally for the educated aristocrat. But it is a persuasive model and one that ultimately yields notions like the autonomy of the self as refracted through the democratizing elements of the radical enlightenment. But this posit of human potential carried with a notion of educating citizens and education presupposed the development habit and more importantly of character. So volition could be learned, character formed and virtuous action intended. Thomas Aquinas, in common with Aristotle and Maimonides, inter alia, held that (Christian) virtue could only result from God's grace and not habit and the character that would express it.

Both the Greeks and the Hebrews stressed moral development and individual responsibility. In *The Republic*, Plato even instructed that children should be removed from parents to socialize them into appropriate social roles. Character and not intent is the central posit here, both for the individual to develop the possibility of living a virtuous life and for the culture to provide the structures to foster that possibility. The (idealized) state was to shape the structures for education and thereby the conditions for virtuous action on the part of the citizenry. Law, that is, was a tool of social engineering from the very outset but one in the service of a harmonious virtuous reality beyond individual greed or desire.

Whatever variant of liberal state theory one offers, the pluralism at the heart of liberalism makes such a dependence on law as a moralizing structure antithetical. It is clear that liberalism, however, is currently contested by those who would conjoin classic philosophic notions of law as necessary power for cultural character building with their very different value base. I do not think we have to stress the fact that generally through human history philosophers have not prevailed. Plato had to write his Laws as second best given the impossibility of instantiating his Republic. Notoriously Socrates was forced to eat hemlock for his crimes of blasphemy and corrupting the morals of minors. (Would a scan of his brain shown much in common with the brain of a contemporary child molester?) The Greek high culture lasted only a short time and its Hellenized versions diverged, particularly in Rome, from any the practical possibility of the citizen in a non-corrupt legal order.

Theological Notions of Responsibility and Free Will

The theological move against tragedy is, perhaps, even more bleak. The sense from the Hebrew (Jerusalem) is that humanity is created from dust and will return to it, and that all human aspiration is grounded on unavailing narcissism (including the writing of books, no less essays). The same tradition, of course, warranted that we are made in the image of God. It also promises the possibility of salvation, though generally only for believers. It might seem then, that we are like unto both God and dust. But if we could aspire to God, the aspiration is shown to have had limited historical actuality. Hebraic prophecy, a high point of revealed ethical demand, was invariably predicated on idolatry and greed of the people of Israel, and thus perhaps chose to highlight the iniquitous turn of humanity's nature.

What do we make of the conflicting revelations? Perhaps ironically, the tendency derived from Christian theology against the rational nature of human existence and against rationality itself could turn that theology on its head. The Hebrews did allow that living according to Torah would warrant a life. But the exemplary Biblical cases, notably prophecy, as stated, demonstrate the incapacity of the people to adhere to the basic standards of decency circumscribed by revealed law. The Christian moment, of course, promised salvation but it undercut the direction to achieve that state by will or act. (This account simplifies the theological struggles, e.g. between St. Augustine and Pelagius.) Christian theology also undercut the power that the philosophers accorded reason.

This dark side of the human soul bequeathed to us as an aspect of our Christian legacy, allied with the dark aspects of Jewish and Greek influences may play out by reinforcing any tendencies negating individual optimism about the nature of moral control. We then have two competing tendencies in the backdrop of Western metaphysics—one that emphasizes the agon or struggle of the human soul over the transgressive and irrational (not necessarily the same things) and another that also demands struggle but affirms that only God, an outside force, can bring grace.

The common aspect I want to emphasize from these various influences that underlie Western philosophic anthropology is the sense of conflict and struggle immanent in the individual and species being. The sense of conflict and struggle, I maintain, makes sense only at the level of an inchoate consciousness, whatever the operation of the brain. This sense of effort and conflict is deeper than the particular intention in any given case—it propels the self toward any integrity, in the sense of wholeness it may conceivably achieve. (It may be characterized as losing as often as winning in the struggle toward a wholeness that may be achievable only momentarily and contingently.) Again Western history certainly, in its theology at least, has always provided an underlying rebuke to individual agency. "The Devil made me do it" has not always been a joke. Christian theology has had a current of anti-rational implication.

Of course, we have to be careful when we ascribe any uncontested set of claims on any of the Western versions of theology. Christianity within Catholicism has its own traditions and conflicts of interpretation. The history leading to the Reformation and the wars in religion's name subsequent to the constituting of the various Protestant confessions makes clear competing notions of Christianity itself. Each version needs explication for its respective position on determinism, choice, responsibility and freedom. No less is the case with Judaism. As fraught as the contemporary question "Who is a Jew?" may be, the history of Jewish thought is itself the subject of tension, struggle, debate and controversy. So any general statement about what Christianity holds, or what Judaism holds, is bound to be problematic. That being said, I will now say that Judaism is philosophically committed to a position of free will.

But what is the position of God in relationship to this posited freedom? Harry Wolfson (1979) claims that all the philosophers of scripture up to and including the Arabic philosophic period, including the Hellenic Jewish philosopher Philo, the Church fathers and all the leading Islamic philosophers, posited that the capacity for human free choice was a God given gift. Affirming the claim that Jewish philosophers held freedom to be a central attribute, Lenn Goodman (1987) argues that Maimonides as well as Aristotle and Spinoza are nevertheless compatibilists. For each, Goodman argues, determinism is central, but human action and character are also self-determining and not merely externally controlled.

What is the rabbinic position on the question of intention if freedom is assumed to be a central value and capacity? How does intention relate to the compatibilism that Goodman posits of Maimonides, who in this sense is in accord with Aristotle and the rabbis? Two concepts are of significance: intention and yeser. The first is what we mean by intention, assuming that we do mean something beyond the firing or arousal of brain mechanism. The second concept is less well known and goes to a claim about tendencies or desires good and evil that motivate the humanity from birth and likely for most to death. Each is immanent in the originary narrative of the exile from Eden, which has dominated Western theology.

The Hebrew Bible has been and continues to be influential, perhaps even more influential than it has been in recent years. The first story, indeed, the original story concerning human creation and anthropology is the story of Eden and the fall from grace in Christian thought or the fall from truth in the thought of Maimonides, the most eminent Jewish medieval thinker. The relationship of humanity to God, of man to woman, of faith and law to desire, of harmony to strife, of the limits of reason for happiness are all folded within the tale of Adam, Eve, the Serpent, and God. Western theologians never exhaust the meanings encapsulated within the story not only because of its originary pedigree but because each generation rightfully appropriates the story for its own cultural needs.

Why does Eve allow the Serpent to seduce her? Why does the Serpent feel the need to do so? Why does Adam so readily allow himself to also comply against God's mandate? What are the differences in punishment that God meets out for the respective transgression by each of the sinning parties? Jewish and Christian thought draw endlessly on elaborating the issues and the consequences of this first human exile. The hermeneutic responses to the story of the fall are at the core of the questions that I am touching on here. They involve the question of God and limit terms, the nature of crime and obnoxious behavior, the limits on desire by self-control, the nature of knowledge, the plasticity of consciousness, the function and nature of punishment, inter alia. The noted Judaica scholar Jacob Neusner (1991) argues that the Serpent because of deliberate, conscious intention is sanctioned by God more severely than either Adam or Eve, each of whom is effectively duped and so punished in a lesser degree. Maimonides, in *The Guide of the Perplexed*, comments that the loss of Eden represented the loss of humanity's capacity, without struggle, to differentiate truth from falsity, and to confuse truth with good and evil, categories unnecessary in the harmony of the garden. So the Serpent, the story goes, must from that point slither and presumably no longer speaks. But on some reckonings humanity lost even more—it lost its instinctual grounding and its tranquility in a hospitable world. The question of severity of punishment is not so clear. From Kant to Gilbert and Sullivan it is easy to talk about the punishment fitting the crime.

Neusner (1991), while analyzing various dimensions of the notion of responsibility and the nature of political theory, also holds that rabbinic Judaism posited free will and attributed responsibility and punishment based to some degree on an assessment of degree of deliberation and intention. He goes so far as to claim that intention even beyond action is central to human fault in rabbinic thought. He attributes the reasons for this position to be the rabbinic theological need to tie human action into relationship to God's commands and to rest all politics and corporate responsibility (of the Jewish people) to what the people have done and might do.

The link between the social order of holy Israel and the cosmic order in Heaven is forged in the shared if ineffable bonds linking God and humanity, the fragile yet firm web of plans, intentions, and attitudes. That accounts, as I just said, for the, to us egregious responsibility that the politics undertakes for not only what people have done but also what they might do, that is, for what their present intentions and plans signal that they are going to do. Why do we kill the potential sinner or criminal before he or she does anything at all? Because the determinant is attitude, which governs all else. And the attitude (it is assumed) now has come to ample demonstration, even though commensurate actions have yet to take place. That that intangible future also forms the object of political sanction-kill him first, before he does anything-we now realize forms the critical indicator of that which the politics bears responsibility. And, I am inclined to think, the individual's attitude, not that of society, is at stake: society cannot form an improper affective intention, only an individual can.

In fact, rabbinic distinctions concerning intention and the attribution of fault for some degree of conscious negligence seem remarkably or perhaps not so remarkably similar to common law development. The concept of yeser is perhaps structurally more basic than even intent to rabbinic thought. Intent must be formed out of the forces that constitute human agency. Yeser are constitutive forces. The rabbis talk of good yeser and evil or bad yeser. So what is yeser? Boyarin (1993) and Schofer (2003) argue that yeser is for rabbinics a given tendency—either one impulse for some rabbis, or two, struggling between good and evil. In some cases bad yeser may have good results, warranting reproduction and sexual satisfaction when properly channeled. But though Boyarin and Schofer find subtlety and the possibility of self-realization in the individual's struggle with yeser some commentators in the tradition have much less optimism for its place in human anthropology. Davidson (2005), in his recent biography of Maimonides, quotes the commentator Jabez:

The "evil inclination . . . loves the commission of sins and despises the negative commandments," and in the same way, "the human intellect . . . loves intellectual thoughts, . . . and despises the true opinions of the Torah, resurrection, and the Great Judgment Day, all of which stand in opposition to intellectual syllogism."

Further, following Kierkegaard and the ordinary man who traveled with the attractive woman without attempting to seduce her or being seduced by her, it would seem that only moral luck (Aristotle), the analogue of the knight of faith (grace), or conscious intellectual struggle will transform the individual, enabling the proper path. And that conscious effort may be inconsequential. Yeser then, like notions of character, intent, rationality and its weakness, vary through the Western history of ideas. There is no warrant that history is or will be progressive.

4 From Intent to Social Danger: Current Trajectory

Intention has been long considered a necessary element for the finding of criminal fault for Western morality and law. But intention is only a marker for a mental or psychological element for moral or criminal fault. Intention should not and cannot be equated with the philosophical notion of intentionality, famously figured by Franz Brentano. The intentional element in criminal jurisprudence differs from what might be generally labeled intention. The intention that constitutes an element of a crime may be an omission, that is, the non-doing of some act that the law demands as duty. Some societies demand a duty to rescue a person at risk if no danger exists for the likely rescuer. Others place no duty on the Samaritan. In any event the question of attribution is cultural, and contested.

The question of whether or not to find criminal fault and attach blame for some degree of unintentional negligence has attracted a good deal of theoretical attention, but suffice it to say that some degree of recklessness has been ultimately enough to provide the necessary mental element for criminal culpability. We also have attached criminal sanctions to corporations beyond the ascription to a particular human being. And there are examples of strict liability in tort law and arguably in criminal practice as well. The point is that intention in this usage is a construct or place holder for a presumption that some undefined awareness should generally exist before the ascription of blame. Intention draws on an intuition of human freedom and agency. We may be cynical or skeptical and claim that the law here rests on notions of soft determinism, i.e., a myth of freedom that the cognoscenti have generally known, at least with respect to others, to be a fiction.

Intention is a marker for a presumed or attributed psychological state. Anglo-American criminal jurisprudence has long insisted on both the finding of both mens rea and actus reus for legitimate ascription of criminal culpability. Actus reus, i.e., the behavioral element of the crime, already has a definitional consequence of finding an action not a behavior. An action for law as for philosophy presumes an actor, one who purposely affected a result in the world—in short an agent.

Let me give a recent and contentious example of definitional reach from recent conceptual politics where a strong case put forward from feminist jurisprudence has altered criminal attribution. The jurisprudence concerning the judgment of the occurrence of rape has gone through various stages in the last generation. Rape had been defined as the forcible, non-consensual vaginal penetration by the penis. But there have been text book cases that clearly indicate that the alleged rapist never realized he did not have such consent or he would not have proceeded. From the woman's experience, she was indeed sexually taken against her will. This is rape, or not, based on cultural and legal definitions, not on the real world consciousness of the alleged perpetrator. Nor do I think that knowledge of the alleged violator's brain state would be of significant help, in this case at least, to make an attribution of blame.

The issue goes to the just balance between potential offender and victim concerning what was actually known or should have been known. A way to lessen the problem is to calibrate the nature of punishment. But can we talk about fair punishment if the offender did not intend rape but did rape by the new formulation? Alternatively is it fair to a victim to tell her she was not raped when she knows she was? The question must be extended-fair for whom? The recent balance has been to recognize the victim's experience as central to the crime.

So what is intention and how does the fact finder ascertain intention? Also should we hold someone criminally liable in the absence of intention even if the offender is negligent to some significant degree? What would that degree be? Further can we legitimately hold someone liable for consequences that are socially dangerous though they were unintended and not negligent? This presents the problem of creating conditions of strict liability and holding someone responsible criminally though they lacked any element of consciousness or fault except the fortuity of initiating a sequence of events that resulted in chargeable social danger. Perhaps equally importantly, do we wish to keep a mental element central to the question of attribution of fault?

My caution is that, despite a robust challenge by jurisprudential commentators who seek to preserve notions of agency the conditions for altering the paradigm of fault attribution, mass society tends away from intention and toward some notion of social insurance and protection against harm, irrespective of the state of mind of the dangerous or objectionable actor. Versions of attribution of fault derived by some commentators now or in the near future may well tip the balance toward mechanisms that rely on indicators other than ascription based on an assessment of the consciousness or as part of that consciousness- the intention of the other.

Philosophically sophisticated analysis has also been advanced to undercut or at least reframe the relationship of that aspect of criminality that we call evil. Hannah Arendt talked about the banality of evil in her controversial analysis of the Eichmann case (Arendt 1963). Arendt was not letting Eichmann off the hook, but she was saying that he was no different from many if not most bureaucrats. The social structure itself can generate evil effects, which in and because of aggregate behaviors have great reach and are well beyond any individual intention. Susan

Neiman (2002), following Arendt, has argued we can no longer place intent as a central category for assessing and ascribing evil to human action.

Where certain medieval and perhaps even contemporary actors blamed the Devil for criminal transgression, some scientists have sought to discover some universal for at least some criminal tendency in individual biology. Phrenologists saw skull formation as indicative of potential criminal tendency. For a while, body type figured into criminological theory. Genetics, notably the xyy chromosomal pattern became associated with a high potential toward violent, potentially criminal behavior.

We have also traversed a social space where scientists and policy makers have had great faith in expertise that could humanely deal with criminal offenders predicate on questions of social dangerousness and not individual intent. Even after public faith in scientific expertise has waned in the criminal justice arena, schemes that would look just at behavior and not intent for social control purposes have been and are very much still a part of our policy armamentarium. So there are competing tendencies in reformulating the jurisprudence of criminal responsibility. One tendency is to focus on assessing dangerousness of the offender and not the intent. Questions of volition, consciousness and ascription of other mental attributes become of little relevance. The question then becomes both epistemological and political. Can social science or biology or more particularly neuroscience provide the criteria to both discover the criminally dangerousness on the one hand and then provide appropriate means of disposition on the other? But an equally significant question is, even if social science or cognitive science, or even ultimately neuroscience can provide concepts to reshape the control of public deviant behavior, would this make for good policy and politics?

The other tendency besides a move toward making intent epiphenomenal or in fact irrelevant is to use social science, psychiatry and now neuroscience to understand offense and perhaps mitigate punishment as *caused* by brain function and not intent. We are then dealing with a causal model and not attempting to discern reason. The distinction is between intent and motivation. But here motivation may be expunged as well in the name of an independent biological variable.

5   Libet and the Potential Paradoxical Assault on Notions of Moral and Legal Consciousness

Benjamin Libet has designed some of the most impressive empirical work we have on brain functioning and its possible relationship to intent and consciousness. In his career he has worked with some of the most influential neurosurgeons, experimentalists and philosophers concerned with mind/body relationships. He is a neuroscientist who has maintained a view that mind cannot be readily collapsed into the brain. So he has remained committed to a notion that individuals can make choices that are differentiable from the operations of brain mechanics. He argues against attempts to identify mind and brain philosophically. He is in fact about as libertarian as a neuroscientist might be. Yet arguably it is his work that might most effectively refute the status of consciousness and more particularly intention as having anything but contingent relationship to brain functioning.

Libet's work is instructional for the question of the potential or even likely possible applications of any neural science work that posits the epiphenomenality of consciousness. The work is important for two reasons. The empirical findings support arguments about consciousness as merely a reflection on and after behavior. Daniel Wegner (2000) argues that this and other work must be understood to mean that intentions are not causal and conscious will illusory. But the work is significant for another reason, beyond its merit as cutting edge neuroscientific research. This concerns not the truth or accuracy of Libet's work or his interpretation of it, but the appropriation of his work by academic lawyers, policy makers and politicians. The question of influence may be as important as the empirical experiments.

Let me turn to some implications of work like Libet's in respect to legal application. Below I reproduce a question that was posed in December 2004 in the final exam given to students in Professor Walter Dickey's Criminal Law course at the University of Wisconsin Law School. Dickey has been an influential contributor to criminal jurisprudence. He interrupted his scholarly work and ran the Wisconsin Department of Corrections for several years. The question is not a speculative flight into theory but a concern that the problem presented is current. Where the concern in this volume is with the causal capacity of consciousness to affect behavior, law assumes such capacity as a matter of folk psychology. In reality law has worked through some of the possible contentious issues that might nullify consciousness as only an observing mechanism. The problem is one of disciplinary misreading. Where this volume is concerned with a confined issue, lawyers, politicians and policy makers could well read misread beyond it intellectual concerns and use neuroscience to reinforce tendencies that already exist to undercut notions of autonomy and advance institutional control mechanisms beyond what neuroscientist contemplate and philosophers think wise.

Here is Professor Dickey's question:

Dr. John is a distinguished scientist at the University of Grace Medical School. His specialty is the brain and he has done years of work on brain imaging. Brain imaging requires the use of computer imaging to see which parts of the brain are activated and when they are activated in relation to various activities. So for example, Dr. John is able to identify when patients are experiencing various emotions, such as grief and fear because particular locations of the brain have been found to "light up" when these emotions are experienced. Indeed, Dr. John has testified in criminal cases as to whether certain situations and activities elicited fear in defendants by duplicating the situations and taking a brain image.

Lately Dr. John has been conducting experiments in which he has plotted timelines reflecting the temporal relationship between the experience of thoughts and feelings, and the subject acting on them. He has developed a substantial body of laboratory and clinical evidence that violent actions often come before the thoughts and emotions which are commonly believed to give rise to violent acts.

Dick has been charged with First Degree Intentional Homicide in violation of 940.01 He killed Vic in a fight in a bar, but claims that Vic broke a bottle and was coming at him with the intention of slashing him with it. Vic was heard by witnesses to say "You're dead meat" before attacking Dick. Dick has pled not guilty and not guilty by reason of mental disease or defect, under 971.15. You are an assistant District Attorney.

The defense lawyer for Dick has indicated that he intends to call Dr. John as a witness. Dr. John will testify that he has conducted extensive brain imaging of Dick and has concluded that, like all people on which he has conducted brain imaging, Dick acts reflexively before experiencing the thoughts or feelings that he (Dick) believes cause him to act. The lawyer says this will show conclusively that his client did not intend to kill. Dr. John will testify further that his research shows that free will is a myth. "My experiments prove we often don't think before we act. It's the other way around," is how the defense lawyer has paraphrased Dr. John. Your boss has asked you to write a memo explaining whether the evidence of Dr. John's testimony is admissible in this criminal case.

Let's assume that the expert testimony is at least partially admissible. The conclusion about free will as myth is certainly problematic, but attempts by appellate courts to constrain experts to "facts" and not conclusions frequently fail. Certainly one way to safeguard the law from any challenge about its assumptions of agency in ordinary cases would be to limit expert testimony. Stephen Morse has spent a significant part of his career marshalling arguments to protect robust legal commitments to the person as agent. He recently responded to the presumed critique of agency from neuroscience in an essay commissioned by the American Association for the Advancement of Science (Morse 2004). Morse significantly relied on Libet's empirical work as setting the conditions for any legal challenge to notions of agency in criminal jurisprudence. Lauding Libet's "exceptionally creative and careful studies," he concludes: "I do not think that they imply, however, that conscious intentionality does no causal work. They simply demonstrate that nonconscious brain events precede conscious experience, but this seems what one would expect of the mind-brain. It does not mean that people can 'veto' the act, which is another form of mental act that plays a causal role." He also argued that attempts to reduce mind and its reasoning processes to brain mechanism were unlikely to diminish the status of agency in criminal jurisprudence.

I know Professor Morse and I generally agree with him on most issues concerning the attribution of legal responsibility. Morse uses words carefully. Here he talks of "mind-brain" and of "intentionality." "Mind-brain" and "intentionality" may not resolve the question put in Dickey's hypothetical. Dick, the defendant, may have a self-defense plea. He may be able to mitigate to something less than what is called in many jurisdictions first degree murder, to a lesser charge of unlawful homicide under several potential theories, depending on the jurisdiction. Manslaughter based on heat of passion and manslaughter based on an unreasonable mistaken response to the alleged attack are possible, but the heat-of-passion defense is unlikely.

What does the definition of intentional homicide require? I have already stated that in most jurisdictions, intent for mens rea can be formed instantaneously. The law is already sensitive to the difference between conscious intent and intentionality. If the criminal element for intentional unexcused homicide is predicated on conscious intent, and if the expert testimony comes in, and if the jury believes the expert that behavior precedes intent in this case, it would seem that there was no intent and therefore no crime. Why an insanity plea might be used is unclear except, unlike Wisconsin, in a capital sanction case. A defendant can be committed on a finding of insanity, and he is likely to be so, and to serve as long or longer time than for a criminal conviction, in a place that is a prison even if called a hospital. But the facts do not show what I think is definitionally required in most states for the successful use of the defense. What can we make of real but inexcusable rage based on threat or a challenge to manhood or just testosterone madness?. There is a significant body of law that makes it clear that uncontrollable rage may in the right case mitigate (as will self-defense) but will not excuse. Criminal jurisprudence cares little for rage even if it can be shown that it precludes the formation of intent.

Morse talks in terms of intentionality and if the mental element for conviction implies intentionality as the standard, the prosecution may face little problem in terms of supporting a burden of conscious intention. Intentionality by all means can be implied in any purposeful behavior. The root of intentionality is full bodied in the sense that it implies directed, purposeful action. If this is what the law requires then in this case and perhaps generally neuroscience poses little new for law. In fact, some commentators think that this is the way the law operates. But if the state must show conscious intent and the expert testimony is admitted and the jury buys the expert, then the state has a problem.

There are several solutions:

• The definition of criminal responsibility could be altered to read that conscious intention is not required for fault; only purposive action—intentionality and not intention.

• The law could turn to character rather than specific, conscious intent as the defining characteristic in criminal attribution. I have no doubt that this happens in sub rosa ways already. But for good reasons the law protects against character as defining responsibility in any particular case. We do not want people on the jury who know the defendant, for fear of prejudice. Propensity or even past behavior may be deadly wrong in terms of attributing fault in a specific case.

• The law could give up on requiring proof concerning consciousness at all. It can demand proof of behavior and then determine appropriate disposition if the sanctioned behavior is proved. But this is not a solid solution because it undercuts folk understanding on the one hand and does not resolve certain cases where the question of crime is not the behavior but the underlying motivation. Such a policy shift could result in disposition placed in the hands of experts (read bureaucrats). In the hypothetical case did Dick defend himself or not? Was his rage justified or excusable under the circumstances?

I have not discussed the place of affect with respect to consciousness and intention. Guilt is the elephant in the room. Legal guilt is a social attribution. The actor may experience the feeling of guilt and the law may find that feeling misplaced, neurotic. Or the actor may experience existential guilt, not misplaced. Such feelings, just like rage, are conscious and may determine future response and may be significant for the affirming meaning in the world. Sterilizing the law of the guilt problematic in the name of efficiency or as a matter of reform to mitigate vengeance undercuts representations of autonomy culturally and perhaps also elides some aspect of the self that is morally real and not mere social construction.

6   Notes toward a Conclusion

Anthony Kronman (1993) has lamented the loss of Aristotelian prudence in either law teaching or in legal research. He asserts that economics has gained hegemony in legal discourse. He means that legal academics think in institutions and complex structures and not individual case by case analysis. Policy suggestions that come from such structural thinking may well involve paradigmatic shift. Kronman echoes Frederick van Friedrich Hayek, who earlier in the twentieth century also warned of the dangers consequent to massive political shift through broad legislation, which given complexity will invariably result in perverse effects. Hayek's "road to serfdom" argument must have been unsettling as well as overwrought for those looking to social change through legislative sweep.

Whatever one thinks of the Hayek or Kronman position I think that it does point to the possibility of paradigm shift more sweeping and radical in any area of social contest than is generally felt possible. Neuroscience research is accompanied with great fanfare in the popular media. It can help the blind to see. I can help us determine if people are lying. It can help differentiate the truly traumatized from malingers—and on and on. The truth for each of these claims is problematic but if the public is dramatically reinforced of the correctness of any of these claims it may well support uses beyond the knowledge base. The first generation of scientific researchers who adduce powerful results are not the people who generally apply those results over the long haul. The institutional rationalization of neuroscience into policy can produce the kind of banality of perverse affects that concern Arendt and Neiman. Even should these people be attentive to the possibilities of abuse of so potentially powerful knowledge, it will be difficult to marshal policy that advances human concerns and is not captured for social control purposes that undermine fragile models of autonomy and dignity.

The Greeks had their dark side, and bad yeser can be appropriated in the discourse of any day as pointing to the irrational, dangerous, and impulsive elements in the anthropology of the species. The Manichean heresy is not well understood today, but I conjecture that Aristotelian prudence is not ascendant in the world, that character is not formed in liberal polities to express virtue, Jewish, Christian, or Greek, and that monotheism has not won the day. I fear that in their recesses, in their synapses if you will, people secretly believe that evil is as powerful as good and that the universe is of the battleground for the struggle of these elemental forces. The best of neuroscientists enjoy the kind of consciousness that Spinoza suggested possible by understanding that the world was constituted by one substance and that substance is called God. Freedom then famously is the joy of understanding and therefore accepting necessity. For most of us, if we refuse the Manichean subversive sentiment, we find only bleak and sterile mechanics. If we are only synapses and sinew programmed in evolutionary logic, why not remove those with propensities toward criminal offense? Of course, the old point always must be raised: who will police such action?

The problem is one of interdisciplinary misreading. While this volume is concerned with a refined issue concerning the current status of consciousness and its relationship to brain mechanism and most see no problem with neuroscience's undercutting notions of individual autonomy, I do not think this is how politicians and policy makers will view this research. During the struggles of the enlightenment, from Descartes through Spinoza and into Leibniz, Wolf, Newton, and Locke, intellectuals were cautious for fear of state or church animus. Much could be said, as long as it was not broadcast. I am not calling for self-censorship here. I am merely cautioning that as with innumeracy, even smart people will confound neuroscience beyond its empirical base.

Acknowledgments

A special thank you to Pam Hollenhorst, Assistant Director of the Institute for Legal Studies. I must also thank Walter Dickey, my colleague at the law school and Guy Lord, my friend and a child psychiatrist each of whom read an earlier draft of this chapter. Laurence Tancredi and Michael Stone each provided me with citations to recent neuroscientific literature for which I am indebted. Susan Pockett deserves my thanks for forcing me toward greater clarity and protecting me from glaring error, any editor can do no more. Thank you as well to Michael Morgalla and Genevieve Zook of the University law Library who as usual provided responsive service.

References

Arendt, H. 1963. *Eichmann in Jerusalem: A Report on the Banality of Evil*. Viking.

Boyarin, D. 1993. *Carnal Israel: Reading Sex in Talmudic Culture*. University of California Press.

Davidson, H. A. 2005. *Moses Maimonides: The Man and His Works*. Oxford University Press.

Goodman, L. E. 1987. Determinism and freedom in Spinoza, Maimonides and Aristotle: A retrospective study. In *Responsibility, Character and Emotions: New Essays in Moral Psychology*, ed. F. Schoeman. Cambridge University Press.

Huigens, K. 2003. The dead end of deterrence. In *Aristotle and Modern Law*, ed. R. Brooks and J. Murphy. Ashgate.

Israel, J. I. 2001. *Radical Enlightenment, Philosophy and the Making of Modernity*. Oxford University Press.

Kronman, A. 1993. *The Lost Lawyer: Failing Ideals of the Legal Profession*. Belknap.

Maimonides, M. 1963. *The Guide of the Perplexed*. University of Chicago Press.

Morse, S. 2004. New neuroscience, old problems. In *Neuroscience and the Law: Brain, Mind and the Scales of Justice*, ed. B. Garland. Dana.

Neiman, S. 2002. *Evil: An Alternative History of Philosophy in Modern Thought*. Princeton University Press.

Neusner, J. 1991. *Rabbinic Political Theory*. University of Chicago Press.

Price, A. W. 1995. *Mental Conflict*. Routledge.

Schofer, J. 2003. The redaction of desire and editing of Rabbinic teachings concerning yeser ("inclination"). *Journal of Jewish Thought and Philosophy* 12, no. 1: 19–53.

Sorabji, R. 1992. Intentionality and physiological processes: Aristotle's theory of sense perception. In *Essays on Aristotle's* De Anima, ed. M. Nussbaum and A. Rorty. Clarendon.

Wolfson, H. A. 1979. *Repercussions of the Kalam in Jewish Philosophy*. Harvard University Press.

Zaibert, L. A. 2003. Intentionality, voluntariness and culpability: A historical philosophical analysis. In *Aristotle and Modern Law*, ed. R. Brooks and J. Murphy. Ashgate.

15 Bypassing Conscious Control: Media Violence, Unconscious Imitation, and Freedom of Speech

Susan Hurley

We are what we pretend to be, so we must be careful about what we pretend to be.
—Kurt Vonnegut Jr., *Mother Night*[1]

Why does it matter whether and how individuals consciously control their behavior? It matters for many reasons. Here I focus on concerns about social influences of which agents are typically unaware on aggressive behavior.

First, I survey research about the influence of viewing media violence on aggressive behavior. The consensus among researchers is that there is indeed a robust causal influence here.

Second, I explain why, in the context of work in cognitive science and neuroscience on imitation, this influence is not surprising. Indeed, it would have been surprising if aggressive behavior had been immune from general imitative influences. Imitation is a topic of intense contemporary scientific interest and of great importance for understanding what is distinctive about human minds. Recent advances in understanding imitation and related processes shed light on the mechanisms and functions that may underlie the influence of media violence on aggressive behavior. Human beings have a distinctive tendency to imitate and assimilate observed or represented behavior, which operates at various levels and is often automatic and unconscious. Automatic imitative influences of which individuals are unaware can compromise their autonomy.

Third, I consider how this bears on the liberal principle of freedom of speech. This principle goes beyond the general liberal principle of freedom of action so long as action does not harm others; speech is given additional, *special* protection from interference, even when it does harm others. Why? Answers often invoke autonomy. In particular, speech is often assumed to engage autonomous deliberative processes in hearers by which they consciously control their responses to speech. Social influences that bypass autonomy are implicitly assumed to be negligible. But what if they aren't? Empirical work on imitation is relevant to both the likely effects of speech and to the character of the processes by which its effects are brought about.

As a result, I suggest, liberals should begin to think about responsibility in eco-logical terms: to rethink issues about the way individual responsibility depends on social environments, and about shared individual and social accountability for the effects of speech when individuals are subject to social influences that compromise their full autonomy. This requires understanding imitation and its implications for issues about media violence, rather than persisting in unscrutinized assumptions about the autonomous character of responses to speech.

Issues about media violence have been relatively neglected in discussions of freedom of speech, compared, say, to pornography and hate speech. This is unfortunate, because media violence raises basic issues about harm to third parties in a simpler way, without also raising the complex issues about paternalism, equality, and silencing effects that are raised by pornography and hate speech. The basic issues are still difficult, and getting clearer about them may help to make progress on all fronts. In particular, there is a large overlap between media violence and pornography, so arguments about media violence may apply to some pornography, in ways that do not depend on the more complex and controversial arguments about equality and silencing effects. My lack of attention here to pornography per se should thus not be taken to imply that I regard my arguments as irrelevant to it. On the contrary.

I want to emphasize that the argument I develop about media violence is not paternalistic: it turns on harm *to others*, not on harm *to self*. Opposition to paternalism is irrelevant to it. Moreover, I am not arguing for any particular policy response; that is a difficult further question. Rather, I am trying to open up a set of issues and to excavate connections that need considerable further thought, at the levels of both theory and legal policy.

1   Does Exposure to Media Violence Tend to Increase Aggressive Behavior?

The Effects of Media Violence: Consensus and Denial

Several hundred research studies have examined the relationship between exposure to violence in the media and aggressive behavior.[2] They have measured the effects of violent entertainment and, to a lesser degree, of news reports of violence, and have focused on whether exposure to media violence tends to increase aggressive behavior. In general, aggressive behavior is defined conservatively in terms of intentional production of physical harm or threats of physical harm (Berkowitz 1993).[3] Responses have been highly politicized, and proponents of each side have often been regarded as selective in their appeals to evidence (Renfrew 1997, p. 161; Huesmann and Taylor 2003; Potter 2003; Bushman and Anderson 2001; Freedman 2002). Unfortunately, this work has been assessed without putting it into the essential context of our growing knowledge of imitation in general, as I shall do here.

Since the Williams (1981) Report, many liberals have felt able to dismiss as unsubstantiated the thesis that exposure to media violence tends to increases aggression.[4] This dismissal is now seriously dated. Surprisingly, there is a strong disconnect between even educated public opinion on this subject and the increasingly convergent majority opinion of researchers.[5] This strong and growing consensus has often not been accurately reported in the media, and has not got across to the public. Here are some quotations from recent textbooks:

... the consensus of research opinion accepts that media violence does cause violence in society. (Howitt 1998, p. 61)[6]

The evidence in support of the hypothesis that viewing violence leads to an increase in aggressive behavior is very strong. (Gunter and McAleer 1997, p. 114)

For most investigators of media violence effects ... there's no longer a question about whether viewing violent events in the mass media enhances the likelihood of further aggression. (Berkowitz 1993, p. 208)

This consensus view was endorsed in 2000 by the American Psychological Association, the American Academy of Pediatrics, the American Academy of Child and Adolescent Psychiatry, the American Medical Association, the American Academy of Family Physicians, and the American Psychiatric Association. (See Bushman and Anderson 2001.)

If readers wish to sample a few of the many studies, some suggestions: An influential meta-analysis published in 1994 by Paik and Comstock found a positive significant correlation between exposure to media violence and aggressive behavior, regardless of research method. (See also Comstock and Scharrer 2003; Anderson and Bushman 2002, p. 2377; Anderson et al. 2003.) *Science* recently published the results of a longitudinal study (Johnson et al. 2002) in which more than 700 families were followed for 17 years. This study linked television exposure to subsequent aggression. Contrary to what might be assumed, the link holds for adolescents and young adults as well as children.[7] Alternate explanations that were statistically controlled for and ruled out include childhood neglect, family income, neighborhood violence, parental education, and psychiatric disorders.[8] Recent evidence shows that exposure to violent video games also tends to increase aggression (Anderson and Bushman 2001).

Effect Sizes

What is the magnitude of the effects of media violence? The effect sizes shown in the 1994 meta-analysis are larger than the effects of calcium intake on bone mass, lead exposure on IQ in children, or asbestos exposure to cancer—all risks we take seriously (Bushman and Anderson 2001, pp. 480–481; Comstock and Scharrer 2003).

Moreover, even small effects are magnified in human significance by the huge viewing audiences of the mass media (as the advertising industry well appreciates). Suppose, for example, that only 10 percent of viewers who see a certain program are influenced to be more aggressive.[9] This may seem a small effect size, but 10 percent of 10 million viewers is still a million people. The effects of increased aggression in a million people, some of which threatens or physically harms third parties, may be highly significant in terms of human suffering (Rosenthal 1986). Whether this is a price worth paying is a further question. Perhaps it is, but we shouldn't duck the question.

Methodologies

The research meta-analysis pulls together is of three main methodological types (Anderson and Bushman 2001, p. 354). First, experimental studies randomly assign subjects to violent or non-violent media and assess them later for aggression. Lab experiments are not merely correlational, but permit rigorous controls and support causal inferences, according to standard scientific criteria. However, they are criticized as artificial in relation to real-world violent behavior, and for focusing on short-term effects (Paik and Comstock 1994, p. 517; Geen 1990, p. 95). The Williams Report pointed out that criminal and antisocial behavior cannot ethically be experimentally produced, so surrogates or related behaviors are often measured; in some cases this involves fictional or pretend contexts, such as hitting a doll, begging the question of the relationship between fictional contexts and real-world aggression (1981, pp. 65–66, 68).[10] Field (as opposed to lab) experiments achieve similar controls while making more naturalistic measurements (though the degree of control may not be as high). For example, institutionalized delinquent boys were first assessed for aggressiveness, and then shown violent or non-violent films for several nights. Those shown violent films were subsequently more violent in daily life, not just in the lab. The effect was especially strong for the boys who had previously rated low in aggressiveness (Berkowitz 1993, pp. 207–208).

Second, there are correlational field studies, which assess types of media consumed and their correlation with aggression at a given time. As is well recognized in this literature, correlational studies alone do not establish causation.

Third, longitudinal studies assess correlations between types of media consumed and aggression across time periods. The cross-lagged longitudinal technique used in some longitudinal studies does support causal inferences.

Correlation vs. Causation

It is worth pausing to focus on the familiar objection that correlation does not show causation, which is often voiced in relation to the thesis that media violence has harmful effects (Renfrew 1997, p. 161; Williams 1981, pp. 65, 71, 84; see also

Chartrand and Bargh 1999, p. 895). Perhaps aggressive tendencies cause people to seek out media violence (the "reverse hypothesis"), or perhaps both have some further common cause. It is important to recognize that media violence research addresses this point effectively.

First, triangulation between different research methods and the mutually supporting results they yield in meta-analyses supports the thesis that exposure to media violence is not merely correlated with increased aggression but tends to cause it. Experimental studies with careful controls and manipulations support causal claims, and they converge with the results of more naturalistic fieldwork and correlational studies (Renfrew 1997, p. 157; Potter 2003, pp. 28–29).[11]

Second, cross-lagged longitudinal studies also support causal inferences (Eron et al. 1972; Renfrew 1997, pp. 156, 161). Here, measures of two variables are made at both an earlier and a later time. If the correlation between A1 and B2 is substantially greater than that between B1 and A2, this indicates that A causes B, not vice versa. For example, viewing media violence by 8-year-old boys is strongly correlated with aggressive behavior by those same boys 10 years later, but aggressive behavior at the earlier age is not strongly correlated with viewing media violence 10 years later.[12] The pattern holds across all levels of aggressiveness in the earlier age group, so is not due to different levels of aggression in the younger children. The result controlled for other variables such as parental socio-economic status, boys' IQ, parental aggressiveness, etc. A similar pattern is found again 12 years further on, at age 30, bridging 22 years. The 8-year-old boys with the strongest preference for media violence were most likely to have been convicted of a serious crime by age 30 (Berkowitz 1993, pp. 227 228).[13] Similar results have been found across five different nations (ibid., pp. 228–229).

As time passes, the relationship between exposure to media violence and aggression may well be reciprocal or circular: exposure may increase aggressive tendencies, which in turn lead those affected to seek out further exposure to media violence. The supposition that those with aggressive tendencies may tend to seek out media violence is consistent with the thesis that media violence increases aggression; aggression and media violence may be in this way mutually reinforcing, in a truly vicious cycle.[14]

Short-Term vs. Long-Term Effects

It is helpful to distinguish short-term and long-term influences of media violence. Berkowitz explains the short-term effects in terms of *priming* (1993, p. 210ff; see also the discussion below of imitation and the chameleon effect). Several studies show that mere exposure to words connected with aggression primes punitive behavior to a fellow experimental subject. Visual images are especially effective primes. Subjects are more aggressive to someone who has earlier provoked them after they watch a video scene in which a villain gets a deserved beating. Berkowitz also gives the example of suicide contagion: combined evidence from 35 US cases shows a significant upward trend in the number of suicides in the month or so after a celebrity's suicide is reported. There are similar findings for the UK (Berkowitz 1993, pp. 204–205).

Huesmann, an author of the influential 22-year cross-lagged longitudinal study cited above, gives a unified account of short- and long-term cumulative effects in terms of the acquisition of cognitive scripts that serve as guides for behavior over the longer term. Scripts can be acquired through social learning or imitation as well as through direct experience of results, and incorporate procedural know-how as well as declarative knowledge (Huesmann 1998, pp. 89, 97; Huesmann 2005, pp. 259–260). Predisposing personal factors and environmental context interact through observational and enactive learning to lead to the emergence of aggressive scripts (Huesmann 1998, p. 96). Repeated exposure to certain behavior patterns does not merely prime short-term copying behavior, but also establishes particular scripts and makes them more readily accessible for use over the longer term. Certain types of media violence are more likely to generate aggressive scripts than others.[15] However (as one would expect from the literature surveyed below on the "chameleon" and related effects), exposure to violent media can increase the accessibility of violent behavioral responses in ways that bypass norms, values and attitudes over which the agent has conscious control (Comstock and Scharrer 2003); such influences can operate even though the agent "officially" has a negative attitude toward violent behavior. (See also Wilson and Brekke 1994.) Both short-term priming and longer-term script effects can be triggered, without awareness on the part of the subject, merely by the presence of apparently irrelevant contextual cues: children exposed to a violent scene in which a walkie-talkie features have been shown to be more likely to behave aggressively later in the presence of a walkie-talkie; the color of a room in which violence is observed can have a similar effect (Huesmann 1998, pp. 82, 83, 97, 98; Berkowitz 1993, p. 222). While priming effects and script activation often *can* be evaluated and inhibited, it is a further question how the evaluative and inhibitory scripts are acquired and activated. Scripts are more likely to be controlled while they are first being established, but in the longer term and with maturity, may become automatic (Huesmann 1998, p. 90). As well as activating aggressive scripts, viewing violence may disinhibit violence through desensitization and changing what is regarded as normal. Children who have just viewed a violent movie are slower than controls to intervene in serious fighting between other children (Berkowitz 1993, pp. 223–224). One often hears the view that media violence may have a cathartic effect, in defusing pent up aggression. Unfortunately, the evidence simply does not support a catharsis effect (Huesmann and Taylor 2003; Potter 2003, p. 39).

In summary, the evidence shows that exposure to media violence causes an increased tendency to aggressive behavior of significant effect size across the population of viewers, in both the short and the long term.

By what mechanisms does exposure to media violence have these effects? I suggest that these may include the evolutionarily useful tendency of humans to imitate actions they observe others performing, which operates in part automatically and unconsciously.[16] Moreover, to the extent an automatic, unconscious tendency[17] to imitate explains the influence of exposure to media violence, we cannot expect introspective assessments of this influence by those subject to it to be accurate. (On the myth that "it may affect others but it doesn't affect me," see chapter 2 of Potter 2003.) Let us now consider what has been learned about human imitative tendencies.

2 Imitation

Background and Distinctions

Imitation is currently a focus of intense interest within the cognitive sciences and neuroscience. In the nineteenth century, and often even today, imitation was often thought of as a low-level capacity, and is often still thought of as such, but scientists now consider this view mistaken. In information-processing terms, imitative learning appears to require solving a difficult correspondence problem: the translation of a novel perceived action into similar performance (Prinz 1990; Nehaniv and Dautenhahn 2002; Heyes 2001, 2005). The capacity to imitate is rare, and is linked in important ways to distinctively human forms of intelligence, in particular to language, culture, and the ability to understand other minds (Rizzolatti and Arbib 1998, 1999; Gallese and Goldman 1998; Gordon 1995; Tomasello 1999; Arbib 2002 and in press; Arbib and Rizzolatti 1997; Gallese 2001, 2005; Meltzoff 2005; Iacoboni 2005; Hurley 2005, 2006; Whiten et al. 2001, 2005, Hobson and Lee 1999). Social learning by imitation is not merely a means by which children acquire culture, but may also have pervasive influence throughout adulthood (Comstock and Scharrer 2003), in ways we are only just beginning to recognize. If so, this has important consequences for our understanding of ourselves, both individually and socially.

It is helpful to distinguish different forms of social learning that are sometimes run together under the generic heading of imitation. In *full-fledged imitation*, a novel action is learned by observing another do it. As well as novelty, there is means/ends structure: you copy the other's means of achieving her goal, not just her goal. In *emulation*, you observe another achieving a goal in a certain way, find that goal attractive and then attempt to achieve it yourself. Through trial-and-error learning you may rapidly converge on the other's means of achieving the goal; this is not imitation in the strict sense, but rather emulation of a goal plus trial-and-error learning. Another contrast is with mere *response priming*, as in contagious yawning or laughing. Here, bodily movements may be copied but there is no means/ends structure; they are not copied as a learned means to a goal. Yet another contrast is with *stimulus enhancement*, whereby another's action draws your attention to a stimulus that then triggers an innate or previously learned response. Emulation, response priming and stimulus enhancement are easy to confuse with full-fledged imitation, and careful experiments are needed to distinguish them.[18] Indeed, goal emulation and response priming can be thought of as the ends and means components, respectively, of full-fledged imitation. The evidence I survey concerns the copying of ends, of means, and of both in full-fledged imitation; all are potentially relevant to issues about the effects of media violence. Some of the evidence I review concerns imitation in the more restrictive sense of full-fledged imitation, while some of it concerns copying in the broader sense, including copying goals or bodily movements and without a requirement of novelty.

Imitation in Animals and Children

Goal emulation and response priming are found in nonhuman animals, but full-fledged imitation has proved difficult to find in any but the most intelligent animals (see Byrne 1995, Heyes and Galef 1996, Tomasello and Call 1997, Galef 2005; etc.): apes (Whiten et al. 2005), cetaceans (Herman 2002), and some birds (Pepperberg 1999; Hunt and Gray 2003; Weir et al. 2002; Akins and Zentall 1996, 1998; Akins et al. 2002). Some argue that it is present only in enculturated animals, raised by and continually with human beings (Tomasello and Call 1997; Tomasello 1999). While the animal results are fascinating, space is limited so I will pass over them to focus on the human evidence, though making some comparisons.

Consider children first. An influential series of papers by Meltzoff and co-workers demonstrate the imitative tendencies of newborn human infants and imply that neonates can equate their own unseen behaviors, such as facial gestures, with gestures they see others perform. Infants also "perfect" actions they see unsuccessfully executed by adult models, apparently discriminating and copying the goal of the unsuccessful action (Meltzoff 1996, 1988, 2005; Meltzoff and Moore 1977, 1999).

Kinsbourne (2005) argues that young children perceive enactively; perception is automatically enacted in imitative (in a broad sense that includes copying of bodily movements) behavior, unless actively inhibited. Arousal increases the strength of the imitative tendency. Inhibition is a function of frontal areas of the brain, but babies and very young children don't yet have well-developed frontal function and cannot inhibit imitative behavior. Overt imitation is the tip of the iceberg of continual covert imitation that doesn't break through inhibition in adults.

Importantly, children don't just emulate goals; they also imitate novel means to attractive goals. One experiment used a touch-sensitive light panel lying on a table at which the experimenter was sitting; the experimenter turned it on in an odd way, by bending over to touch it with his forehead. 14-month-olds who see this demonstration, after one week's delay, also turn it on by touching it with their foreheads (Meltzoff 1988, 2005). They do not do this unless they have seen the model do it first. While children do not always imitate unselectively (Gergely et al. 2002), they have a greater tendency than chimps to imitate rather than to emulate when the method imitated is transparently inefficient (Tomasello 1999, pp. 29–30). For example, after seeing a demonstrator use a rake inefficiently, prongs down, to pull in a treat, two-year-old children do the same; they almost never turn the rake over and use it more efficiently, edge down, instead. In contrast, chimps given a parallel demonstration tend to turn the rake over (Nagell et al. 1993). When it is obvious that the observed action is causally *irrelevant* to the goal, or highly *inefficient*, chimps try another means to achieve the goal—they emulate. Children, in contrast, tend to be strongly conventional and conformist: "imitation machines" (Tomasello 1999, p. 159).

Chimps seem to be better off in this comparison, at least in the short run. Why might it be beneficial to humans in the long run to imitate (as opposed to emulate) with such determination? Tomasello (1999) explains this in terms of the *ratchet effect*: a tendency to imitation preserves rare one-off insights about how to achieve goals, which would not be rediscovered readily by independent trial-and-error learning, and so lost without imitation. Imitation makes these advances available to all as a platform for further development. Via the ratchet effect, imitation is the mechanism that drives cultural and technological transmission, accumulation and evolution.

Imitation in Adults

Adults with damage to certain areas of cortex imitate (also in the broader sense) uninhibitedly, even counter to instructions. (See Luria 1973, discussed in Kinsbourne 2005.) Lhermitte and co-workers study patients with damage to a frontal brain area, which they suggest normally inhibits automatic connections between similar perceptions and actions. Damage to this inhibitory area releases the underlying imitative patterns of behavior (Lhermitte et al. 1986; Lhermitte 1986; Stengel et al. 1947). Lhermitte's imitation syndrome patients persistently imitate gestures the experimenter makes, although they have not been instructed to do so, and even when these are socially unacceptable or odd: putting on glasses when already wearing glasses. When asked why they imitate, since they had not been asked to, patients indicate that they feel they have to, that it is their duty, that the gestures they see somehow include an order to imitate them, that their response is the reaction called for; they do not disown their behavior and may attempt to justify it.

However, the human tendency to imitate is not confined to the young and the brain-damaged.[19] Various experiments demonstrate the way similarity between stimulus and response can affect responses. For example: normal adult subjects instructed to point to their nose when they hear the word 'nose' or point to a lamp when they hear the word 'lamp' performed perfectly while watching the experimenter perform correctly. But they were unable to avoid mistakes when they observed the experimenter doing the wrong thing: they tended to copy what they saw done rather than follow the instruction heard, even though they were trying to follow clear instructions to obey the verbal command (Eidelberg 1929; Prinz 1990). Although the underlying tendency to imitate is inhibited in normal adults under many conditions, it is still there, and it can easily be released.

Ideomotor Theory and the Chameleon Effect

Wolfgang Prinz explains such observations in terms of what William James called *ideomotor theory*: every representation of movement awakes in some degree the movement that it represents. The representation of an action's goal can elicit movements that would be means to that end; it has effects even when movements do not break through overtly. Watching an action sequence speeds up your own performance of the same sequence, even if you cannot explicitly distinguish and recognize it; merely imagining a skilled performance, in sport or music, improves your own performance: constitutes a kind of practicing, as many athletes and musicians know (Jeannerod 1997, pp. 117, 119; Pascuale-Leone 2001). Moreover, neurophysiologists have shown recently that observing a particular action primes precisely the muscles that would be needed to perform the same action (Fadiga et al. 1995). Prinz (1990, 2005) argues, from the tendency to imitate and the reaction time advantage of imitative tasks, that perception and action share a common neural code that enables and facilitates imitation. On the traditional view of perception and action as separate, imitation requires a complex translation between unrelated input and output codes. A common code would avoid this correspondence problem; no sensory to motor translation is needed.

Bargh, Chartrand, Dijksterhuis, and other social psychologists contribute further evidence of an automatic, unconscious tendency to imitate in normal adult subjects. They demonstrate that the mere perception of another's behavior automatically increases, in ways subjects are not aware of, the likelihood of the perceiver's behavior that way himself. This is an imitative tendency in a broad sense, applying to goals of action as well as bodily movements that are the particular means employed; modeled personality traits and stereotypes automatically activate corresponding behavior in us. We automatically tend to assimilate our behavior to our social environment; Chartrand and Bargh (1999) call this the *chameleon effect*.

Here are some examples. External representations of hostility seem to prime mental representations of hostility, making participants significantly more likely to follow experimenter instructions to give shocks. And, *even with no instruction to be rude*, people are, spontaneously, significantly more rude when primed with words representing rudeness; ditto for politeness. Given subliminal exposure to words associated with the elderly, such as 'sentimental', 'gray', and 'bingo', people get slower, their memories get worse, and their attitudes become more conservative. Participants who interact in an unrelated task with someone who rubs her foot rub their own feet significantly more; transferred to another partner who touches his face, participants start to touch their faces instead; they are unaware of the model's behavior or its influence on their own. (See Bargh et al. 1996; Bargh 2005; Bargh and Chartrand 1999; Chartrand and Bargh 1996, 1999, 2002; Carver et al. 1983; Chen and Bargh 1997; Dijksterhuis and Bargh 2001; Dijksterhuis and van Knippenberg 1998; Dijksterhuis 2005.)

One study measured performance on multiple-choice factual questions (Dijksterhuis and van Knippenberg 1998; Dijksterhuis 2005). Some participants were primed, before doing the multiple-choice test, by doing some ostensibly unrelated exercises about college professors; other participants were not. The participants primed by thinking about this stereotype, generally associated with intelligence, got significantly higher scores. In another session different participants were primed by an unrelated exercise about soccer hooligans, while a control group was not. The participants primed by thinking about this stereotype, generally associated with stupidity, got significantly lower scores. It doesn't matter whether the primes are conscious or subliminal: people don't see any relation between the priming stimuli and the effects on their own behavior, even when they are conscious of the primes. Such priming works also for thinking about general traits as well as stereotypes, for aggressive as well as benign behaviors.[20] The results are highly robust, across dozens of different stereotypes and dependent variables, and using a variety of different priming methods. The chameleon effect is automatic and unconscious, applies to meaningful and meaningless acts, to ends and to means, and does not depend on the subject's volition or any relevant independent goal that would rationalize the primed behavior. External visual and verbal representations of behavior have a remarkable direct ability to control action, as Bargh (2005) concludes from a survey of converging lines of research.[21]

Ideomotor theory is also invoked by these scientists to explain their results. They hold that there is a direct link between perception and action; just thinking about or perceiving a certain kind of action has a tendency to lead to behavior in line with the thought. When? All the time. The chameleon effect is the default underlying tendency for normal humans adults; it needs to be specifically overridden or inhibited— as it often is in normal adults, for example, by being engaged in an intentional goal-directed activity that makes different demands. Nevertheless, the underlying default tendency remains, covertly even when inhibited; and often it is not inhibited.[22]

Bargh emphasizes how hard it is for people to accept that these imitative influences apply to themselves: because they are unconscious and automatic, so people are not aware of them, and because such external influences threaten their conception of themselves as in conscious control of their own behavior.[23] But, as Bargh argues (personal communication), to gain control over external influences on their behavior people need first to recognize that they are subject to them, instead of denying this. Otherwise, people won't attempt to control such external influences, and they'll have a field day (Bargh 1999; Wilson and Brekke 1994; Potter 2003, p. 101). Of course, a person can autonomously decide to enter an environment in which he will be subject, in ways he will not be conscious of, to influences that alter his behavior[24]—but only if he recognizes when making the decision that he will become subject to such influences. Otherwise, his choice to enter the environment of such influences would not be autonomous.

Mechanisms and Functions of Imitation: Mirror Neurons, Language, Understanding Other Minds, Cultural Transmission

What kind of neural processing might explain the preceding observations? Mirror neurons seem relevant here. These are a particularly intriguing type of sensorimotor neuron, which have matching perceptual and motor fields: they fire when the agent perceives another acting in a certain way or when the agent does the same type of act herself. They can be very specifically tuned. For example, certain cells fire when a monkey sees the experimenter bring food to the mouth with his own hand *or* when the monkey does the same (even in the dark, so that the monkey cannot see its own hand). The correspondence is not just visual: hearing an expression of anger increases activation of muscles used to express anger.[25]

The function of mirror neurons, and their relation to imitation, is a focus of current interest. Mirror neurons are arguably necessary, though not sufficient, for full-fledged imitation. They were discovered in macaque monkeys, but while these monkeys can emulate, they have not been shown to be able to imitate in the strict sense.[26] In monkeys, the mirror system appears to code for the ends rather than the means of action. In humans, in contrast, the mirror system has means/ends structure: some parts of it code for the goals of actions, others for specific movements that are means used to achieve goals. Rizzolatti, one of the discovers of mirror neurons, suggests that the human mirror system can be used to imitate and not just to emulate because it codes for means as well as ends, unlike the macaque's (2005).[27]

There is also much current interest in whether mirror neurons can illuminate the relationships among imitation and two other distinctively human capacities: for language, and for identifying with others and understanding the mental states that motivate the actions of others. The greatest differences between chimp and human brains are precisely in the significant expansion of the areas around the Sylvian fissure that subserve imitation, language, and the understanding of action (Iacoboni 2005). This is also where mirror neurons are concentrated.

An hypothesis gaining support among scientists and philosophers is that mirror neurons are part of the mechanism for understanding observed actions by inter-subjective identification with others, empathy and simulation.[28] When you see someone do something, your own motor system is primed to imitate, even if imitation is inhibited, or taken "off line": such simulation can be regarded as off-line imitation. This enables you to regard yourself and others as similar, to identify with others, and to understand the motivation of others' actions in a means/ends structured way. Simulation may also enable you to consider counterfactual possibilities or the results of alternative possible actions, and may in this way be among the mechanisms that enable deliberation. (For further details see Hurley 2005.)

Mirror neurons coding for the goals of action are found in Broca's area,[29] one of the primary language areas of the human brain and among those activated when imitative tasks are performed. Transient "virtual lesions" to Broca's area (created by transcranial magnetic stimulation) interfere with imitative tasks (Iacoboni 2005). Now a nativist view of language could motivate a kind of protectiveness about Broca's as the best candidate for an innate language area in the brain.[30] But recently scientists have developed new arguments about how language could develop, via neural mirror systems, out of capacities for imitation and identification with others (Arbib 2002 and forthcoming; Arbib and Rizzolatti 1997; Iacoboni 2005; Rizzolatti and Arbib 1998, 1999).[31] Whether the mirror properties of neurons in Broca's area are innate, acquired, or both is a question for further work.[32]

Finally, consider why evolution might favor neural structures that facilitate response priming, emulation, and imitation. Suppose variations in the behavioral traits of adults that are not genetically heritable slightly favor some members of a generation over others, so that some reproduce successfully and others do not. Their offspring may benefit if they can acquire the behavioral traits of their successful parents through response priming, emulation, and imitation as well as through genetic inheritance. A young creature that tends to copy its parents will tend to pick up the nonheritable behaviors of creatures that have survived long enough to reproduce, and to form associations between such behaviors and the environmental conditions in which they are appropriate. Depending on how costly or error-prone individual learning is, such social learning may contribute more to genetic fitness.[33]

Later in life, the ability to turn imitation on and off selectively can be a Machiavellian social advantage: by imitating the behavioral signs used by a group of cooperators to identify members, you may be able to obtain the benefits of cooperation from others, but then inhibit your own cooperative behavior before it comes time to reciprocate (a behavioral analogue of free-riding "greenbeard genes"; see Dawkins 1982, p. 149).

Once the capacity for imitation has evolved genetically, imitation provides a mechanism for the cultural transmission of information and for cultural accumulation and evolution, as Tomasello (1999), Boyd and Richerson (1982, 1985), Blackmore (1999), Baldwin (1896), and others have argued in various ways. Issues arise here about how genetic and cultural evolution constrain and influence one another: must genes keep culture on a leash or can "memes" drive genetic evolution? But for present purposes my survey of recent work on imitation and its implications must end here.

Summing Up: Applying Imitation Science to the Imitation of Aggression

I have surveyed the striking convergence of different lines of research on imitation, in cognitive neuroscience, neuropsychology, social psychology, and theories of cultural evolution. Recent evidence and opinion strongly favor of the view that human beings have pervasive imitative tendencies; these are, at least in significant part, automatic and unconscious, not the result of autonomous deliberative processes. However, our imitative tendencies may also be essential to the way our distinctively human minds are built and to their distinctive social ecology. The importance of imitation in molding human behavioral patterns has not yet been widely assimilated, not its social significance widely appreciated. Perhaps when the roles and mechanisms of imitation in general are better known and understood, so will be the risks associated with the imitation of media violence in particular. Consider how some of the specific points about imitation surveyed above apply to the imitation of observed aggression.

We share with some other social animals capacities for social learning, expressed in the short-term priming of observed bodily movements and the emulation of attractive goals other agents are observed to obtain. Observed aggressive action does not have a special exemption from these general tendencies. Thus, observing aggression should tend to prime similar bodily movements in the short term, which may or may not be inhibited, and, when the results of observed aggression are attractive, emulation of goals should be expected. Moreover, the strong human tendency not just to emulate, but to imitate novel observed actions—even when the observed means are inappropriate means of obtaining the goal—applies to aggressive actions along with others. Children, whose frontal functions aren't fully developed, should be expected to have particular difficulty in inhibiting the tendency to imitate observed aggression (Philo 1999). But according to ideomotor theories, a tendency to imitate observed aggression should also be expected in normal adults, and to have

effects even when it is inhibited. For both adults and children, observing or imagining violent behavior constitutes a kind of *practicing* for violence, a honing of the
skills of violence, just as in sporting or musical activities. The chameleon effect indicates that mere perception of aggression automatically increases the likelihood of
engaging in similar behavior, in ways subjects are not conscious of. Exposure to representations of violent stereotypes or traits, like others, should be expected to prime
unconscious automatic assimilation, mental as well as behavioral. These automatic
effects require specific overriding and inhibition for aggression as much as for other
kinds of action. If there is a direct link between perception and action, then observing violence should be expected to increase the likelihood of doing violence. The
link between representations of aggression and similar actual behavior should be
no less strong and direct[34] than the link is for other types of behavior, a link on
which powerful evidence from various disciplines converges. With the discovery of
the mirror system and currently developing theories of its function, we may be on
track to understanding the causal mechanisms that subserve human imitative tendencies at large, including the tendency to imitate observed aggression.

Since human imitative tendencies often operate automatically and unconsciously,
they can bypass processes of autonomous deliberation and control, and are least
accessible to control when they are unacknowledged. This bypass will threaten
people's sense of deliberative autonomy and control, hence be hard to accept, in
general (as indeed Bargh has found)—and especially so when the influence is
toward behavior the subjects may consciously disapprove of, such as aggression.
Ironically, denial reduces subjects' ability to control such influences. Evidence of
the effects of media violence doesn't just threaten financial interests in the media
industry, but also challenges the conception many people have of themselves as
autonomous, a conception that also plays important roles in political theory.

But while at one level our automatic tendency to imitate may threaten our autonomy, recall also that strong imitative tendencies are distinctively human and are
arguably connected, neurally and functionally, with other distinctively human capacities: for language, for identifying with and understanding other agents, for assessing counterfactual possibilities (Iacoboni 2005; Gallese 2001, 2005; Meltzoff 2005;
Hurley 2005, 2006; Gordon 1995, 2005; Arbib 2002; Gallese and Goldman 1998;
Rizzolatti and Arbib 1998; Williams et al. 2001; Whiten and Brown 1999; Hobson
and Lee 1999; Meltzoff and Gopnik 1993; Meltzoff and Decety 2003), which are in
turn arguably fundamental to our capacities for rationality and responsible action.
Even though imitative tendencies may often be automatic and unconscious and
bypass autonomous deliberation, these tendencies arguably also contribute, in both
evolutionary and developmental terms, to our having our distinctively human capacities in the first place. If so, we would not be more rational or responsible or
autonomous without these underlying imitative tendencies; the human style of

imitative social learning may well be a deeply functional feature of human nature. We may only possess our distinctively human abilities to make up our own minds, as deliberative, responsible agents, because of the distinctively imitative way in which our minds are made up.

But this rethinking of the nature and social ecology of autonomy has political implications. Different ways of understanding the nature and basis for our distinctively human deliberative autonomy may affect the roles this trait plays in political philosophy, and how best to foster, protect, and respect it.

3   Freedom of Speech

Assumptions

I want finally to bring the preceding lines of research into contact with issues about freedom of speech. Suppose for the sake of argument that three things are true. First, exposure to media violence tends to increase aggressive or violent behavior, with resulting significant harm to third parties. The increase holds statistically, across a population of viewers, which is of course consistent with causation.[35] Second, human beings have a tendency to imitate observed or represented actions that often operates automatically and unconsciously. Three (putting the first and second points together), the tendency for exposure to media violence to increase aggressive or violent behavior in harmful ways often operates automatically, in ways that the affected agent is unaware of and that bypass his autonomous deliberative processes. Exposure to media violence can have harmful effects in ways that bypass autonomous deliberative processes (*bypass effects*) as well as in ways that operate via autonomous deliberative processes (*non-bypass effects*). The third assumption is that, even setting aside non-bypass effects, bypass effects still increase aggressive or violent behavior significantly across a population of viewers, resulting in significant harm to third parties.[36]

The work surveyed above should make these empirical assumptions plausible, but let us now consider the implications for freedom of speech IF they are true. How do these empirical propositions bear on traditional views of why freedom of speech should have special protection and of how resulting harms should be dealt with? I will first set out sketch the relevant theoretical background and apply it to violent entertainment. Then I will consider a handful of possible objections.

Liberalism and the Special Protection Principle

A background principle in liberal societies is that government should not interfere with our actions, except to prevent harm to others (Mill 1859; Williams 1981, chapter 5). The principle of freedom of speech makes an exception to this exception. It is important to recognize that the principle of freedom of speech does *not* depend on denying that speech causes harm to others; speech is not plausibly viewed as self-regarding action. If speech did not harm others, it wouldn't need *special* protection; it would fall under the general liberal protection of liberty except where harm to others is caused.[37] But even speech that is admittedly likely to harm others is given special protection from interference. Thus the principle of freedom of speech makes an exception to the general principle that government can regulate conduct likely to harm to others. People are permitted to do more harm to others through speech than through other conduct. Why?

The nutshell version of the justifications for special protection of speech distinguishes three main categories of argument[38]: *arguments from truth* (Mill 1859), *arguments from democracy* (Meiklejohn 1948; Bullinger 1985), and *arguments from autonomy* (Mill 1859). The arguments from truth and democracy are consequentialist, but arguments from autonomy can take consequentialist or deontological form, according to whether autonomy is seen as a good to be promoted (Scanlon 1979) or as a constraint on justifications of government interference (Scanlon 1972). There are subtle variations on each theme: for example, populist and egalitarian and distrust versions of arguments from democracy (Meiklejohn 1948; Fiss 1998, 1991, 1987; Ely 1981). Different conceptions of autonomy and related ideas are invoked (Brison 1998a). The autonomy interests of speakers and of audience are distinguished (Scanlon 1979). The three types of argument can be related in mutually supporting ways, yielding pluralist accounts of freedom of speech. Each type of argument has also been roundly criticized (Schauer 1982, 1984; Alexander and Horton 1984; Brison 1998a). However, for present purposes I do not argue against these three rationales for giving special protection to speech, but rather query the extent to which they capture violent entertainment.

'Speech' is a term of art for present purposes. Not everything that is normally regarded as speech (talking in libraries) gets special protection, and some things do that are not normally regarded as speech (exhibiting photographs). The question "What counts as speech?" is closely connected to the question "Why give special protection to speech?" According to what I call *the special protection principle*, conduct of a certain kind counts as *specially* protected speech to the degree it is captured by the rationales for special protection. That is, the justifications for letting people to more harm to others through speech than nonspeech determine what counts as speech and distinguish it from nonspeech. The distinction needn't be sharp; the rationales for special protection may capture different kinds of conduct to different degrees and thus yield different degrees of special protection. For example, political argument is arguable captured by the rationales to a higher degree than nude dancing, and so warrants a greater degree of special protection.

Should We Extend the Special Protection Accorded to Speech to Violent Entertainment?

To what degree, then, is violent entertainment captured by the rationales for special protection? My answer is "To a very low degree."

Even if violent entertainment can at times serve truth or democracy, most violent entertainment—as opposed to the representation of actual violence in the news— is not well captured by the arguments from truth or from democracy. (I will return to the distinction between news and entertainment.) The strongest case for special protection of violent entertainment would have to be made under the heading of arguments from autonomy.

Consider speaker autonomy first. Violent entertainment is predominantly commercial, and aims at economic profit (Hamilton 1998). It only weakly engages interests in speaker autonomy, unless speaker autonomy has already been associated, in a way that would be question-begging here, with a right to freedom of speech that extends to producing violent entertainment for commercial motives. Moreover, it is important here not to confuse autonomy with self-expression (for example, through art). Self-expression per se is not the beneficiary of special protection and does not justify harming others. There are many ways of expressing oneself that may harm others but do not count as speech or warrant special protection. Nero was presumably expressing himself aesthetically when he (perhaps apocryphally) spilled fresh human blood on green grass. Violent entertainment is thus only very weakly captured by rationales concerned with speaker autonomy.

It fares even worse under rationales concerned with audience autonomy, because of the extent to which the effects of violent entertainment on viewers bypass autonomous processes, and because it does not aim primarily to convey truthful information (as news does). Audiences may want violent entertainment, but not everything people want respects or serves their interests in autonomy, especially if wants have been cultivated and manipulated by powerful financial interests to create a profitable market. The power of the media industry over the public should be compared to the power of government as a potential threat to autonomy (Fiss 1998; Brison 1998a, p. 334). Moreover, as we have seen, there is good reason to believe that many effects of violent entertainment on audiences are unconscious and automatic and bypass autonomous deliberative processes. Audience autonomy would arguably be increased, not decreased, if such influences were reduced.

Does my argument about audience autonomy here become paternalistic? No. I am *not* arguing that it is better for audience's autonomy for them not to be subjected to certain influences, even if audiences want to subject themselves to such influences. Recall the posture of the argument at this point. I asked why we are freer to harm others through speech than through other forms of conduct; the harm concerned is harm to third parties, not to speaker or to audience. The answer most relevant to violent entertainment is "Because giving special protection respects or promotes autonomy." I then ask "But does violent entertainment in fact respect or promote autonomy?" And I consider why it may not do so, but may in fact decrease audience autonomy. I am rebutting a justification of special protection in terms of autonomy, not putting forward autonomy as a positive justification for anything. I am certainly not arguing that audiences should be deprived of the violent entertainment they want because it decreases their autonomy and hence is bad for them. Rather, I am arguing that if violent entertainment causes harm to third parties in ways that bypass autonomous deliberative processes, such harm cannot be justified in terms of audience autonomy.

Scanlon (1979) explains, in developing his second version of an argument from autonomy for free speech, that we tend to assume that an audience is free to decide how to react: what belief or attitude to form. It is thus able to protect itself against unwanted long-range effects of speech. "If we saw ourselves as helplessly absorbing as a belief every proposition we heard expressed, then our views of freedom of expression would be quite different from what they are." (Scanlon 1979, pp. 524–525; cf. Wilson and Brekke 1994; Gilbert 1991; Gilbert et al. 1993). But in fact our control is incomplete. "Expression," Scanlon writes, "is a bad thing if it influences us in ways that are unrelated to relevant reasons, or in ways that bypass our ability to consider those reasons" (1979, p. 525). Scanlon considers how subliminal advertising can affect our beliefs about the means to our goals, and can make us think we have reasons even when we don't. And he considers the possibility that it might also have a deeper effect, and change us by giving us new desires and goals. His point is that any such manipulative, unreliable processes of belief and desire production, of which audiences are unaware and hence uncritical, do not enhance audience autonomy, especially if they exploit audiences for the speaker's gain. In his view, the "central audience interest in expression" is an autonomy interest: "the interest in having a good environment for the formation of one's beliefs and desires" (ibid., p. 527).[39] This suggests that autonomy requires more than non-interference; it makes positive demands on social environments. Scanlon asks whether expression must take a sober, cognitive form in order to gain protection. After all, visual images may be more effective than words in inducing desired behavior in an audience. But it does not follow that speakers should be allowed to use such means, even if they are the only means to create the desired effect: audiences have an interest in avoiding manipulative changes, as in subliminal advertising, which bypass their deliberative control and operate independently of reasons (ibid., p. 547).[40]

The evidence of automatic and unconscious imitative and chameleon effects I cited earlier is highly relevant to these remarks by Scanlon.[41] To paraphrase: if we realized that we tend to absorb and imitate patterns of behavior we observe auto-matically and unconsciousness, then our views of freedom of expression would be quite different from what they are.[42] Perhaps they should be. Here, however, I have argued from within existing views that violent entertainment should not receive much in the way of special protection as speech.

As a result of the low degree of capture by rationales for giving special protec-tion to speech, the degree of special protection given to violent entertainment should be correspondingly low. On the assumptions made above, exposure to violent entertainment produces through unconscious, automatic processes significant harm to others as a result of increased levels of aggressive or violent behavior across the population of viewers. Prevention of such harm to third parties provides a strong reason (or "compelling interest") for liberal government to interfere with violent entertainment, and is not effectively blocked by the rationales for giving special protection to freedom of speech, since these are very weakly engaged by violent entertainment.

Some immediate qualifications: First, no particular policy response or way of interfering is recommended. There are different options here: civil liability and effective self-regulation are alternatives to direct censorship. Second, the third-party-harm reason for interference may be outweighed by other values, including values other than free speech values. We strike balances that permit harm to inno-cent third parties in other contexts, after all: consider the use of cars. Perhaps the harm suffered by third parties is the price we have to pay to have great art that rep-resents violence, since there is no practical way to regulate just the dross[43] and the great art at issue is worth the cost in harm to third parties. I do not argue against this position here, but if that is what it comes down to we should own up to this bal-ancing judgment and not dress it up as something else. Third, note again that my argument is *not paternalistic in any way*. It does not turn on any paternalistic claim to be for the good of those who would prefer to produce or consume violent enter-tainment, but turns purely on harm to third parties. Fourth, it is not offered as an argument within any particular jurisdiction or specific existing jurisprudence, such as US jurisprudence, but as a general normative argument within a liberal democ-ratic context that deserves to be taken seriously by courts.

I expect this argument to be controversial. I now consider six of the possible objections.

News versus Entertainment: Why Does News Deserve Special Protection?

Doesn't my argument prove too much? Doesn't it also show that violent news should not be protected as speech against showings of harmful effects?[44] If media violence has effects that bypass audience autonomy, why protect violent news any more than political acts with harmful effects, such as dumping a pollutant that will cause a number of deaths into a lake in order to protest environmental regulation? Alternatively, why not protect violent entertainment as well as violent news, and just punish the agents of violent acts?[45]

In responding, I draw on the truth and democracy rationales as well as the autonomy rationale for special protection. The line between news and political speech, on the one hand, and entertainment, on the other, is difficult to draw in practice. It may not be sharp, especially given commercial incentives to edit and present the news in ways that maximize its entertainment value. Nevertheless, I believe a distinction between news and entertainment should be drawn in this context by reference to the thought that the primary purpose of news is to report events truthfully. Violent news thus engages the argument from truth directly, in a way that violent entertainment and pollutant dumping do not; if it doesn't, it isn't news. Of course, entertainment often conveys truths; but entertainment needn't aim to report truths, and the reporting of truth need not be entertainment. In contrast, news must aim to report truths, even if it has other, commercial aims as well; and a true report just is news. Moreover, violent news, along with other news, is plausibly regarded as essential to the operation of a democracy. Voters must have access to reasonably accurate information for a democracy to function; information about actual violent events is often of great political significance. In contrast, the primary aim of violent entertainment is not to report actual violent events. Finally, just because the primary aim of violent news is to report actual violent events (unlike violent entertainment), it at least contributes information for autonomous deliberation, even if it also has effects that bypass autonomous deliberation. So its effects at least run along parallel tracks, autonomous and nonautonomous (see below).[46]

Thus representations of violent events in responsible news media are captured by all three types of argument for special protection. Even if they are sometimes misleading, such representations arguably make an important net contribution to the evidence people have for arriving at true beliefs about the state of society, which voters in a democracy need for democracy to function well, and which provides reasons for autonomous, deliberative decision making. So violence in the news is specially protected to a high degree against any further harmful bypass effects it may have, as in suicide contagion.

Statistical Causation, Probability of Harm, and Degree of Protection

Is my argument undermined by the statistical character of the harmful effects? Though exposure to media violence doesn't necessarily cause increased aggression in particular cases, I have assumed that it does so across a population of viewers. Causation is still causation, even when it operates statistically, across populations.[47] And causation at the population level is all that is needed for a showing of significant harm, given the size of modern viewing audiences.

However, it would be sufficient for my application of the special protection principle to make an even weaker assumption at the population level, namely, of a significant probability of causing harmful effects across the population. If the degree of special protection is low because the degree of capture is low, then the probability that conduct will cause serious harm need not be conclusive to provide a compelling reason to regulate that conduct.

To see why, consider what it means, operationally, for the degree of special protection of certain conduct to be higher or lower. Not all nonspeech conduct that can cause harm to others is regulated by liberal governments, even though nonspeech is not specially protected. Whether regulation is justified depends in general on the expected harm, which is a product of the seriousness of harm and the probability the conduct will cause it. A compelling government interest in regulation of potentially harmful nonspeech conduct does not require that the probability of causing harm is conclusive. If given nonspeech conduct must have expected harm to others of level X to create a sufficient government interest in regulation to justify interference, then speech with the same level of expected harm will not justify interference, in virtue of special protection. But if expected harm to others from speech is much higher than X, either because of the seriousness of the harm, or the high probability of this harm resulting, or both, then the special protection given to speech can be overcome.

The degree of special protection can thus be understood as the additional degree of expected harm to others that is required to warrant interference with speech (Schauer 1984, p. 1303). Centrally protected speech such as political argument, falling squarely under all rationales for special protection, receives high-level special protection: overcoming special protection requires a very high probability of catastrophic resulting harm. Less centrally protected speech receives lower-level special protection, and so may be vulnerable to demonstrations of a somewhat lower probability of somewhat less catastrophic harm, which nevertheless provides a compelling governmental interest in regulation; the probability need not be conclusive. There is no basis for requiring conclusive proof of harmfulness, beyond reasonable doubt.[48]

Can "More, Better Speech" Remedy Bypass Effects?

The traditional remedy for harmful speech, under freedom of speech doctrine, is "more, better speech." Can't more, better speech remedy the harmful bypass effects of media violence, without calling the special protection of media violence into question? If the additional speech argues that violence is bad and gives reasons why, the answer is probably No, since the relevant influences operate unconsciously and automatically. However, if the additional speech provides people with scientific evidence that their behavior actually is subject to such direct, automatic imitative influences, including influences toward aggression (however unpalatable that is), so that they can take steps to guard against such influences, then perhaps the additional speech will have some tendency to mitigate the harmful effects (Wilson and Brekke 1994). That would depend on the answers to various questions, which may not be known.

First, will enough people understand and accept the evidence of direct imitative influences on behavior, despite the widespread tendency to deny such influences? Second, will they be able to take effective steps as individuals to counter such influences? Or will the influences tend to persist, like many visual illusions, even when they are recognized as such? Recognition of such influences may be necessary but not sufficient for controlling them. How much harm will result from imitative influences that are resistant in this way? Third, will enough individuals in fact choose to take such steps in relation to media violence, even if they are able to? Or will they prefer to allow themselves to be subject to such influences, perhaps because it is pleasant to do so, or too much trouble to do otherwise?

Furthermore, if many individuals choose not to take steps to counter the influence of media violence on their behavior, despite recognizing this influence, does that absolve others of any accountability for resulting harms to third parties? What of those who market and profit from media violence? Consider several possible parallels. Some choose to smoke, despite recognizing its potential harmful effects on third parties via passive smoking. Does the smoker's choice to endanger third parties absolve those who profit from cigarettes of any accountability for passive smoking harms to third parties? Some choose to drink and drive, despite recognizing the potential harmful effects on third parties. Does the drinker's choice to endanger third parties absolve those who profit from selling alcohol of any accountability for drunk driving harms to third parties? How analogous are these cases to media violence? They raise, at any rate, some general questions about accountability.

The Intervening Accountable Parties Exception; Autonomy versus Shared Accountability

Perhaps, contrary to the way I have set the problem up, media violence doesn't need special protection as speech. Even when nonspeech is in question, there are exceptions to the principle that there is good reason to restrict activities that cause harm to third parties, when the harm is caused via the acts of a second party who is regarded as solely accountable. Selling alcohol to second parties may predictably cause harm to third parties, but if the second parties are sober when they choose to buy and drink alcohol knowing they must later drive, then the behavior of the second party may be regarded as the relevant cause of harm to third parties, not the activity of selling alcohol. If speech is merely subject to this exception for intervening accountable parties, this does not constitute special protection. Of course, this requires it to be shown for speech as much as for nonspeech that the intervening second parties are indeed responsible for the relevant choice (not already drunk, for example) and hence accountable.[49] In the case of media violence, it would have to be shown that the choice to behave aggressively or violently was one for which the agent was responsible and accountable.

However, speech is being given special protection if this exception is *automatically* triggered by speech, in a way that it is not for nonspeech activity. It may be assumed that responses to the content of speech necessarily reflect autonomous choices, so that if responses by hearers to the content of speech intervene between speech and harm to third parties, then hearers rather than speakers are responsible and hence accountable for the harm. To assume that speech automatically gets the benefit of this intervening accountable parties exception is just to assume special protection for speech, on grounds of hearer autonomy.

But to the extent the evidence I have discussed brings the assumption of "hearer" (or viewer) autonomy into question, there is no shortcut to an automatic exception to the third-party-harm principle for speech, on grounds of intervening accountable parties. For harmful speech to get the benefit of the intervening accountable parties exception, there would have to be some reason other than an automatic assumption of autonomy to regard the hearers as accountable for their harmful choices.

This reply raises another important concern about recognizing the harmful bypass effects of media violence: a worry about undermining individual accountability for aggression by allowing aggressors to blame media violence. If we recognize that harmful effects may result from speech in ways that compromise audience autonomy, does that not threaten the accountability of individual hearers of speech for harmful acts they are thus influenced to do?

Not necessarily. Care is needed concerning the relationships between autonomy, responsibility, and accountability, which I cannot explore fully here. But more is required for autonomy than for responsibility or for accountability. An inference from autonomy to responsibility and hence to accountability may be valid, but it would not follow that the reverse inference was also valid: accountability does not require autonomy. Autonomy is an ideal that we often fall short of in making choices and acting intentionally. We do not regard people has not responsible or accountable for their choices whenever they fall short of autonomy. If we did, the world would be transformed beyond recognition. People often intentionally enter into contractual relationships, make purchasing decisions, commit crimes, get married, have children, and so on, under influences that compromise their autonomy. Nevertheless, they are often rightly regarded as responsible and accountable for the sub-autonomous choices they make and their consequences. When people are influenced by media violence toward aggression in ways that compromise their autonomy, it does not follow that they are not responsible or accountable for their intentional actions and the harm they cause. There is no automatic inference from account-ability to autonomy, or from lack of autonomy to lack of accountability. The specter of proliferating insanity defenses based on the bypass effects of media violence can be laid to rest: the argument would prove too much.

Let me take stock of the last few paragraphs. On the one hand, I argued that special protection of speech cannot be justified by assuming audience autonomy, so that speech would automatically trigger the intervening accountable parties excep-tion to the third-party-harm principle. Even if autonomy implies responsibility and hence accountability, audience autonomy cannot be assumed, given the prevalence of bypass effects, and thus does not justify assuming that "hearers" who mediate harmful bypass effects must be accountable; that question remains open. On the other hand, I argued that accountability does not require autonomy; so that influ-ences that compromise autonomy do not necessarily undermine individual respon-sibility or accountability for harmful acts. We are thus back to where we started: individuals subject to bypass effects may still be responsible and accountable for the harms they cause, despite their lack of autonomy. Conduct that responds to speech, like other conduct, is often subject to influences that compromise autonomy, but the agents are often nevertheless responsible for such conduct and rightly held account-able for its effects—though accountability may be shared. Speech is not special in respect of intervening accountable parties.

Further argument would be needed to show that certain ways of compromising autonomy do undermine accountability for resulting harmful acts. In contrast, while I cannot argue for it here, I favor a compatibilist conception of responsibility that upholds the responsibility and accountability of individual agents for many bypass effects—*at least given knowledge of the prevalence of such effects*—without thereby exonerating others of a duty to try to avoid such harms. It is important for purposes of *upholding* individual responsibility and accountability for bypass effects that the evidence concerning such effects become more widely known. Suppressing it is just the *wrong* thing for friends of individual responsibility to do.

More generally, I suggest that it is a serious mistake to assume that if an individ-ual agent is responsible for his action and rightly held accountable its harmful effects, then no further questions arise about how others might *also* be responsible and accountable or how those harmful effects can most effectively, and should, be avoided. While rightly holding individuals accountable for what they do, we should at the same time consider the social and cultural environment in which they act, and the influences it has on their action. Holding individuals accountable for the harms their acts cause should not exempt others further back in the causal chain from sharing accountability for avoidable harms to third parties. As a society, we are obligated to try to prevent serious harms to innocent members of society, to change the social environment in ways that predictably reduce such harms, while at the same time rightly holding individuals accountable for their actions. There is no incompatibility here. Responsibility for certain effects is not exclusive; nor is there a fixed quantity of it, which once allocated to an individual agent is somehow used up.[50] Rather, responsibility is a kind of normatively constrained causality that does not begin and end with individuals but emerges from dynamic and continuous interactions between individuals and their social environments. What is needed is an ecological approach to responsibility that spells out the way responsible individual agency is causally embedded in and grows out of social reason-giving practices and cultural norms. Governments cannot escape their own accountability for shaping such practices and norms in harm-avoiding ways by simply allocating accountability solely to individuals, as if individual responsibility were somehow independent of social context.

Parallel Tracks and Black Leather

Media violence may both engage autonomous deliberative processes and have effects that bypass such processes. As with pornography, "messages" may be inserted into violent entertainment to protect it against criticism and give it "speech value," and to make it easier for people to justify their enjoyment of it to themselves and others. If an instance of speech operates along parallel tracks in this way, does it engage the audience autonomy rationale for special protection or not? Does it rate a net positive or negative score for audience autonomy? Can special protection for violent news that operates along parallel tracks be defended in a way that also extends to violent entertainment?

Consider the recent film *The Matrix*. It has enough intellectual content to have inspired a number of philosophical essays. It also has a certain distinctive style, which involves lots of sunglasses, black leather, and violence. The sunglasses and black leather appear to be purely cosmetic; you could peel them off, or replace them with wire-rims and tweeds, without affecting the intellectual content of the film. Is the level of violence like this also? This *black leather test* might be developed to provide one possible response to the parallel tracks problem.

The Dangers of Censorship[51]

Empowering direct government censorship is itself dangerous; we are wise to distrust such power. If government routinely has power to decide degree of capture and of special protection, it seems inevitable that such power will be used politically. For example, films showing the horrors of war and implicitly critical of government policies on war could be censored on grounds that their violent content is likely to lead to harm to third parties.

However, direct government censorship is not the only regulative possibility. More effective self-regulation can be explored (Potter 2003, chapter 11). Civil product liability in tort, perhaps class-based, is another possibility (ibid., pp. 163–166), which raises further issues. Entertainment products aren't supposed to lead to violence; but is an entertainment product defective if it does? Has the entertainment industry misled the public concerning the effects of violent entertainment? It could also be argued that civil liability just distributes the power to decide degree of special protection across courts as a function of private litigation. Is that any less worrying than direct government censorship? On the other hand, is manipulation of the content of entertainment by the financial interests of the entertainment industry ("more powerful than many governments," as the refrain goes), or simply by market forces, any less worrying (Hamilton 1998)?

Concluding Remarks

There are many other relevant issues that I cannot pursue here. My aim has been to break ground by bringing recent research about imitation into contact with issues about media violence and freedom of speech.

The cognitive and social sciences have not yet put their heads together over imitation. In particular, work on imitation in cognitive science and neuroscience has not yet been assimilated or appreciated by the social sciences and philosophy, even though it raises fundamental questions, both theoretical and practical. How do the important roles of imitation for human being bear on our view of ourselves as autonomous, on individualistic values of liberal societies such as freedom of expression, on the relationship between violence in the media and aggression in society and related policies, on the social ecology of responsible agency?

Assumptions about autonomy and responsibility embedded in liberal political theory need rethinking in light of emerging evidence about the nature of human minds. A better understanding of what is distinctive about human minds may change our views of what threatens our autonomy and how best to protect it. If liberal values are survive and flourish in the face of these new discoveries about imitative learning, we need to begin to link questions about how we make up our minds with questions about how minds are made up.

Acknowledgments

This chapter revises and updates "Imitation, Media Violence, and Freedom of Speech" (*Philosophical Studies* 117, 2004: 165–218).

For helpful comments and discussion, I am grateful to Larry Alexander, Dick Arneson, John Bargh, Simon Blackburn, Susan Brison, Guy Claxton, George Comstock, Mark Greenberg, Celia Heyes, Rowell Huesmann, Rae Langton, Harry

Litman, Philip Pettit, Sue Pockett, Lawrence Solum, Wayne Sumners, Tillmann Vierkant, various anonymous referees, and members of audiences on various occasions when I have presented this paper. I am also grateful to the Gatsby Foundation, London, and to the Lifelong Learning Foundation, Manchester, for making possible the 2002 conference on imitation at Royaumont Abbey, discussions at which influenced my ideas for this article.

Notes

1. Thanks to Guy Claxton here.

2. The meta-analysis by Paik and Comstock (1994) covered 217 studies; Potter (2003) uses a rough figure of 300. Adding in reviews and analyses, it has been claimed (Potter 2003, pp. ix, 26), brings to figure up to about 3,000.

3. Cf. Potter 2003, chapter 5, on different understandings of violence.

4. While this focused on pornography rather than media violence, since much pornography represents violence, issues about whether pornography and media violence have harmful effects are closely related. See Comstock and Scharrer 2003 for the increased effect sizes of violent stimuli with erotic content.

5. Or perhaps not so surprisingly? It appears that many people simply do not want to believe that media violence has harmful effects. The disconnect between the strong consensus of scientific opinion and media reports on this question is documented methodically by Bushman and Anderson (2001, p. 485): "As it became clearer to the scientific community that media violence effects were real and significant, the new media reports actually got weaker." They consider possible explanations: vested financial interests in the media that influence public opinion (the motion picture industry has financed literature skeptical about the evidence that media violence causes aggression; see also Hamilton 1998), misapplication of fair reporting criteria that give disproportionate weight to vocal minority views, the failure of the scientific research community to argue its case effectively to the public. Bushman and Anderson also list six parallels between die-hard resistance to the evidence of harmful effects of media violence and of smoking, including efforts by holders of vested financial interests to influence public perceptions of the evidence. See also Huesmann and Taylor (2003) on the psychology of denial involved here. Potter 2003 insightfully analyzes and debunks the myths that keep various interest groups talking past one another on this subject.

6. For a different earlier view, see Howitt and Cumberbatch (cited by Williams 1981, p. 67). See also Potter 2003, pp. 28–29. (Howitt says that about 80 percent of the studies support this thesis.)

7. See also Berkowitz 1993, p. 201; see also Potter 2003, chapter 4, on the myth that the harmful effects of media violence are confined to children; Comstock and Scharrer 2003 on age. Cf. Williams 1981, pp. 88–89, who seems to assume that sexual maturation, if it could only be made precise, would imply that children would no longer need special protection from pornography.

8. The Johnson study did not directly measure viewer's exposure to TV violence, but rather how much TV different viewers watched. Arguably, there is so much violence on TV that the higher viewers can be assumed to have been exposed to more TV violence than the lower viewers. If this inference is regarded as problematic, see supporting longitudinal studies that look specifically at exposure to media violence: Huesmann et al. 2003; Eron et al. 1972. Cf. Renfrew 1997, p. 162, referring to older, less comprehensive data. Thanks here to Rowell Huesmann.

9. See Smith and Donnerstein 1998, p. 178 for the very conservative 10 percent figure, derived from the Huesmann longitudinal study. See also Berkowitz 1993, p. 233. See Comstock and Scharrer 2003 for a discussion of effect sizes; the overall effect size in the Paik and Comstock meta-analysis was 0.31, which is equivalent to aggressive behavior being exhibited by 65.5 percent of those above the median in exposure, but only by 34.4 percent of those below the median (Bushman and Huesmann 2001, p. 234).

10. However, pace Freedman (2002), evidence of aggressive play cannot simply be dismissed as irrelevant to real-world aggression; imagination and play contribute significantly to learning (see Pascuale-

Leone 2001; Jeannerod 1997, pp. 117, 119). Moreover, as Potter argues (2003, p. 73), "most people over-estimate the ability of adults to distinguish between reality and fantasy. Many adults exhibit the same problems that are attributed to children." See also Gilbert 1991; Gilbert et al. 1993.

11. Freedman's skeptical review (2002) is distorting in various ways, including that he assigns weights to results on the basis of how many tests were included in a given "study" (p. 54), fails to distinguish carefully lack of significant effect from significant evidence for no effect (see the slide in his categorizations from p. 55 to p. 57), misunderstands the causal role of arousal as a mechanism (pp. 51–52, 77, 80, 91, 102, 195; see also discussion below), wrongly dismisses play aggression as irrelevant (pp. 101, 105), shifts assumptions without justification (for example, compare p. 63 and p. 164 on whether children are more susceptible than adults to the influence of media violence, and pp. 81–83 and p. 207 on whether and in what contexts the content of movies carries social messages), employs varying standards of argument (see for example his claims on p. 132; p. 210; compare also his claims about advertising, p. 204, with, say, the evidence about its unwanted effects reviewed in Wilson and Brekke 1994; see also Gilbert 1991, Gilbert et al. 1993).

12. The statistical techniques for comparing these correlations have become more sophisticated over time. It is now considered good practice to compute structural or regression models to compare possible causal models, rather than simply comparing correlations (see Kline 1998). However, for present purposes this does not matter, because the conclusions of the studies under discussion have been shown to be the same with the more sophisticated techniques (Huesmann and Miller 1994). Thanks here to Rowell Huesmann.

13. In this study the same pattern did not hold for girls. See Geen 1990, pp. 97–99, 111.

14. Although the pure "reverse hypothesis" fares badly in light of the evidence: see Comstock and Scharrer 2003. See also Potter 2003, p. 120; Geen 1990, pp. 94, 99–100; Renfrew 161; Smith and Donnerstein 176.

15. See and cf. Smith and Donnerstein; Berkowitz 1993, pp. 209ff; Potter 2003. Such modulation may be useful in guiding regulatory approaches to media violence.

16. This may interact with an arousal mechanism; see Kinsbourne 2005 and discussion below. Freedman's (2002) argument concerning the role of arousal in relation to the influence of media violence is unpersuasive. He regards it as discrediting the influence of media violence on aggression. But of course exposure to media violence has effects via one or another mechanism; arousal may be one of these (as researchers have argued; see Huesmann and Taylor 2003), and arousal may also increase, as Kinsbourne claims, imitative tendencies. If media violence is almost invariably arousing and arousal tends to increase aggression (as Freedman suggests), then far from discrediting the influence of media violence, arousal may be among the mechanisms by which media violence has its effects, perhaps interacting with imitative tendencies. Knowing what the mechanism is by which media violence has its effects does not show that it does not have them.

17. On the relation between automatic processes and unconscious processes, see Wilson 2002, pp. 226: although there are certainly exceptions, "in general, it is fair to characterize most nonconscious thinking as automatic and most conscious thinking as controlled." I will go along with this generalization for present purposes.

18. There is more complexity here than I can indicate in this brief compass. *Imitation* is a contested concept; the various criteria proposed for full-blooded imitation do not always coincide, even with carefully controlled experiments (see Heyes 2001, 2005; Heyes and Galef 1996). See also Rizzolatti 2005 on possible neurophysiological correlates of means/ends structure within the mirror system.

19. Bargh (2005) comments on the striking similarities between the externally controlled behavior of Lhermitte's patients with frontal brain damage and of normal college students in priming experiments (described in the text).

20. Priming with specific exemplars (e.g. Albert Einstein) produces contrast or comparison effects, while priming with a generic category (e.g. scientists) produces assimilation effects.

21. Freedman (2002) appears to be unaware of these lines of research or their direct application to representations of violence, along with representations of other behaviors. For example, his unpersuasive comparisons of the effects of advertising with the effects of media violence, p. 204, are not informed by the results of this research or other related work, such as in Wilson and Brekke 1994.

22. Gordon (1995) argues that it takes a special containing mechanism to keep the emotion-recognition process from reverting to ordinary emotional contagion, and this mechanism is not fail-safe. If simulation theory is right, he holds, only a thin line separates one's own mental life from one's representation of the mental life of another, and "off-line" representations of other people have an inherent tendency to go "on-line."

23. See also chapter 2 of Potter 2003.

24. Thanks here to Dick Arneson and Larry Alexander.

25. See also the discussion of emotional mirroring in Gallese 2005 and Iacoboni 2005.

26. But see Voelkl and Huber 2000 for evidence of imitation in marmosets.

27. Mirror neurons appear to code for means in parietal areas, for goals in Broca's area—one of the main language areas of the brain (Iacoboni 2005).

28. See e.g. Gallese 2001, 2005; Hurley 2005; Gordon 1995; Goldman 2005, discussing autistics' deficiency at imitation in early years; Williams et al. 2001 on mirror neurons as basis for imitation and mindreading and autism as a deficit in an ontogenetic cascade. Consider also the finding of Chartrand and Bargh 1999, experiment 3, that those high in dispositional empathy imitated more than those low in empathy. Thanks here to John Bargh.

29. Or the homologue thereof in other primates.

30. A remark to this effect was made by Marco Iacoboni at the Royaumont conference (2002) on imitation. See Iacoboni 2005.

31. See also Christiansen 1994; Christiansen et al. 2002; Deacon 1997; Tomasello 1999 on establishing shared reference to an object through joint attention, established by gaze following and role-reversal imitation. Arbib (2002) has emphasized the recombinant decompositional structure of full-fledged imitation and the way it establishes a kind of first-person/third-person parity or intersubjectivity, which may help to explain how related features of language emerge.

32. Heyes (2005) explains how they might be acquired.

33. Mirror neurons may have originated in motor control functions, and been exapted for imitation (Rizzolatti 2005 and remarks at the Royaumont conference 2002; Gallese 2001; Hurley 2005, 2006). See also Boyd and Richerson 1985; Blackmore 1999.

34. In *Ashcroft v. Free Speech Coalition*, the US Supreme Court struck down a statute banning virtual child pornography (produced without using actual children). The *Ashcroft* Court assumed without substantial argument that any causal links between images of child abuse and actual child abuse are "indirect" and "remote," not "strong," and that the criminal act "does not necessarily follow" but "depends upon some unquantified potential for subsequent criminal acts." However, a robust causal link does not become indirect merely because it operates over a large population statistically rather than without exception. The Court in *Ashcroft* appears to be worryingly ignorant of the scientific research surveyed here. First Amendment jurisprudence is in danger of wedding itself to the now-exploded myth that the content of external representations, words or pictures, does not normally have "direct" effects on behavior but only effects that are under the actor's conscious control.

35. Causation is regularly established in science and medicine statistically, though the cause does not guarantee the effect in particular cases: consider the effects of drugs.

36. Brison (1998b) criticizes a spurious argument for giving special protection to freedom of speech, which assumes that either speech is causally inert, or, if it has harmful effects, does so only through autonomous rational processes. As she argues, speech is not causally inert, and has harmful effects that do not operate only through autonomous rational processes.

37. "Given that a background assumption of our constitutional democracy is a general principle of liberty stating that the government may justifiably interfere with individual liberties only to prevent people from harming others, if speech is harmless there is no need to give it special protection." (Brison 1998b, p. 40) See also Brison 1998a, pp. 314–316; Schauer 1982, pp. 63–65; 1984 1292–1293.

38. See also Barendt 1985.

39. Note that a response can be sensitive in nonautonomous, undeliberated ways to the content of information. Specific contents may trigger direct, automatic responses. If so, regulating certain contents can protect autonomy, and avoiding the regulation of certain contents can threaten autonomy. Again, the

idea of content-regulation does not line up cleanly with issues of autonomy in the way that is often presupposed in free speech jurisprudence.

40. See also Brison 1998a, pp. 327–328. In his later article Scanlon retracts his earlier Millian principle of freedom of speech. Its basic flaw, in his later view, was to regard autonomy as constraint on justifications for governmental interference rather than as a good to be promoted; doing so gave the audience interest in autonomy too great and constant a weight. I do not think that the distinction between consequentialist and deontological autonomy arguments for free speech affects the use I make of Scanlon's points here. Even if special protection is understood in deontological terms as a constraint, as in his older view, I am discussing the extent to which special protection can be justified in terms of autonomy to begin with. Scanlon also distinguishes categories of interests protected by freedom of speech (speaker, audience, bystander) from categories of acts of expression or kinds of speech. He is wary of the latter: the purposes and content of speech can be controversial, such distinctions are likely to be misapplied, and it is difficult hard to regulate one category of speech and not another and to avoid overbroad regulation. See also Alexander and Horton 1984; Alexander 1989, pp. 549–550.

41. Though Scanlon's emphasis on subliminal perception may be misplaced; recall that that consciously as well as subliminally perceived stimuli have robust priming effects on behavior.

42. Cf. the assumptions made by Alexander and Horton 1984, p. 1333, on mental mediation of harmful effects.

43. As things are in the US, the way the balance is struck depends critically on whether the harm in question flows from the content of speech or not. Compare: "[T]he possible harm to society in permitting some unprotected speech to go unpunished is outweighed by the possibility that protected speech of others may be muted. . . ." (*Broadrick v. Oklahoma*, 413 U. S. at 612). Here, third-party harm is outweighed. However, when images of child abuse are produced from actual child abuse, and the production rather than the content of the work was the target of a statute, "[T]he fact that a work contained serious literary, artistic, or other value did not excuse the harm it causes to its child participants" (*Ashcroft*, paraphrasing *New York v. Ferber*, 458 U. S. at 761). Here third-party harm outweighs literary or artistic value. The scientific work summarized above provides reason to doubt that the distinction between harm flowing from the content of speech and other harm can bear this much weight, since the content of speech often has *direct* influence on behavior that the actor is nevertheless unaware of and does not control. That is, the distinction between content and noncontent as the source of direct influence distinction does not align with the issue of whether the agent is aware of and in control of the influence. This point emerges clearly from the psychological literature, but appears to contradict an underlying jurisprudential assumption that effects that flow from content operate through autonomous processes.

44. Consider suicide contagion (Berkowitz 1993, pp. 204–205), or copycat crimes.

45. This argument was put to me by Larry Alexander.

46. See Potter 2003, p. 114.

47. Projecting statistical causation onto an individual case can produce an increased probability of causing harm in that case. Similarly, if a drug causes harmful side effects in one third of those who take it and we don't have any differentiating information about a particular case, there will be some probability of the drug causing harm in the particular case.

48. On standards and burdens of proof, see Schauer 1982; Alexander and Horton 1984, pp. 1335, 1339; Langton 1990, pp. 341–342, 347–348; Williams 1981, p. 59. Note that standard of proof beyond reasonable doubt in criminal law applies to proof that the accused has committed the illegal act, not to proof that the illegal act, on the assumption he has committed it, produces harm. The harmfulness of criminal acts is judged by the legislature when they decide to make them criminal. The normal standard governing civil liability is the preponderance of the evidence.

49. However, a relevant difference is in the level of general knowledge of the risks to third parties posed by drinking as opposed to those posed by viewing violent entertainment.

50. Here I am indebted to discussions with Susan Brison; see Brison 2005. See also Potter 2003, p. 52, on accountability vs. influence, and chapter 13, on sharing responsibility and the need for a public health perspective.

51. Thanks to Mark Greenberg for discussion of these points.

References

Akins, C., Klein, E., and Zentall, T. 2002. Imitative learning in Japanese quail (*Conturnix japonica*) using the bidirectional control procedure. *Animal Learning and Behavior* 30: 275–281.

Alexander, L. 1989. Low value speech. *Northwestern University Law Review* 547–554.

Alexander, L., and Horton, P. 1984. The impossibility of a free speech principle. *Northwestern University Law Review* 1319–1357.

Anderson, C., Berkowitz, L., Donnerstein, E., Huesmann, L. R., Johnson, J., Linz, D., Malamuth, N., and Wartella, E. 2003. The influence of media violence on youth. *Psychological Science in the Public Interest* 4, no. 3: 81–110.

Anderson, C., and Bushman, B. 2001. Effects of violent video games on aggressive behavior, aggressive cognition, aggressive affect, physiological arousal, and prosocial behavior: A meta-analytic review of the scientific literature. *Psychological Science* 12, no. 5: 353–359.

Anderson, C., and Bushman, B. 2002. The effects of media violence on society. *Science* 295: 2377–2378.

Arbib, M. 2002. The mirror system, imitation, and the evolution of language. In *Imitation in Animals and Artifacts*, ed. C. Nehaniv and K. Dautenhahn. MIT Press.

Arbib, M. Forthcoming. From monkey-like action recognition to human language: An evolutionary framework for neurolinguistics, behavioral and brain sciences. *Behavioral and Brain Sciences*.

Arbib, M., and Rizzolatti, G. 1997. Neural expectations: a possible evolutionary path from manual skills to language. *Communication and Cognition* 29: 393–424.

Ashcroft v. Free Speech Coalition, 122 S. Ct. 1389 (2002).

Baldwin, J. 1896. A new factor in evolution. *American Naturalist* 30: 441–451, 536–553.

Bandura, A., Ross, D., and Ross, S. A. 1963. Imitation of film-mediated aggressive models. *Journal of Abnormal and Social Psychology* 66: 3–11.

Barendt, E. 1985. *Freedom of Speech*. Clarendon.

Bargh, J. 1999. The most powerful manipulative messages are hiding in plain sight. *Chronicle of Higher Education*, January 29: B6.

Bargh, J. 2005. Bypassing the will: Towards demystifying the nonconscious control of social behavior. In *The New Unconscious*, ed. R. Hassin et al. Oxford University Press.

Bargh, J., and Chartrand, T. 1999. The unbearable automaticity of being. *American Psychologist*, July: 462–479.

Bargh, J., Chen, M., and Burrows, L. 1996. Automaticity of social behavior: Direct effects of trait construct and stereotype activation on action. *Journal of Personality and Social Psychology* 71, no. 2: 230–244.

Berkowitz, L. 1993. *Aggression: Its Causes, Consequences, and Control*. McGraw-Hill.

Blackmore, S. 1999. *The Meme Machine*. Oxford University Press.

Boyd, R., and Richerson, P. 1982. Cultural transmission and the evolution of cooperative behavior. *Human Ecology* 10: 325–351.

Boyd, R., and Richerson, P. 1985. *Culture and the Evolutionary Process*. University of Chicago Press.

Brison, S. 1998a. The autonomy defense of free speech. *Ethics* 108, no. 1: 312–339.

Brison, S. 1998b. Speech, harm, and the mind-body problem in first amendment jurisprudence. *Legal Theory* 4: 39–61.

Brison, S. 2005. Comment on Kinsbourne. In *Perspectives on Imitation: From Neuroscience to Social Science*, volume 2, ed. S. Hurley and N. Chater. MIT Press.

Broadrick v. Oklahoma (1973), 413 U.S. 601.

Bullinger, M. 1985. Freedom of expression and information: An essential element of democracy. *Human Rights Law* 6 J. 339.

Bushman, B., and Anderson, C. 2001. Media violence and the American public: Scientific facts vs. media misinformation. *American Psychologist* 56, no. 6–7: 477–489.

Bushman, B., and Huesmann, L. R. 2001. Effects of television violence on aggression. In *Handbook of Children and the Media*, ed. D. Singer and J. Singer. Sage.

Byrne, R. 1995. *The Thinking Ape: Evolutionary Origins of Intelligence.* Oxford University Press.

Carver, C., Ganellen, R., Froming, W., and Chambers, W. 1983. Modelling: An analysis in terms of category accessibility. *Journal of Experimental Social Psychology* 19: 403–421.

Chartrand, T., and Bargh, J. 1996. Automatic activation of impression formation and memorization goals: Nonconscious goal priming reproduces effects of explicit task instructions. *Journal of Personality and Social Psychology* 71: 464–478.

Chartrand, T., and Bargh, J. 1999. The chameleon effect. *Journal of Personality and Social Psychology* 76, no. 6: 893–910.

Chartrand, T., and Bargh, J. 2002. Nonconscious motivations: Their activation, operation, and consequences. In *Self and Motivation*, ed. A. Tesser et al. American Psychological Associatiion.

Chen, M., and Bargh, J. 1997. Nonconscious behavioral confirmation processes: The self-fulfilling nature of automatically-activated stereotypes. *Journal of Experimental Social Psychology* 33: 541–560.

Christiansen, M. 1994. Infinite Languages, Finite Minds: Connectionism, Learning and Linguistic Structure. PhD dissertation. University of Edinburgh.

Christiansen, M., Dale, R., Ellefson, M., and Conway, C. 2002. The role of sequential learning in language evolution: Computational and experimental studies. In *Simulating the evolution of language*, ed. A. Cangelosi and D. Parisi. Springer.

Comstock, G., and Scharrer, E. 2003. Meta-analyzing the controversy over television violence and aggression. In *Media Violence and Children*, ed. D. Gentile. Praeger.

Dautenhahn, K., and Nehaniv, C. 2002. *Imitation in Animals and Artifacts.* MIT Press.

Dawkins, R. 1982. *The Extended Phenotype.* Oxford University Press.

Deacon, T. 1997. *The Symbolic Species: The Coevolution of Language and the Human Brain.* Penguin.

Dijksterhuis, A. 2005. Why we are social animals: The high road to imitation as social glue. In *Perspectives on Imitation: From Neuroscience to Social Science*, volume 2, ed. S. Hurley and N. Chater. MIT Press.

Dijksterhuis, A., and Bargh, J. 2001. The perception-behavior expressway: Automatic effects of social perception on social behavior. *Advances in Experimental Social Psychology* 33: 1–40.

Dijksterhuis, A., and van Knippenberg, A. 1998. The relation between perception and behavior, or how to win a game of Trivial Pursuit. *Journal of Personality and Social Psychology* 74: 865–877.

Eidelberg, L. 1929. Experimenteller beitrag zum Mechanismus der Imitationsbewewung. *Jahresbücher für Psychiatrie und Neurologie* 45: 170–173.

Ely, J. H. 1981. *Democracy and Distrust.* Harvard University Press.

Eron, L. D., Huesmann, L. R., Lefkowitz, M. M., and Walder, L. O. 1972. Does TV violence cause aggression? *American Psychologist* 27: 153–263.

Fadiga, L., Fogassi, L., Pavesi, G., and Rizzolatti, G. 1995. Motor facilitation during action observation: A magnetic stimulation study. *Journal of Neurophysiology* 73: 2608–2611.

Fiss., O. 1987. Why the state? *Harvard Law Review* 100: 781–94.

Fiss, O. 1998. *The Irony of Free Speech.* Harvard University Press.

Fiss, O. 1991. State activism and state censorship" *Yale Law Journal* 100 2087–2106.

Freedman, J. L. 2002. *Media Violence and Its Effect on Aggression.* Toronto University Press.

Galef, B. 2005. Breathing new life into the study of animal imitation: What and when do chimpanzees imitate? In *Perspectives on Imitation: From Neuroscience to Social Science*, volume 1, ed. S. Hurley and N. Chater. MIT Press.

Gallese, V. 2001. The shared manifold hypothesis: From mirror neurons to empathy. *Journal of Consciousness Studies* 8: 33–50.

Gallese, V. 2005. "Being like me": Self-other identity, mirror neurons and empathy. In *Perspectives on Imitation: From Neuroscience to Social Science*, volume 1, ed. S. Hurley and N. Chater. MIT Press.

Gallese, V., and Goldman, A. 1998. Mirror neurons and the simulation theory of mind-reading. *Trends in Cognitive Science* 12: 493–501.

Geen., R. 1990. *Human Aggression.* Open University Press.

Geen, R., and Donnerstein, E., eds. 1998. *Human Aggression.* Academic Press.

Geen, R., and Thomas, S. L. 1986. The immediate effects of media violence on behavior. *Journal of Social Issues* 42, no. 3: 7–27.

Gergely, G., Bekkering, H., and Király, I. 2002. Rational imitation in preverbal infants. *Nature* 415: 755.

Gilbert, D. 1991. How mental systems believe. *American Psychologist* 46, no. 2: 107–119.

Gilbert, D., Tafarodi, R., and Malone, P. 1993. You can't not believe everything you read. *Journal of Personality and Social Psychology* 65, no. 2: 221–233.

Goldman, A. 2005. Imitation, mindreading, and simulation. In *Perspectives on Imitation: From Neuroscience to Social Science*, volume 2, ed. S. Hurley and N. Chater. MIT Press.

Gordon, R. 1995. Sympathy, simulation, and the impartial spectator. *Ethics* 105: 727–742.

Gordon, R. 2005. Intentional agents like myself. In *Perspectives on Imitation: From Neuroscience to Social Science*, volume 2, ed. S. Hurley and N. Chater. MIT Press.

Greenawalt, K. 1989. Free Speech Justifications. *Columbia Law Review* 1989: 119–155.

Gunter, B., and McAleer, J. 1997. *Children and the Faces of Television*, second edition. Routledge.

Hamilton, J. T. 1998. *Channelling Violence: The Economic Market for Violent Programming.* Princeton University Press.

Herman, L. 2002. Vocal, social, and self-imitation by bottlenosed dolphins. In *Imitation in Animals and Artifacts*, ed. K. Dautenhahn and C. Nehaniv. MIT Press.

Heyes, C. 2001. Causes and consequences of imitation. *Trends in Cognitive Sciences* 5, no. 6: 227–280.

Heyes, C. 2005. Imitation by association. In *Perspectives on Imitation: From Neuroscience to Social Science*, volume 1, ed. S. Hurley and N. Chater. MIT Press.

Heyes, C., and Galef, C. B., eds. 1996. *Social Learning in Animals: The Roots of Culture.* Academic Press.

Hobson, R. P., and Lee, A. 1999. Imitation and identification in autism. *Journal of Child Psychology and Psychiatry* 40, no. 4: 649–659.

Howitt, D. 1998. *Crime, the Media, and the Law.* Wiley.

Huesmann, L. R. 1998. The role of social information processing and cognitive schema in the acquisition and maintenance of habitual aggressive behavior. In *Human Aggression*, ed. R. Geen and E. Donnerstein. Academic Press.

Huesmann, L. R. 2005. Imitation and the effects of observing media violence on behavior. In *Perspectives on Imitation: From Neuroscience to Social Science*, volume 2, ed. S. Hurley and N. Chater. MIT Press.

Huesmann, L. R., and Miller, L. 1994. Long term effects of repeated exposure to media violence in childhood. In *Aggressive Behavior: Current Perspectives*, ed. L. Huesmann. Plenum.

Huesmann, R., and Malamuth, N. 1986. Media violence and anti-social behavior: an overview. *Journal of Social Issues* 42, no. 3: 125–140.

Huesmann, L. R., Moise, J., Podolski, C. P., and Eron, L. D. 2003. Longitudinal relations between children's exposure to television violence and their aggressive and violent behavior in young adulthood: 1977–1992. *Developmental Psychology* 39, no. 2: 201–221.

Huesmann, L. R., and Taylor, L. D. 2003. The case against the case against media violence. In *Media Violence and Children*, ed. D. Gentile. Praeger.

Hunt, G., and Gray, R. 2003. Diversification and cumulative evolution in New Caledonian crow tool manufacture. *Proceedings of the Royal Society London* B 270: 867–874.

Hurley, S. 2005. The shared circuits model: How control, mirroring and simulation can enable imitation and mindreading. Available at www.interdisciplines.org.

Hurley, S. 2006. Active perception and perceiving action: The shared circuits hypothesis. In *Perceptual Experience*, ed. T. Gendler and J. Hawthorne. Oxford University Press.

Hurley, S., and Chater, N., eds. 2005. *Perspectives on Imitation: From Neuroscience to Social Science*. Two volumes. MIT Press.

Iacoboni, M. 2005. Understanding others: Imitation, language, empathy. In *Perspectives on Imitation: From Neuroscience to Social Science*, volume 1, ed. S. Hurley and N. Chater. MIT Press.

Iacoboni, M., Woods, R., Brass, M., Bekkering, H., Mazziotta, J., and Rizzolatti, G. 1999. Cortical mechanisms of human imitation. *Science* 286: 2526–2528.

Jeannerod, M. 1997. *The Cognitive Neuroscience of Action*. Blackwell.

Johnson, J., et al. 2002. The effects of media violence on society. *Science* 295: 2468.

Kinsbourne, M. 2005. Imitation as entrainment: Brain mechanisms and social consequences. In *Perspectives on Imitation: From Neuroscience to Social Science*, volume 2, ed. S. Hurley and N. Chater. MIT Press.

Kline, R. G. 1998. *Principles and Practice of Structural Equation Modeling*. Guilford.

Langton, R. 1990. Whose right? Ronald Dworkin, women, and pornographers. *Philosophy and Public Affairs* 19, no. 4: 311–359.

Lhermitte, F. 1986. Human autonomy and the frontal lobes, part II. *Annals of Neurology* 19, no. 4: 335–343.

Lhermitte, F., Pillon, B., and Serdaru, M. 1986. Human autonomy and the frontal lobes, part I. *Annals of Neurology* 19, no. 4: 326–334.

Luria, A. 1973. *The Working Brain*. Penguin.

Meiklejohn, A. 1948. *Free Speech and Its Relation to Self-Government*. Harper.

Meltzoff, A. 1988. Infant imitation after a 1-week delay: Long-term memory for novel acts and multiple stimuli. *Developmental Psychology* 24: 470–476.

Meltzoff, A. 1996. The human infant as imitative generalist: A 20-year progress report on infant imitation with implications for comparative psychology. In *Social Learning in Animals*, ed. B. Galef and C. Heyes. Academic Press.

Meltzoff, A. 2005. Imitation and other minds: The "like me" hypothesis. In *Perspectives on Imitation: From Neuroscience to Social Science*, volume 2, ed. S. Hurley and N. Chater. MIT Press.

Meltzoff, A., and Decety, J. 2003. What imitation tells us about social cognition: A rapprochement between developmental psychology and cognitive neuroscience. *Philosophical Transactions of the Royal Society of London* B 358: 491–500.

Meltzoff, A., and Gopnik, A. 1993. The role of imitation in understanding persons and developing a theory of mind. In *Understanding Other Minds: Perspectives from Autism*, ed. S. Baron-Cohen et al. Oxford University Press.

Meltzoff, A., and Moore, M. 1977. Imitation of facial and manual gestures by human neonates. *Science* 198: 75–78.

Meltzoff, A., and Moore, M. 1999. Persons and representation: Why infant imitation is important for theories of human development. In *Imitation in Infancy*, ed. J. Nadel and G. Butterworth. Cambridge University Press.

Meltzoff, A. N., and Prinz, W., eds. 2001. *The Imitative Mind: Development, Evolution, and Brain Bases*. Cambridge University Press.

Mill, J. S. 1849. *On Liberty* (Hackett, 1978).

Nagell, K., Olguin, R., and Tomasello, M. 1993. Processes of social learning in the tool use of chimpanzees (*Pan troglodytes*) and human children (*Homo sapiens*). *Journal of Comparative Psychology* 107: 174–186.

Nehaniv, C., and Dautenhahn, K. 2002. The correspondence problem. In *Imitation in Animals and Artifact*, ed. K. Dautenhahn and C. Nehaniv. MIT Press.

New York v. Ferber 1982), 458 U.S. 747.

Paik, H., and Comstock, G. 1994. The effects of television violence on anti-social behavior: A meta-analysis. *Communication Research* 21, no. 4: 516–546.

Pascual-Leone, A. 2001. The brain that plays music and is changed by it. *Annals of the New York Academy of Sciences* 930: 315–329.

Pepperberg, I. 1999. *The Alex Studies: Cognitive and Communicative Studies on Grey Parrots.* Harvard University Press.

Philo, G. 1999. *Message Received.* Longman.

Potter, W. J. 2003. *The 11 Myths of Media Violence.* Sage.

Prinz, W. 1990. A common coding approach to perception and action. In *Relations between Perception and Action*, ed. O. Neumann and W. Prinz. Springer.

Prinz, W. 2005. An ideomotor approach to imitation. In *Perspectives on Imitation: From Neuroscience to Social Science*, volume 1, ed. S. Hurley and N. Chater. MIT Press.

Renfrew, J. 1997. *Aggression and Its Causes.* Oxford University Press.

Rizzolatti, G. 2005. The mirror neuron system and imitation. In *Perspectives on Imitation: From Neuroscience to Social Science*, volume 1, ed. S. Hurley and N. Chater. MIT Press.

Rizzolatti, G., and Arbib, M. 1998. Language within our grasp. *Trends in Neuroscience* 21: 188–194.

Rizzolatti, G., and Arbib, M. 1999. From grasping to speech: Imitation might provide a missing link: Reply. *Trends in Neuroscience* 22: 152.

Rizzolatti, G., Fadiga, L., Fogassi, L., and Gallese, V. 2002. From mirror neurons to imitation: Facts and speculations. In *The Imitative Mind*, ed. A. Meltzoff and W. Prinz. Cambridge University Press.

Rizzolatti, G., Fogassi, L, and Gallese, V. 2001. Neurophysiological mechanisms underlying the understanding and imitation of action. *Nature Reviews: Neuroscience* 2: 661–670.

Rosenthal, R. 1986. Media violence, antisocial behavior, and the social consequences of small effects. *Journal of Social Issues* 42, no. 3: 141–154.

Scanlon, T. 1972. A theory of freedom of expression. *Philosophy and Public Affairs* 1: 204.

Scanlon, T. 1979. Freedom of expression and categories of expression. *University of Pittsburgh Law Review* 40: 519.

Schauer, F. 1982. *Free Speech: A Philosophical Inquiry.* Cambridge University Press.

Schauer, F. 1984. Must speech be special? *Northwestern University Law Review* 1284–1306.

Smith, S., and Donnerstein, E. 1998. Harmful effects of exposure to media violence./ In *Human Aggression*, ed. R. Geen and E. Donnerstein. Academic Press.

Stengel, E., Vienna, M., and Edin, L. 1947. A clinical and psychological study of echo-reactions. *Journal of Mental Science* 93: 598–612.

Tomasello, M. 1999. *The Cultural Origins of Human Cognition.* Harvard University Press.

Tomasello, M., and Call, J. 1997. *Primate Cognition.* Oxford University Press.

Voelkl, B., and Huber, L. 2000. True imitation in marmosets. *Animal Behaviour* 60: 195–202.

Vonnegut, K. 1966. *Mother Night.* Delacorte.

Weir, A., Chappell, J., and Kacelnik, A. 2002. Shaping of hooks in New Caledonian crows. *Science* 297: 981.

Whiten, A., and Brown, J. 1999. Imitation and the reading of other minds. In *Intersubjection Communication and Emotion in Early Ontogeny*, ed. S. Braken. Cambridge University Press.

Whiten, A., and Byrne, R., eds. 1997. *Machiavellian intelligence II: Extensions and evaluations.* Cambridge University Press.

Whiten, A., Horner, V., and Marshall-Pescini, S. 2005. Selective imitation in child and chimpanzee: A window on the construal of others' actions. In *Perspectives on Imitation: From Neuroscience to Social Science*, volume 1, ed. S. Hurley and N. Chater. MIT Press.

Williams, B., ed. 1981. *Obscenity and Film Censorship: An Abridgement of the Williams Report.* Cambridge University Press.

Williams, J., Whiten, A., Suddendorf, T., and Perrett, D. 2001. Imitation, mirror neurons, and autism. *Neuroscience and Biobehavioral Reviews* 25: 287–295.

Wilson, T. 2002. *Strangers to Ourselves: Discovering the Adaptive Unconscious.* Harvard University Press.

Wilson, T., and Brekke, N. 1994. Mental contamination and mental correction: unwanted influences on judgements and evaluations. *Psychological Bulletin* 116, July: 117–142.

16 Neurosociety Ahead? Debating Free Will in the Media

Sabine Maasen

Prologue: Is Mrs. Smith's Limbic System in Love?

Brain researchers may say "such and such neurophysiological processes in such and such brain area indicate that the subject is in love or sees green objects." However, it is inadmissible to say "being in love, seeing green objects or wanting something is nothing but activation of such and such neurons," as being in love, seeing green objects, and wanting something is in need of a certain subjective experience.
—Roth 2004, p. 80

1   The New Fad

High time for a new vogue in science: About 20 years after chaos theory was embraced as *the* new theory of the nonlinear, valid for science, society, and understanding selves alike, brain research is about to conquer our visions. Earlier, chaos theory, too, made it into the media and evoked breathtaking discussions on far more than just theoretical issues. It soon assumed the status of a worldview called "chaotics" (Hayles 1991), applicable to the explanation of almost everything: the shape of clouds, the behavior of crowds, the management of stocks, and the therapy of traumata and shocks (Maasen and Weingart 2000).

The dust has long since settled. Nowadays, it is brain research that is hailed as the ultimate answer to understanding science, society, and selves. Again, yet another unity of science seems in sight, the neurosciences taking the lead this time. Yet another way of governing societies appears to suggest itself: neurodidactics, neurotheology, neuroeconomy, and neurotechnology stimulate respective endeavors, be they industrial, spiritual, educational, or "neuroceutical." Finally, one more illusion is about to be unmasked: the self, formerly held to be governed by free will, which is now revealed as fiction, albeit of a useful kind. Call it hype or horror: the recent fad, provocatively stated, is ultimately about brainy selves happily living in neurosociety explained by the neurosciences and largely regulated by neurotechnologies.

In truth, while this abbreviated story line is, as yet, only a daydream of single entrepreneurs in the domain of consulting (Lynch 2004), it has already had its effects on the general media discourse, at least in Germany. Various applications of the neurosciences have attracted the journalists' interest. More often than not, the findings have been glossed over in a more humoristic note. Neuro-marketing, for instance, is being mocked as revealing insights that are not really new with the help of costly experimentation and instrumentation. For example, neuro-marketing seems to have found out that favorite brands are favored by our brains, too (Schnabel 2003).

The debate becomes far more serious, however, once other applications are discussed: Should we conceive of criminals as responsible and guilty, or "just" as deviant and dangerous? Should we educate our children according to their self-proclaimed needs and talents as their developing brains always know best what they need (Singer 2002, Roth 2003)? Issues such as these are not treated as more or less probable *applications* of brain research. Rather, they are debated as highly questionable, albeit as yet only thinkable, *implications* of brain research for notions of person, responsibility, and, last but not least, free will. The latter implication in particular proves disquieting for most.

Thus, the self (that is, the conscious, volitional individual and its agency) has come under attack—and not for the first time! About 20 years ago, postmodernists had already declared the death of the subject. In this view, the self is a fiction invented post hoc. Rather than acting on the basis of "own" intentions, motives or habits, the subject came to be thought of as driven by relations of power and knowledge. To postmodernists, these very intentions, motives or habits are not the source of a pure and self-conscious individuality, but the result of subconscious desires and discourses external to the self. The subject is merely a crossing of these structures.

Although this debate has not been resolved, other issues such as agency and empowerment (or lack thereof) have become more prevalent concerns. These debates rest on the assumption that the self, the acting, willing and reflecting self, needs to be more than just a crossing of desires and discourses. At least, the self is said to have, and indeed cultivate, a capacity to reflect and sort out inner and outer conditions for his or her actions, rather than being fully determined by them. To this end, all kinds of educational, therapeutic and self-instructing practices emerged, currently flooding Western societies: This recent hype of self-help offers indicates the creed that the self can be advised to determine his or her own actions—within the limits of inner or outer constraints, of course. This call for self-regulating, willing selves is a political one. Indeed, juridical and moral practices ascribing guilt, or the organization of everyday life attributing responsibilities, for instance, can hardly be understood without taking recourse to a subject who consciously steers his or her own courses of action.

However, as social practice arrives at this kind of position, another challenge occurs: this time, the self, the conscious, volitional individual and its agency, are being attacked by the neuro-cognitive "front." In their view, the self and its free will are fictions invented by the brain. Consciousness as well as "free will" and volitional decision making are but observations post factum, recollections of something already accomplished by the brain. Accordingly, neuroscientific findings claim the concepts of self, free will and consciousness to be scientifically untenable, specifying that it is our brain rather than our "self" who decides what we want, what we do, and who it is who says 'I'.

Today, free will and consciousness have become the focus of a concerted scientific effort. Inspired by the "cognitive turn" in psychology, the "decade of the brain," and the institutionalization of the "cognitive sciences," neurobiologists, cognitive psychologists and cognitively inclined philosophers all counter our long-cherished intuitions about what volition and consciousness are, thus challenging this "inner feel," this special quality accompanying perception, volition, reflection, and action. Notably, they insist on consciousness and the notion of free will (or the representation thereof) as being nothing but the name for the interplay of various regions in the brain on which cognitive functions operate. Willing and doing are fully determined by the brain. Other than that, talking about experiential or phenomenal aspects of consciousness and free will is relegated to folk psychological wisdom. Now that heuristics, techniques, and instruments are available, the issues proper (that is, the neural correlates of consciousness and free will) can and should be addressed (Crick and Koch 1998; Milner 1995; for an overview, see Zeman 2001).

Yet the skeptics, it seems, are not convinced. Are we indeed, and do we simply act on, an assembly of neurons and cognitive functions? In fact, as most philosophers keep reminding the neuroscientists, we are still discussing the age-old paradox of the "mind-body problem": while we believe ourselves to be physical beings, we also believe that we are conscious, willing entities whose awareness of physical beings cannot be physical. Thus it appears that we are both physical and non-physical. This brings up the problem as to how the physical and non-physical relate? After all, the two dimensions have no means of "communication."

In view of all the challenges and tensions the notion of free will, selves and societies faced with, it is about time to sort out the debate following the neuro-cognitive challenge. With respect to what the debate is essentially about, the recent discussion staged in Germany's leading feuilletons (magazine or essay pages of a newspaper) is revelatory. From a discourse analytical perspective, the debate, while still being highly controversial, gives rise to the conviction that the dominant views of volition and selves have to be reconsidered. It is not so much the empirical findings that cause the stir, but the at times far-reaching conclusions brain researchers derive from them. While the leading proponents of the debate still advance their positions in the service of public enlightenment (e.g. to free us from the illusionary concept called free will) and hope for consensus among scholars from the sciences and the humanities, a discourse analytical approach arrives at a different conclusion. Discussing free will in the media is not only an important way of popularizing the issue but also a way to promote brain research in general. It enforces the adoption of strong, opposing views: in this instance, the notion of free will as an illusion versus the plea not to mix neurophysiological and personal levels of description. Given this basic opposition, the key proponents argue about more detailed theoretical, but most of all, about implications concerning science policy and politics as well as specific societal consequences. A quick glance at everyday practices concerning the exertion of free will may give hints as to how to further the debate. In view of what lies ahead (neuro society), we are badly in need of an all-encompassing and ongoing debate about what follows for science, societies, and selves. In fact, this debate has only just begun.

2   Why Talk about Free Will in the Media?

The debate about the (possible) implications of forefront brain research reached the general public only late. Although a number of more popular accounts of the human brain have been issued in the 1990s, and despite the fact that it became a topic in talk shows, internet chats, radio features and brain researchers were also welcomed at Lion's Club meetings or at public panels, not very many people seemed to have been interested in discussing the consequences of novel findings in brain research—neither with respect to human self-understanding nor to social practice at large (Kuhlmann 2004).

Starting in mid 2003, three major German newspapers (*Der Spiegel, Frankfurter Allgemeine Zeitung* (*FAZ*), and *Die Zeit*) drew attention to this research.[1] *FAZ*, in particular, staged a debate that otherwise may never have surfaced on the more general agenda.[2] In fact, a marked distinction remained: unlike many of the preceding controversies (gene technology, stem cell debate etc.) the debate about brain research did not so much arouse much general interest as take place largely within the self-contained forum of expert discourse. Neuroscientists, philosophers, theologians, lawyers, and pedagogues enacted a debate that might have a deep impact on understanding ourselves (free will), and applied branches of brain research proclaimed bold consequences on didactics and on economics—but only a few insiders seemed to care. Most profoundly, neuroscientific findings were said not only to alter our understanding of individual responsibility but also society's ways of dealing with deviant behavior—but even at this point, only a few criminologists concerned themselves with these issues. All in all, the debate as a whole was characterized by a considerable academic standard, but made a somewhat sterile impression. Without any backing by protest movements (ecologically minded, women, handicapped persons, as in the Human Genome Project), non-governmental organizations, or citizen's juries, the key discussants simply replaced the academic ivory tower with the magazine pages of the leading print media (Kuhlmann 2004, p. 143).

As is usual in media discussion, the debate was characterized by opposing factions, strong views and far-reaching conclusions. Owing to the lack of resonance in the broader public, the setting of the agenda with regard to what might be foreseeable consequences was largely left to the key spokesmen, notably Wolf Singer, Gerhard Roth, and, on the sidelines and more moderately, Wolfgang Prinz. In their view, the neurosciences revealed free will as being non-existent. While Singer and Roth convey the message "Free will is an illusion—let's rebuild societies accordingly" (e.g., let's refrain from ascribing will and guilt to persons), Prinz is careful to distinguish two different spheres: the neurophysiological and the political sphere: In his perspective, free will is an illusion in the neurophysiological sphere, yet necessary in the political sphere. In the latter, we can ill afford to let go of notions such as free will and guilt as they regulate social life. True to this reasoning, Prinz (2004) pleads for keeping the two spheres apart, taking both of them and their logics of functioning seriously.

Although this debate took place in inner circles of scientific, mostly interdisciplinary, conferences and journals as well, it never reached there the resonance and prominence it assumed in the media. One reason for this difference may be found in the fact that free will is ultimately conceived of as an academic question, to which there are many and decisive answers, but no consensus in sight. Within the sciences as well as between the sciences and philosophy and other more culturally oriented disciplines, "free will" seems to afford no more (but no less) than boundary work (Gieryn 1983, p. 405). All factions feel challenged to negotiate, that is, they either take to defending the neurocognitive challenge or they object to it. It is worth noting that boundary work is more than just an academic enterprise. In modern knowledge, society negotiations of this kind often actively look for public attention. This is more than an exhibition bout, however. Convincing the public (political, industrial, general) means enlisting public acceptance for one's discipline, which in turn may pay off in political and financial support for research.

Negotiating science in the media is characterized by two basic dilemmas. The first dilemma is about popularization and accuracy. Time and time again, scientists complain of sensationalism, inaccuracy, and oversimplification. As Stephen Hilgartner has convincingly shown, popularization and accuracy are not strict opposites. Rather, they are connected by a continuum of intermediate forms (Hilgartner 1990), ranging from more simplistic accounts in science (i.e., textbook knowledge) to scientific presentations in public spaces (e.g., science museums). The same is true for the debate about free will—it ranged from high-standard expositions in the feuil-leton to easy-to-understand introductions in scientific journals.

Another dilemma pertains to the relation of knowledge and non-knowledge. As early as 1966, Julius Lukasiewicz observed that exponential growth in the volume and complexity of information creates the prospect of "instant antiquity." In addi-tion, one's degree of grasp "is quickly diminishing while one's (degree of) ignorance is on the fast side" (Lukasiewicz 1966, p. 122). One should note, though, that an overall rise in ignorance indicates neither how it is constructed or distributed nor whether it is intentional, amounting to a refusal to know things. However, it does point to the increasing necessity to use one's span of attention economically. As is well known, attention economy puts a premium on entertainment. Given this so-called knowledge-ignorance paradox, free will is quite an esoteric topic. The debate on free will uses two main strategies to win the public over: (a) "infotainment" in order to render serious issues "hot news" (see, e.g., articles on neuromarketing) or present the challenge as new although it is not (Hagner 2004), and (b) "visible sci-entists" who "stand for" a certain idea, position or vision. Visible scientists are gen-erally said to be articulate, colorful, and more or less "controversy-prone" (Goodell 1977) as is the case with Singer and his colleagues.

3   Public Understanding of the Brain Sciences

In a certain sense, debating scientific issues in the media, particularly if the break-throughs announced are still pending rather than factual, may seem a risky endeavor—a risk the neurosciences share with other key technologies, such as nan-otechnology, for instance. Yet in modern knowledge cum media society, there are scarcely better ways to keep oneself on the agenda. Even more so, given today's calls for science to enlighten the public. Since the lay public has not only become more and more alienated from specialized research performed in the "ivory tower," but has equally grown aware of risks connected to certain technologies (e.g. gene technology), it is increasingly reluctant to lend unconditional support without any knowledge about the issues at stake. In this vein, the discussion about "free will" is also an example of PUS, short for "public understanding of science."

Since 1985, as indicated by the so-called Bodmer Report, scientists have a duty to communicate with the public about their work (Bodmer 1985). In order to counter the lamented "scientific illiteracy" of the general public, scientists were called to "pour" knowledge from the lab-world to the life-world, employing enlight-ening presentations as the prime vehicle (see, e.g., Miller 2001). Although ranging from oral to written or performative (as in science museums), and from blunt information to edutainment, most attempts adhered to a one-way-street type of communication.

This model of science communication soon turned out to be deficient in itself. Notably, historians, philosophers, and sociologists of science showed that the scientific process departed markedly from the hypothesis-experiment-falsification/ verification method usually put forward in public as the way science progresses (see, e.g., Collins and Pinch 1993; Latour 1987). Rather, it has been considered vital for the public to realize that much of the science it is confronted with (e.g., Human Genome Project, stem-cell research; brain research) is "science-in-the-making." Secondly, while it is clearly more difficult to report on ongoing as opposed to established research, there are, however, ways to attract the lay audience. Much current research raises a number of social, ethical, and policy issues (e.g., labeling of genetically modified food, cyber crime, environmental legislation and an individual's right to privacy). Typically, these types of ongoing research are laden with promises and fears, despite the lack of certification by the scientific communities involved (Weingart 2001, chapter 6). "If we are entering a new age for public understanding of science," Gregory and Miller write (2001, p. 119), "it is important that citizens get used to scientists arguing out controversial facts, theories, and issues. More of what currently goes on backstage in the scientific community has to become more visible if people are going to get a clearer idea of the potential and limitations of the new wonders science is proclaiming." (See also Hilgartner 2000.) Hence, engaging a wider audience into science-in-the-making may actually sensitize the public for both cognitive and non-cognitive aspects of scientific claims. By changing the ways in which we interact with one another, science and technology influence how we define the general welfare, our views on the role of government, and the approach we take in exercising our rights as citizens. Today, technological advances are giving humans the ability to intervene in spheres they could not attain earlier. Consequently, average citizens are faced with choices of which they had no knowledge previously.

Indeed, the changes in knowledge about living organisms, particularly the human organism, and the ability to manipulate and tinker with life, raise a host of ethical, legal, and social issues. The most pressing fall into six general categories: privacy, handling of prenatal life, manipulation of germ lines, free will and individual responsibility, genetic reductionism and determinism, and genetic enhancement. Fundamental to all six is the realization that there is no perfect or ideal human genetic constitution to which all others are inferior, as well as the recognition that genetic information should not be used to advance ideological or political agendas. In order to assess risks and chances, a knowledgeable public is considered a prime prerequisite.

In this vein, the recent neuroscientific challenge in which free will is cast in the guise of a mere illusion can be read as an instance of public understanding of science. Neuroscientists eagerly enlighten the general public about their field. Above all, this pertains to the hybrid and complex range of neuroscience itself. The complexity of the brain is so great that understanding even the most basic functions will require that we fully exploit all the tools currently at our disposal in science and engineering and simultaneously develop new methods of analysis. While neuroscientists and engineers from varied fields such as brain anatomy, neural development and electrophysiology have made great strides in the analysis of this complex organ, there remains a great deal yet to be uncovered. Not surprisingly, this calls for more research, more funds, and last but not least, for public acceptance of a costly type of research.

To this end, it is useful to draw attention to potential applications and remedies. For example, by understanding how neuronal circuits process and store information, one may be able to design computers with capabilities beyond current limits. By understanding how neurons develop and grow, we could develop new technologies for central nervous system repair following neurological disorders and injuries. Moreover, discoveries related to higher-level cognitive function and consciousness could have a profound influence on how humans make sense of their surroundings and interact with each other. The ability to successfully interface the brain with external electronics would have enormous implications for our society and facilitate a revolutionary change in the quality of life of people with sensory and/or motor deficits.

Indeed, there is hardly any domain of science that does not attempt to present itself as a key technology—consider, for a few examples, gene technology, nanotechnology, or stem-cell research pointing to therapeutic cloning.[3] This strategy is highly ambivalent, however, given that it regularly produces bifurcated responses as to the feasibility and desirability of these apparatuses, procedures or treatments. In Germany as well as in other European countries, the public debate over embryonic stem cells not only gave rise to a heated discussion of whether or not therapeutic cloning could ever become a reliable form of treatment, it also provoked an irresolvable controversy over the "dignity of man."

The lessons learned from these experiences are that public acceptance is hard to attain. Even more so, as both promises and perceived threats strongly interfere with pre-existing "knowledge" (false or correct), habits, and positions gained from preceding debates. While the issue of free will seems fairly abstract at first sight, it did hold the attention for a number of months (neglecting pre- and after-publications). Although it never became a lively debate backed by other forums of deliberation (e.g., social movements; see above), it connected to the fear of "being determined," this time by neurophysiological processes; it dealt with allegedly promising technological possibilities (e.g., neurodidactics); and most importantly, it bore on the critical concepts of responsibility and free will underlying legal decisions (on public perception of genetic determinism, see Dreyfus and Nelkin 1994 and Nelkin 1994), and was highly informative on an astounding scientific and philosophical standard—in fact, it was a debate addressing the *Bildungsbürgertum* (the educated middle class). No wonder perhaps: is the attack on the free will not an attack on the *citizen*?

4   Free Will: Is There Really Something to Talk About?

It all started with Benjamin Libet's experiments in 1985. While brain and nerve impulses were being monitored, subjects were asked to make some trivial choice—e.g., to move a finger up or down and to report the moment of decision making. What Libet found was that the nerve impulse from the brain to the finger was on its way *before* subjects reported having made the choice. Fact is, the difference is less than half a second—but since nerve impulses propagate at finite maximum speeds, once the impulse to move the finger one way or the other is on the way, it appears that no later decision can derail it, nor can the finger's movement depend upon the later decision (Libet 1985). These findings are still being investigated. (See Haggard and Eimer 1999.)

Does the finding that everything we will and actually do is based on neurophysiological conditions really challenge our long-cherished notions of what it means to exert free will? What, in fact, do we mean by free will in everyday knowledge? Peter Bieri, an analytical philosopher, sets out boldly to counter the challenge—drawing on a "clear mind" and conceptual analysis rather than insisting on bold claims unjustified by empirical findings, as he scathingly comments (2005).

What is the challenge? First, we regularly conceive ourselves as the authors of our volition and actions, second, we tend to think we are headed toward an open future, for which we can always decide between various options, and third, we hold ourselves and others responsible for our actions. However, the finding that everything we do and experience does have a neurophysiological basis seems to cause a complete u-turn: first, we seem to be no more than vehicles of our brain activities, second, our future appears open because we do not know about the brain processes ultimately guiding our actions, and third, the attribution of responsibility therefore seems meaningless.

Bieri, less involved in the general media debate, gives a convincing account of what must have happened: those who felt challenged by the neurocognitive redescription and the neuroscientists alike hold positions that, after a closer look, are based on severe misconceptions of what could possibly be meant by "free will."

Misconception 1: unmoved mover   Do we really believe that our will is free in the sense of being entirely independent of any condition, that it keeps initiating ever-new chains of causality? To be sure, such a will would be purely accidental, it would neither belong to anybody's life or character, nor would it lend itself to learning. In other words: We would be talking about "chaotics" (Hayles 1991), rather than freedom.

Misconception 2: will as non-physical phenomenon   Do we really believe that experiential phenomena are causally autonomous, hence, completely detached from physiological conditions? Quite clearly, most of us do not (fully) understand the material processes giving rise to psychological phenomena. However, not understanding those processes does not imply independence of neurophysiological processes. In other words: No psychological change without physiological change.

Misconception 3: Omniscience of experience   Do we really believe that there is nothing "behind our backs" ruling our lives? Since we tend to think of our volition as spontaneous, we actually infer it to be free. However, not being aware of those processes does not imply independence of the neurophysiological machinery bringing it about. In other words: no perceiving, feeling, thinking, in short, no experiential event without neurophysiological processes.

In Bieri's perspective, the result is unequivocal: Only if there really is a belief in one or more of the aforementioned (mis-) conceptions will it lead to the conclusion that brain research does in actual fact undermine the idea of free will and freely deciding individuals. Those misconceptions, however, are not only highly implausible within the framework of everyday experience, they are also based on an "adventurous metaphysics." Bieri insists that we can describe ourselves (our paintings, hair dryers, philosophical accounts) on various levels or in different dimensions: aesthetic, mechanic, impact, etc. When it comes to humans, we should differentiate between two dimensions. In one of them, we make use of a physicalist account, including neurophysiological narratives about how the brain regulates what happens "inside." This is a mechanistic and deterministic account, given of our (neuro-)biological bodies. In the other dimension, there is a psychological narrative given about ourselves as persons. On this level, we talk about description telling about actions performed by a person, about reasons for these actions, about what this person believes and wishes, what he or she thinks and feels, what he or she remembers and imagines. Freedom can only be thought of, denied, or deliberated on this very level of personhood. Only acting individuals can be "objects" of the search for freedom or the lack thereof.

On the physical level, brain research can tell us about neurophysiological processes and their deterministic nature—or microphysicalist indeterminacies, for that matter. What we will not find on this level, however, is not free will or free action, as the conceptual framework simply does not allow for it. That is, we need the conceptual framework of personhood in order to talk about freedom. This holds for neuroscientists as well—their research is in need of a concept of free will that cannot be derived from brain research itself. In sum, Bieri accuses the neuroscientists of being misled by a category mistake.[4]

What exactly is a conceptually sound account of free will? Our will is free if it is guided by good judgment on what to do in a given situation. Our will is not free if judgment and will fall apart—if, for instance, I act on impulse. In this view, we can also stick to the deep-rooted notion of being able to act otherwise. However, this does not give rise to the approach known as "anything goes." Rather, it means that I could have acted otherwise had I judged things differently. On this account, freedom is the plasticity of our will in relation to our judgment. And this is why we hold someone responsible for their actions: "We judge what you did in relation to what you wanted, and what you wanted, we judge in relation to certain norms."

In this sense, one can acknowledge both the breath-taking findings of the neurosciences and a meaningful sense of free will for volitionally acting and responsible persons. While we understand more fully the neurophysiological machinery instantiating our volition and actions, the latter is also in need of a conceptual framework residing in the categorical systems of personhood—and sociality.

5   What Is Left to Talk About?

It is self-evident that no single contribution ends a debate, however plausible its stance may seem. From a discourse-analytical perspective, Bieri's position, backed by many colleagues in this debate (e.g., Wingert, Kettner, Schockenhoff), is the exact counterpart of the claims made by the neuroscientists. Hence it is bound to provoke further arguments. By focusing on the main dimensions, the neuroscientific challenge becomes amenable to three lines of discussion: theoretical, science political, political.

Theoretical Dimension

As stated before, brain researchers claim that all conscious activities are ultimately based on unconscious processes. Both the personality profile of a person and their individual modes of reaction and actions are determined by genetic factors and early childhood experiences (Roth 2003, p. 526). Accordingly, all perceptions and imaginations, but also concrete action plans are submitted to evaluations in the limbic system. In this selfsame system, the brain checks whether the action's effects are bound to lead to good emotions or not. According to Roth, the limbic system has the first and the final word. The first, when it comes to a wish and a goal, the last, when reason and its reasoned judgment are checked for the emotional acceptability of its advice. Hence "there is rational deliberation of actions, alternative actions and their respective consequences, however, there is no acting rationally" (ibid.).

While hardly anyone would deny such material underpinnings of all thoughts, deliberations, and emotions, many authors do, in fact, reject the claim that by uncovering those physical processes, symbolic processes just vanish into thin air. Like Bieri, Lutz Wingert insists on clearly separating the levels of description. When it comes to thoughts or social devices, such as assertions, money, or political constitutions, we talk about meaningful things and we talk about objects conveying sense. Wingert pointedly states, that saying "nothing *without* my brain" does not at all imply "nothing *but* my brain" (Wingert, in Assheuer and Schnabel 2000). Rather, he confronts the neuroscientists with a paradox: in order to identify the very experiential phenomena (e.g., free will) for which neurophysiological correlates are sought, one needs to rely on symbolic notions of those phenomena. In this way, neuroscientific accounts remain inextricably linked to everyday knowledge or knowledge provided by the humanities.

The Dimension of Science Policy

Whether this calls for a shifting of boundaries with respect to the respective explanatory power of the two vocabularies remains an as yet open question. However, in the dimension of science policy the debate can indeed be regarded as another instance of the science wars *en miniature*. Hardly concealed, the debate articulates a power play between the natural and the cultural sciences. It is about "who is in charge" when explaining age-old problems such as the free will, until now firmly in the hands of the humanities. In Singer's view, the natural scientists, break out of the decreed ghetto and, albeit humbly, begin to think about issues so far reserved for the cultural sciences. In a complementary fashion, philosophers concede that they have become far more irritable by empirical phenomena; an outlook calling for intensified conceptual analysis, rather than (unproven) surrender to bold claims (see the quotation from Bieri above). The battle is not only defined from within. As Wingert points out, there are further favorable conditions. Among others, it seems as if things social do not lend themselves to impatient fantasies. In fact, anything labeled "social" is not of interest any more. This development entails a devaluation of sociology and social philosophy. Biology and economics are the new leading disciplines (see Wingert in Assheuer and Schnabel 2000, p. 2). It is only fair to add, however, that social scientists seem to have actively excluded themselves from this as well as neighboring debates (e.g., on consciousness, see Maasen 2003). Therefore, the field is open not only for adventurous metaphysics (see remarks on Bieri above) but also for adventurous social science (see remarks on Kuhlmann below).

First and foremost, the science wars are confined to brain researchers versus philosophers. Armed with bright brain scans and an impressive array of data, the brain researchers self-assuredly claim priority in explaining volition by way of neurophysiological processes and cognitive mechanisms operating upon them. The neuroscientists claim they will soon find causal explanations showing why certain material, neurophysiological processes give rise to specific states of consciousness. While conceding the reality of psychic states and cultural phenomena, they distance themselves from crude reductionisms, calling for "bridging theories" (Singer 2002, p. 177), uniting both worlds, the material and the cultural, instead. Indeed, this "euphoria of uniting" (Vereinigungseuphorie) (Kettner et al. 2003) smacks of a revival of a "unity of science" program, a reductionist explanatory framework, this time led by the neurosciences. All the more so, as objects of social and cultural systems of description entail descriptions and relations to rule-driven practices. The latter form part of what it means to be a certain thought or action, e.g., whether waving one's hand is just a bodily behavior or part of a greeting ritual. Hence, bridging the gap between biological and physical theories is worlds apart from bridging the gap between neurophysiological theories and sociological ones. Objects of culture are not independent of the way in which we conceive of them. It is difficult to see how the brain-centered naturalism that Singer and colleagues (2002, 2003) seem to advocate might allow for the (multiplicity of) meanings attached to (the same) objects (Kettner et al. 2004, p. 24).

Political Dimension

The debate follows its trajectories in a society enlightened by neuroscientific insights. Two examples, namely jurisdiction and education, may suffice to illustrate the visions and pitfalls of neuroscientific reform. As far as jurisdiction is concerned, Gerhard Roth provides a new approach to delinquency. Given that human personality is built by genetic factors and early childhood experiences, the concept of guilt and the criminological concept of retribution are to be bidden farewell too (see Roth 2003, p. 541). The sentencing of offenders should only be based on repulsion and re-conditioning. In this respect, whether or not measures taken toward improvement are effective depends on the individual's personality profile. Again, early and ubiquitous testing becomes necessary. Likewise, seemingly reformist thought (refrain from guilt) allies with technocracy.

Even a general espousal of this cause inevitably means that criminals will be locked up or given therapy. This time, however, we do it because we deem them dangerous, not because we also consider them guilty. So, would this neurobiological way of treating criminals really be more "humane," as Singer and others suggest? Kettner et al. remind us of Stanley Kubrick's film *A Clockwork Orange*. Those no longer acknowledging sociopaths as persons capable of responsibility and guilt but as objects of re-programmable behavioral repertoires possibly create more suffering than they are able to prevent. Moreover, externalizing the systems of behavior-control by way of neuro-technical programming is far less subtle and efficient than

regulating oneself by way of insight and reasons. The latter is typical of action regulated by socio-cultural norms. Finally, regarding the re-programmers, the question
arises to whom they are responsible, and on what grounds? (Kettner et al. 2004, p.
17)

With regard to education, neurodidactics provides novel insights, too. The neurocybernetic program is based on the insight that brains are highly influenced and
individualized by both genetic constitution and early childhood experiences (Singer
2003, p. 56). Thus the basic advice is to wait and see what questions children have,
"for the young brains know best what they need at specific stages of their development and are capable of critically evaluating and selecting among different options"
(Singer 2002, p. 57). The flip side of this seemingly anti-authoritarian statement is a
technocratic program for timely selection of the best: "To optimize education, one
would have to test children at a very early stage, identify talents, and channel educational activities along the spectrum of talents. One needs to free oneself from the
illusion that all can become equal. This assumption makes no sense at all and contradicts elementary biological laws: my postulate leads to a strong differentiation"
(Singer 2003, p. 116f.)

Kuhlmann counters that in stating this, it is in reality no longer *the child* but *the
neuron* Singer is addressing. As a consequence of his postulate, one can save all
efforts at providing a child with attractive offers so that it may find its own way. In
Kuhlmann's view, we are about to change the criteria for judging such a decision. If
it all depends on material causal factors rather than the insight and experience of
an adolescent, why should we not manipulate the young brain? (Kuhlmann 2004,
p. 152).

Arguing against Neuro Society?

Given that their ideas were on the verge of becoming social reality, Roth and his
neuroscientific colleagues strongly advise discussing their social and ethical implications. (See Roth 2003, p. 543.) While this call for technology assessment is
laudable in principle, it falls short of its self-proclaimed aim. Modern technology
assessment is no longer only concerned with the consequences of a certain technology, but also with the conditions giving rise to it and providing the scope of its
uses or abuses, its acceptance or rejection. Moreover, a technology assessment of
this scope should be performed, in which the broader public should be involved.
Interestingly enough, the media did attempt to stage such a debate. As has been
said earlier, while they succeeded in initiating a serious and high-standard debate
among German intellectuals, they failed utterly to involve a larger audience, attract-
ing none of its representatives. Neither politicians, nor corporate actors, nor pro-

fessionals in the culture business or civil movements, were seen or made themselves heard. The same applies to representatives of industry, notably the pharmaceutics business.

The opposition implicit in most arguments countering the neuroscientific, and above all, the neurotechnical challenges lying ahead, is both obvious and moralistic. The opposition is between "neurotechnical manipulation" and "exercise of free will based on insight and experience." While evident to many, this very distinction and its discussion in the media deserves closer scrutiny.

First, giving no quarter to those who try to counter in a temperate manner, the philosopher Holm Tetens severely questions the fear of neurotechnical manipulation. Following the neurocybernetic model of behavior, he explains that it is the brain which produces the observable behavior of a person. As a consequence, some people hold that all that is needed is to gear into the brain and achieve certain brain states in order to trigger any behavior one wishes to generate. This is why the neurocybernetic model of behavior is invariably confronted with the verdict of presenting humans as being manipulable at pleasure. However, Tetens is eager to emphasize that this is a fallacy. In point of fact, the brain is in need of permanent and rich stimuli—natural or cultural—in order to become "a machine" capable of understanding and producing language and to communicate with others. Only under these conditions are humans able to live and actively shape their natural and cultural environment. In the perspective of a stimuli-demanding brain, the effects of neuro-technical manipulation would be rather limited. The interaction of humans with their highly complex environment can hardly be substituted by laboratory conditions. We should therefore not be afraid of neuro technically trimmed laboratory monsters. Moral verdicts of such kind simply run idle (Tetens 1999, p. 24).

Second, there are those (and, indeed many) who cry out against the end of a liberal ethos stipulating that humans are endowed with the possibility of leading their lives in accordance with their self-gained values (Kuhlmann 2004). Moralizing, however, is a characteristic not uncommon in media debates. At first sight, one might be led to search for the reasons in the issue itself: Denying free will and cultures based on it justly evokes not only level-headed arguments (see Tetens) but also strong emotions and normative reactions. Yet, the question as to why this is happening remains. Would we not, for the most part, act as before, happily sacrificing the notion of "free" will (Tetens 2005)?

Indeed, there are media-specific reasons for this pervasive tendency to moralize controversial issues. To begin with, it is the media who set the agenda altogether (brain research), who put the issue on the agenda (free will) and stage the main controversy (free will: yes or no). In this medialized way, society engages in increased self-observation. It sees "problems" (free will) to which it seeks "solutions" (free will as illusion) that, in turn, produce new "problems" (manipulable brains), and so on. On the one hand, moralizations help to structure the "reality" thus constructed in the media. Moralizing discourse appeals to the code of good-or-bad, and typically media debates try to enrich the controversy with protagonists of both normative stances (Luhmann 1996, p. 64f.). Given the intellectuality of the discussion on free will (see above), Singer and Roth appear to their opponents to be on the bad side, yet far less evil than they would have been in a more popularized debate. . . . On the other hand, moralizing is about rendering this construction "more real." Discarding free will in media debate may be easy, but what about real life? To moralize an issue conveys the impression that this very issue is in need of normative accentuation, because in "real reality" things are different. (Luhmann 1996, pp. 202–204) Moralizing thus compensates the reality deficit of the media discourse.

Third, all factions seem to agree that individuals and societies are rapidly changing as a result of science and technology. Böhme, one of the rare representatives of the cultural sciences engaged in this debate, specifically welcomes the fact that problems deriving from technical-scientific developments are increasingly discussed in public while initiating research in the humanities by the same token (Böhme 2000, p. 49). Natural scientists, in turn, should acquire cultural competencies as their influence on modern societies grows. We need neither the delirious messages of salvation nor the apocalyptic prayers, unsuspecting paintings of scientific progress or helpless invocations of cultural autonomy that have lately filled the feuilletons. Böhme avers that underlying those rhetorical aberrations are either real economic interests or deep-rooted fears, both of which have to be taken seriously and discussed as such. Moreover, in order to understand the human being, a zoon symbolicon living in a world strongly influenced by science and technology, there is no via regia of knowing. Rather, Böhme pleads for a trans-disciplinary cooperation of all sciences, technologies and humanities involved in order to make sense of the neuro-socio-technical complex called neuro-world.

On a methodological note, Christian Geyer, too, warns against a culture of incommensurable perspectives, for it forecloses the chance to learn and understand. He suggests adoption of Davidson's "anomalous monism" (1980) as a methodological device. As opposed to material monism proper, anomalous monism holds all things mental to be material, whereas the reverse, a "panpsychism" is inadmissible (Geyer 2004, p. 89). This stance may help to further the debate—even more so, as Singer himself seems ultimately undecided. If the social and the cultural are indeed not identical with the underlying neurophysiological processes, as Singer concedes, the energetic impotence of the mental he so often claims appears to be a contradiction in terms. Hence no strict material monism with Singer, after all? (Geyer 2004, p. 90f.)

Free Will: The Wisdom of Everyday Practice

Shifting the perspective for a moment may help: Since we did not happen to meet the "lay public" during the feuilleton debate, what do we know about every-day practice? It might be of use to point to two phenomena likely to further the debate.

Self-Help

In (post-) modern societies, the volitionally acting self is taking center stage. Contemporary Western societies are not only highly individualistic, they are regarded as highly differentiated, thus confusing, demanding, and risky. Accordingly, modern selves have the task of sorting out desires and demands representing internal and external constraints for the very act of shaping decisions on what to do. More often than not, these constraints are quite as contradictory as they are manifold and thus have to be balanced. The reverse of the coin named reasoned choice is continuous monitoring of oneself and others. In fact, neo-liberal societies increasingly rely on this capacity of self-regulation. As this is by no means easy, we get help from a host of more or less rationalized programs and policies by which we learn how we govern ourselves and others.

One such program is called self-management. Countless books, brochures, seminars, web sites, and newsletters are at the disposal of all interested parties. Offers concerning time and self-management abound. Their promise seems to be irresistible. Change is possible. You just have to do it! This undertaking demands a conscious, active disposition. To state it bluntly, in the course of your self managing efforts, you have to find out what you really want, for only what you really want, you actually do (Sprenger 1997, p. 71). The practices on offer address individuals and institutions. "Competence-enhancing seminars" as well as coaching for managers, students, politicians, or secretaries are all the rage. Nowadays, quality and change management are routine procedures aimed at improving the efficiency of administrations or companies. In brief: We are surrounded by a culture of efficiency and efficiency-enhancing procedures, all of which are more or less visibly connected to the conscious effort of working on oneself.

Accordingly, training our capacity to decide, exerting our "free will," to put it more precisely, is an important feature of modern life. It should be incorporated into the more abstract discussions we had so far in order to attract a broader audience. The latter may be interested to learn that, neurophysiologically speaking, free will is an illusion. Meanwhile, socially speaking, it is highly knowledgeable in volitionally *reflecting about* and *practicing* volition.

Neuroceuticals

As for volition, we are observing a split usage in current self-management practices: On the one hand, "becoming conscious of something" is treated as prime vehicle of volitional self-monitoring. In order to enhance individual efficiency, the manuals make use of all techniques known in psychology and other domains of thought to monitor and educate oneself, hence to become conscious of one's behavioral patterns and options for changing it: questionnaires, tests, check lists, exercises to relax. On the other hand, there is a strong tendency to perform another type of self-shaping. The best selling drugs these days are not those treating acute illnesses, but those prescribed to counteract chronic pain or disability—Premarin, Prozac, Viagra. The power to volitionally reshape one's life, including one's states of consciousness, seems to extend way beyond what we previously understood as illness. In fact, drugs such as Alazopram set to treat "panic disorder," for instance, are rewriting the norms of what it should feel to be a normal self, capable of effective social interaction. On a general level, pharmacological intervention redefines what is amenable to correction or modification, i.e., amenable to shaping one's self by *volitional use of drugs altering one's state of volition*. As Nikolas Rose maintains, this is not so much about widening the net of pathology. No, "we are seeing an enhancement in our capacities to adjust and readjust our somatic existence according to the exigencies of the life we wish to aspire"—and the self we wish (others) to be (Rose 2003). In the course of this these happenings, the scientific and the general discourse converge on a more somatic, more brainy concept of the self. While a deep-seated distrust or anxiety concerning drug intervention into one's states of consciousness might have been suspected, this is not the case. Volitional pharmacological intervention in particular thus aligns with a neo-liberal regime of individuals who have to govern themselves and who do this employing self-management practices of various kinds. In this respect, why should neurochemicals not be an option? The general public, hence we, as competent members of Western societies, are experts in living with seemingly incommensurable stances. We *both* exert free will and we know that our brain regulates our volitional states and processes whenever we take neuroceuticals—yet another reason to differentiate levels of description and refrain form loose talk regarding incommensurability, at the same time.

Neither scholars of the sciences nor the humanities can afford to ignore ethical (Kempermann 2004), social, cultural and political conditions and consequences of neurotechnically co-shaped selves and societies (Schwägerl 2004). Supported by broad media coverage and extended marketing campaigns, the neuroscientific image of a brainy (neurochemical) self living in a neuro society becomes ever more plausible. Hence it should be subject to ongoing and expanded deliberation among individuals who are not only brains but also members of communicative communities.

Epilogue: Is Mrs. Smith's Limbic System in Love?

No, it is activated, but *she is* in love nonetheless. Neither she nor her significant other would know from her brain state—so much seems to be clear for Roth, Singer, Bieri, and Wingert. Does this not provide a splendid argument to restart the debate right here?

Notes

1. Why such a debate has not (yet) happened in the Anglo-American world is still open for discussion.

2. Many of the contributions have been collected in Brain Research and Free Will. On the Interpretation of the Newest Experiments (2004), a booklet edited by Christian Geyer, chief editor of the *FAZ-Feuilleton* and one of the main stage managers of this debate. Geyer's message is hardly neutral. He sets out to reconcile forefront brain research with a full-blown anthropology—neuroscience with a humanist touch, so to speak.

3. A "manifesto of brain research in the 21st century" initiated by the popular journal *Gehirn und Geist* [mind and brain] revealed an astounding modesty. Eleven brain researchers, asked about the future of their field, were confident about progess (e.g., in the domain of specifically operating pharmaceuticals) and cautious, at the same time (do not expect too much). Hence, the very visibility of such (rather binding) statements by way of a 'manifesto' contributes to moderating the discussion (*Gehirn und Geist* 6, 2004: 30–16)—so did statements following this article in later issues of *Gehirn und Geist*, e.g., by both "insiders" (Prinz, Kettner, Rösler) and a sociologist of science (Peter Weingart).

4. In this vein, Roth offers two ways of "talking cleanly" about causes and reasons. First, reasons are the conscious experience of reasons that in the neurobiological experiment present themselves as complex concatenations of neurophysiological events. Second, reasons are ways of explaining our behavior to ourselves and to others. That is, we act on the basis of causes but we explain those actions with reasons (Roth 2004: 82). This differentiation only helps if one sticks to two levels of description.

References

Assheuer, W., and Schnabel, U. 2000. Wer deutet die Welt? Ein Streitgespräch dem Philosophen Lutz Wingert und dem Hirnforscher Wolf Singer. *Die Zeit* 50: 43.

Bodmer, W. 1985. *The Public Understanding of Science.* Royal Society.

Böhme, H. 2000. Wer sagt, was Leben ist? Die Provokation der Biowissenschaften und die Aufgaben der Kulturwissenschaften. *Die Zeit* 49: 41–42.

Bieri, P. 2005. Untergräbt die Regie des Gehirns die Freiheit des Willens? Manuscript.

Collins, H. M., and Pinch, T. 1993. *The Golem: What Everyone Should Know about Science.* Cambridge University Press.

Crick, F., and Koch C. 1998. Consciousness and neuroscience. *Cerebral Cortex* 8, no. 2: 97–107.

Davidson, D. 1980. Mental events. In *Essays on Actions and Events.* Clarendon.

Dreyfus, R., and Nelkin, D. 1992. The jurisprudence of genetics. *Vanderbilt Law Review* 45: 313–348.

Geyer, C. 2004. Hirn als Paralleluniversum: Wolf Singer und Gerhard Roth verteidigen ihre Neuro-Thesen. In *Hirnforschung und Willensfreiheit,* ed. C. Geyer. Suhrkamp.

Gieryn, Thomas F. 1983. Boundary work and the demarcation of science from non-science: Strains and interest in professional ideologies of scientist. *Amercan Sociological Review* 48: 781–795.

Gregory, J., and Miller, S. 1998. *Science in Public: Communication, Culture, and Credibility* Perseus.

Goodell, R. 1977. *The Visible Scientist*. Little, Brown.

Haggard, O., and Eimer, M. 1999. On the relation between brain potentials and the awareness of voluntary movements. *Experimental Brain Research* 126: 128–133.

Hagner, M. 2004. Homocerebralis: Eine wissenschftsgeschichtliche Einschätzung. In *Hirnforschung und Willensfreiheit*, ed. C. Geyer. Suhrkamp.

Hayles, K. N. 1991. *Chaos Bound. Orderly Disorder in Contemporary Literature and Science*. Cornell University Press.

Hilgartner, S. 2000. *Science on Stage: Expert Advice as Public Drama*. Stanford University Press.

Hilgartner, S. 1990. The dominant view of popularization: Conceptual problems, political uses. *Social Studies of Science* 20: 519–539.

Kempermann, Gerd. 2004. Infektion des Geistes. In *Über philosophische Kategorienfehler*, ed. C. Geyer. Suhrkamp.

Kettner, M., Neumann-Held, E., Röska-Hardy, L., and Wingert, L. 2004. Die Vereinigungseuphorie der Hirnforscher: Acht Nachfragen. In Jahrbuch 2002/2003 des Kulturwissenschaftlichen Instituts Essen, Bielefeld.

Kuhlmann, A. 2004. Menschen im Begabungstest. Mutmassungen über die Hirnforschung als soziale Praxis. *Westend* 1: 143–153.

Latour, B. 1987. *Science in Action: How to Follow Scientists and Engineers through Society*. Cambridge University Press.

Libet, B. 1985. Unconscious cerebral initiative and the role of conscious will in voluntary action. *Behavioral and Brain Sciences* 8: 529–566.

Luhmann, N. 1996. *Die Realität der Massenmedien*. Westdeutscher Verlag.

Lukasiewicz, J. 1966. *The Ignorance Explosion: Understanding Industrial Civilization*. Carlton University Press.

Lewenstein, B. 2002. Editorial. *Public Understanding of Science* 11: 1–4.

Lynch, Z. 2004. Brain waves: Overview of our emerging neurosociety. Corante Tech News (www.corante.com), March 27, 2004.

Maasen, S. 2003. A view from elsewhere: The emergence of consciousness in popular discourse. In *Voluntary Action*, ed. S. Maasen et al. Oxford University Press.

Maasen, S., and Weingart, P. 2000. *Metaphors and the Dynamics of Knowledge*. Routledge.

Milner, A. D. 1995. Cerebral correlates of visual awareness. *Neuropsychologia* 33: 1117–1130.

Monyer, H., et al. 2004. Das Manifest. Elf führende Neurowissenschaftler über Gegenwart und Zukunft der Hirnforschung. *Gehirn and Geist* 6: 30–37.

Nelkin, D. 1994. Promotional metaphors and their popular appeal. *Public Understanding of Science* 3: 25–31.

Sapp, G. 1994. Science at the ethical frontier. *Library Journal* 1: 3.

Schnabel, U. 2003. Der Markt der Neuronen. Hirnforscher werden zu Werbefachleuten. Sie wollen enthüllen, was Käufer zum Konsum treibt. *Die Zeit* 47: 41.

Schwägerl, C. 2004. Neurodämmering. Wer den Geist schützen will, sollte seine Moleküle kennen. In *Hirnforschung und Willensfreiheit*, ed. C. Geyer. Suhrkamp.

Prinz, W. 2004. Der Mensch ist nicht frei. Ein Gespräch. In *Hirnforschung und Willensfreiheit*, ed. C. Geyer. Suhrkamp.

Rose, N. 2003. Neurochemical selves. *Society* 6: 46–59.

Roth, G. 2004. Worüber dürfen Hirnforscher reden—und in welcher Weise? In *Hirnforschung und Willensfreiheit*, ed. C. Geyer. Suhrkamp.

Roth, G. 2003. *Fühlen, Denken, Handeln. Wie das Gehirn unser Verhalten steuert*. Suhrkamp.

Singer, W. 2003. *Ein neues Menschenbild. Gespräche über Hirnforschung*. Suhrkamp.

Singer, W. 2002. *Der Beobachter im Gehirn. Essays zur Hirnforschung*. Suhrkamp.

Sprenger, R. K. 1997. *Die Entscheidung liegt bei Dir. Wege aus der alltäglichen Unzufriedenheit.* Campus.

Tetens, H. 1999. Die erleuchtete Maschine. Das neurokybernetische Modell des Menschen und die späte Ehrenrettung für den Philosophen Julien Offray de La Mettrie. *Die Zeit* 24: 51.

Ungar, S. 2000. knowledge, ignorance and the popular culture: Climate change versus the ozone hole. *Public Understanding of Science* 9: 297–312.

Weingart, P. 2001. *Die Stunde der Wahrheit? Zum Verhältnis der Wissenschaft zu Politik, Wirtschaft und Medien in der Wissensgesellschaft.* Velbrück.

Zeman, A. 2001. Consciousness. *Brain* 24: 1263–1289.

Contributors

William P. Banks
Department of Psychology
Pomona College
550 Harvard Avenue
Claremont CA 91711
WPB04747@pomona.edu

Timothy Bayne
Department of Philosophy
Macquarie University
Sydney NSW 2109
tbayne@scmp.mq.edu.au

Sarah-Jayne Blakemore
Institute of Cognitive Neuroscience
Department of Psychology
University College London
17 Queen Square, London WC1N 3AR
s.blakemore@ucl.ac.uk

Suparna Choudhury
Behavioural and Brain Sciences Unit
Institute of Child Health
University College London
30 Guilford Street, London WC1N 1EH

Walter J. Freeman
Department of Molecular and Cell
Biology
LSA 129
University of California
Berkeley CA 94720-3200
drwjfiii@berkeley.edu

Shaun Gallagher
Department of Philosophy
University of Central Florida
gallaghr@mail.ucf.edu

Susan Hurley
University of Warwick
Coventry CV4 7AL

Marc Jeannerod
Institut des Sciences Cognitives
67 Boulevard Pinel, 659675
Bron, France
jeannerod@isc.cnrs.fr

Leonard V. Kaplan
University of Wisconsin Law School
Madison WI 53706-1399
lvkaplan@wisc.edu

Hakwan Lau
Department of Experimental
Psychology
University of Oxford
South Parks Road
Oxford OX1 3UD

Sabine Maasen
Program for Science Research
University of Basel
Missionsstrasse 21, CH-4003
Bascl
sabine.maasen@unibas.ch

Bertram Malle
Department of Psychology and Institute
of Cognitive and Decision Sciences
University of Oregon
Eugene OR 97403-1227
bfmalle@uoregon.edu

Alfred R. Mele
Department of Philosophy
Florida State University
Tallahassee FL 32306-1500
almele@mailer.fsu.edu

Elisabeth Pacherie
Institut Jean Nicod
CNRS-EHESS-ENS
Paris
pacherie@ehess.fr

Richard E. Passingham
Department of Experimental
Psychology
University of Oxford
South Parks Road
Oxford OX1 3UD
dick.passingham@psy.ox.ac.uk

Susan Pockett
Private Bag 92019
Department of Physics
University of Auckland
s.pockett@auckland.ac.nz

Wolfgang Prinz
Department of Psychology
Max-Planck-Institute for Cognitive and
Brain Sciences
Amalienstr. 33, D-80799
Munich
prinz@cbs.mpg.de

Peter W. Ross
Department of Philosophy
California State Polytechnic University
3801 W. Temple Avenue
Pomona CA 91768
pwross@csupomona.edu

Index